Item Interpretation
of the Luria-Nebraska
Neuropsychological
Battery

Charles J. Golden
University of Nebraska
Medical Center
Thomas A. Hammeke
Medical College
of Wisconsin
Arnold D. Purisch
East Orange
Veterans Administration
Medical Center
Richard A. Berg
St. Jude Children's
Research Hospital
James A. Moses, Jr.
Palo Alto Veterans
Administration
Medical Center and
Stanford University
School of Medicine
David B. Newlin
Indiana State University
Greta N. Wilkening
University of Nebraska
Medical Center
Antonio E. Puente
Northeast Florida
State Hospital

Item Interpretation

of the Luria-Nebraska

Neuropsychological

Battery

University of Nebraska Press   Lincoln & London

Copyright 1982
by the University of Nebraska Press
All rights reserved
Manufactured in the United States of America

Library of Congress
Cataloging in Publication Data

Main entry under title:
Item interpretation of the Luria-Nebraska
neuropsychological battery.
Includes index.
1. Neurologic examination. 2. Psychometrics.
3. Neuropsychology.
I. Golden, Charles J., 1949- . II. Title:
Luria-Nebraska neuropsychological battery.
[DNLM: 1. Nervous system diseases—Diagnosis.
2. Neurologic examination—Methods.
3. Psychological tests—Methods.
4. Psychophysiologic disorders—Diagnosis.
WM 145 188]
RC348.183   616.8'0475   81-16393
ISBN 0-8032 2105-3   AACR2

Dedication

We owe an enormous debt to the genius of A. R. Luria, whose work inspired the development of the Luria-Nebraska Neuropsychological Battery and has enriched all of neuropsychology. We are also indebted to the work of Anne-Lise Christensen, whose publication of *Luria's Neuropsychological Investigation* (1975) allowed what was an interesting idea to become a practical reality. Without her work the attempt to devise this battery would have been much more difficult or even impossible. This book is dedicated to Drs. Luria and Christensen and to their work.

Contents

Preface

This book is the first in a series designed to aid the neuropsychologist in interpreting the Luria-Nebraska Neuropsychological Battery. Although the Luria-Nebraska battery is relatively new compared with other neurodiagnostic tests, neuropsychologists have shown great interest in it, and there is a large and growing demand for interpretive material on the more advanced aspects of its interpretation. This book is the first response to that demand and will serve, we hope, to give the reader a greater understanding of the psychological skills that underlie each item on the test, a knowledge absolutely necessary to employing the more advanced techniques of "syndrome analysis" as described in the writings of Luria (1966, 1973).

The book is not intended either as an introduction to neuropsychology or an introduction to the Luria-Nebraska battery. We assume that the reader is familiar with the test and the test items, along with the test manual and the basic research data available on the test. We also assume a grounding in basic areas of neuropsychological interpretation and specifically with the skills involved in the objective analysis of the Luria-Nebraska battery.

For those without such a background, we strongly recommend gaining familiarity with the *The Luria-Nebraska Neuropsychological Battery: A Manual for Clinical and Experimental Uses* (Golden, Purish, & Hammeke, 1980), *The Working Brain* (Luria, 1973), *Diagnosis and Rehabilitation in Clinical Neuropsychology* (Golden, 1978), *Clinical Interpretation of Objective Psychological Tests,* (Golden, 1979), as well as obtaining a background in basic aspects of neuropsychology.

The reader should also be familiar with the administration and scoring of the items of the Luria-Nebraska and should have given the test frequently enough to be familiar with the items as they are referred to in the text. (Appendix A describes the items briefly to help readers refresh their memories in specific cases.) Except for special instructions and reminders of item content, there is no reference to topics covered in the test manual.

The major part of this book is an analysis of the

Luria-Nebraska scales. Where appropriate this involves item-by-item analysis; in other scales the items are considered as a uniform group. The technique selected in each case depends greatly on the nature of the items in the scale: we have attempted to present them in the way that best fosters an understanding of the battery.

Each chapter is divided into three parts. The first examines the theoretical intent of each item and the significant underlying skills according to Luria's theory, adapting Luria's major works (Luria, 1966, 1973) to the specific items selected for the test battery. Even where Luria is not directly referred to, the theories and ideas, unless otherwise noted, are based on his work. The second section in each chapter presents the results of a series of intercorrelation analyses between the items using a population of 70 normal controls, 70 psychiatric patients, and 198 neurological patients with a wide range of disorders. The study investigated empirically which items on the battery correlated with one another, to determine whether they tapped common skills. These sections offer another view of some of the same information provided in the theoretical analyses. While they also relate the findings to theoretical concepts, we have made no attempt to force agreement between the two methods or to necessarily address the same issues. Rather, we have concentrated each method on those areas where it can give the greater understanding of the items, providing alternative views of the same items.

The third section of each chapter has been similarly organized, describing the factor structures of the Luria-Nebraska scales. These factor analyses are based on a population of 270, evenly divided between brain-injured, psychiatric, and normal patients. The factor analysis performed on each scale was a principal axis procedure with rotation by the Varimax method. Number of factors was determined by Cattell's Scree Test. Appendix B gives more details of the sample and procedure for the factor and correlational experiments. Here we look at the interrelationship of items within each scale to see if they group together in ways useful to understanding them. Evidence is presented independent of the other two sections, thus providing a third perspective for each of the test items.

In addition to discussing the evidence from correlation and factor analysis, we provide detailed tables of the intercorrelations between Luria-Nebraska items and the factor structure of the Luria scales. These tables enable readers to make their own analysis of these data, to discover new insights, and to assess the potential behind hypotheses about interrelationship of items that they may generate while giving the test.

This approach of three separate analyses has been adopted for several reasons. Foremost is our own experience that each technique does indeed present a unique view of the items and their interpretations within or across scales. The theoretical system devised by Luria offers a consistent and logical way to analyze each item from a comprehensive viewpoint. The item intercorrelations reveal actual patterns of interaction that arise either out of the ways the items are constructed or out of their underlying theoretical structure. Finally, the factor analysis groups items in largely logical combinations that indicate which ones within a scale are most closely related. This allows us to discern factor patterns that may describe a specific deficit area in an individual's skills, as well as to identify clusters of well-performed items that represent strengths. Separately or together, these approaches offer insight into patterns of items missed on the test.

In addition to presenting basic chapters on each behavioral scale of the Luria, we review a number of empirical scales that particularly aid interpretation. Of special importance here are the experimental localization scales, which combine items that, when missed together, suggest focal deficits in specific areas of the brain. These scales offer another way of hypothesizing basic deficits that may underlie item performance. Although these scales cannot be considered definitive because they are based on small samples—since it is difficult to find patients with highly localized lesions—they can be used to generate hypotheses in clinical diagnosis—hypotheses that are then confirmed or disproved by the items.

Chapter 13 offers a synopsis of the information in the previous chapters. For each item we list the input modality, output, purpose, and special scales (such as the Localization scales) that the item appears on. This is intended as a quick reference to generate hypothesis about patterns of items for the reader familiar with the basic presentation.

Chapter 14 illustrates the possibilities of the Luria-Nebraska scales and items in diagnosing patients who receive a series of Luria-Nebraska batteries during the course of their treatment for given disorders. This excellent chapter, prepared by coauthor James A. Moses, Jr., illustrates the potential of the Luria-Nebraska in documenting the changing nature of a neurological problem.

The final chapter briefly discusses an issue often ignored in clinical neuropsychological testing—subcortical disorders. Its purpose is to make readers aware of the problems caused by subcortical disorders on tests of cortical skills like the Luria-Nebraska. Several case examples illustrate these effects.

We hope this book will be a useful guide for understanding the battery as a whole and the role of the individual items in advanced diagnosis. We cannot, of course, supply here the necessary familiarity with the test or give experience with accurate feedback, nor can we provide the skills of logic and analysis needed in applying this information, but we hope to give the reader a start in this direction.

As noted above, we consider this book only one step in providing material for the Luria-Nebraska user. We hope that future books will supply more case histories, case analyses and profile interpretation material that will allow the user more practice in using the information in this volume.

It would be inappropriate to end this preface without acknowledging our debt to Dr. A. R. Luria and Dr. Anne-Lise Christensen. Readers familiar with the history of the Luria-Nebraska battery are aware that the test was derived largely from the work of Christensen (1975), which in turn was derived from Luria's works and from her personal observations and correspondence with Dr. Luria. Thus, without Christensen's work it is highly doubtful that the Luria-Nebraska could have been developed as rapidly as it was. Our theoretical discussion (aside from the empirical data and other sources cited in the text) is derived largely from Luria's work (especially the 1966 and 1973 books) as well as from Christensen's summary of it in her 1975 presentation. Some of our discussion does deviate from that material; our own work and that of others has suggested areas where some of Luria's specific conclusions seem to require modification (as opposed to the more general outline of his theory, with which we fully concur). However, we have clearly identified the sources of such speculations or have included them in the empirical sections of each chapter.

We are also grateful to Frances K. Conley, M.D., chief of the Neurosurgery Section at the Palo Alto Veterans Administration Medical Center, for permission to work with her patients, for the cases reported in Chapter 14; and to Connie Heidelberg Sanders for assistance with Chapter 15.

1. Introduction

When we first embarked on the task of standardizing a test based on the theories of A. R. Luria, we were met with incredulity from some, who pointed out that Luria was an intuitive genius whose diagnostic work depended on insight and on the observation of small differences in a patient's behavior under a variety of unstandardized conditions, using a variety of unstandardized scoring procedures. "How," they asked, "could such a procedure become a standardized test battery without destroying the essence of what was Luria?"

Indeed, if one sees the essence of Luria's work as his intuitive skills and experience, this question is quite reasonable. But in our eyes it was not Luria's intuition and experience that made his work so appealing: there have been many neuropsychologists (as well as users of the Rorschach, the Bender, the Draw-a-Person, and so on) and psychologists who have performed feats of intuition that few if any of us can match. However, none of their works suggested the possibility of a standardized test. The aspect of Luria's accomplishment that made his work and theory so useful was not his intuition but his ability to explain complex brain processes in terms of a simple and comprehensive model that could account for the mass of seemingly unrelated data that has been collected in neuropsychology. This was coupled with an assessment system that could be applied intuitively but actually followed a rigorous scientific and logical approach to detailed analysis of the patient's deficits through what Luria called "syndrome analysis."

At the heart of Luria's theory and assessment procedure was the notion of a functional system. Luria (1966, 1973) differentiated between the many ways we use the word "function." As he pointed out, we can talk about the specific function of a small part of a machine (a gear may turn another gear) or about the function of the machine as a whole (to produce *Star Wars* dolls). This dual use of the word has led to a great deal of trouble in neuropsychology. As time progressed we began to confuse the function of a small area of the brain (such as phonemic discrimination) with the function of a larger whole such as receptive speech. Thus we came to see "receptive speech" as a function of one small brain area, whereas receptive speech was actually the result of many areas working together. As in the machine we discussed, no one area of the brain is able to operate alone; all must work in concert. This pattern of cooperation is called a "functional system."

In Luria's theory, all observable human behavior springs not from one part of the brain but from the cooperation of several parts, each necessary but not alone sufficient to produce the behavior. Thus, when one part of the functional system was incapacitated the whole system was lost. (We will not discuss recovery mechanisms or similar topics.) But the neuropsychologist could observe only the loss of the whole system. Thus, though we knew something was injured, we did not know what.

Each area of the brain participates in multiple functional systems, the number depending on learning history and similar factors. If a given area is injured, we would expect every functional system using that area to be destroyed, creating a unique pattern of deficits. The discovery of this pattern lay at the heart of Luria's "syndrome analysis." Once a syndrome was identified, one could deduce the basic deficit underlying it and, by knowing the role of each geographical part of the brain, infer the locus of a neurological problem.

This is not very different from the approach Reitan adopted in analyzing the Halstead-Reitan neuropsychological battery. Reitan (1966) differed from Luria in that, rather than adopting a theoretical system of relationships, Reitan gave the same battery of tests to patients with different injuries in order to empirically establish the pattern of results on a standardized battery that corresponded with each injury. Indeed, this pattern of results corresponds closely to Luria's syndrome arising from a specific lesion. The methods differed not in the goal but in how they went about reaching it. Indeed, Luria's method of analysis can be combined with the Halstead-Reitan approach (see Golden, Osmon, Moses, & Berg, 1980).

It was according to this theory that we attempted to devise a standardized battery. We used Luria's tests as the basis of the items because they lend themselves easily to the syndrome analysis approach and can be administered quickly and efficiently. Also, by retaining the same or similar items, one could employ Luria's qualitative approach to the test while at the same time developing empirical and experimental support for the process.

To develop a usable battery, it was necessary to include items that tested all parts of the brain in different combinations. Thus, if we let capital letters represent parts of the brain, we might use a procedure that tapped ABCDE, ABCDF, ABCXF, ABCXE, WBCDE, WBCDF, and so on through each possible combination. By then analyzing the results, we could identify the area of deficit. For example, if a person missed ABCDE, ABCXE, and WBCDE and nothing else except items in which E was included (to give a simplistic example), we could infer an injury in area E.

Luria, of course, did not go through every possible combination to test his hypothesis. He might, for example, test ABCDE and then, because he observed a small difference in the patient's behavior, skip to XYZWE, in an intuitive jump based on his insight and experience. This of course cannot be done in a standardized test. We are forced to systematically sample all the major combinations of brain areas that might aid in diagnosis: the test will eventually get to XYZWE, not by intuition but by systematic evaluation. The procedure does not necessarily match what Luria might do with a given patient (though in some cases it might), but in the end it should allow the same comparisons in making a final decision.

The procedure differs from Luria's approach in a number of other ways. Obviously, an objective scoring system cannot measure all possible nuances of behavior—which are nearly infinite—but must concentrate on certain major dimensions. We measure fewer things on each item than Luria did because we cannot objectively take advantage of the rare performance. Although such observations cannot be included in the objective scoring system, however, this does not hinder the user from making the same observations Luria made and considering them in interpreting the test battery. Indeed, the structure of the items makes it almost impossible to miss such qualitative observations when the patient gives radically different performances on two tasks that differ only slightly as we systematically explore functional systems.

Thus the analysis of performance across the Luria-Nebraska is the same process of syndrome analysis Luria employed. We have changed the material used to a set of responses to a standardized battery, but we have not changed the process of analysis. Nor, in our experience, have we changed the range of information that can be gained from the test by an experienced and knowledgeable neuropsychologist. Combining the actual test answers with the observer's qualitative inferences provides a powerful tool that can be analyzed on both quantitative and qualitative levels, producing something more useful than either alone (at least for those of us who want objective validation of what we do).

As a consequence, advanced interpretation of the Luria-Nebraska requires a working knowledge of those parts of the brain that contribute to the functional systems represented by the items in the test. Moreover, it is important to recognize how the items or series of items differ in the underlying skills they tap and in their relationships to one another. This volume examines these basic questions and provides some tentative answers.

Before turning to the following chapters, readers should be aware of some cautions to observe in using this approach. First, syndrome analysis always depends upon a pattern of deficits, not deficits on only one or two items. Once one forms a hypothesis of a specific deficit, one must show that most other items using the same skill also show deficits. It is this pattern that defines the problem, not just

missing a given item. We find that overgeneralizing from a single item is a common mistake of novices.

Another problem is the presence of alternate functional systems—there is often more than one way to do a task. The items and scoring information in the battery have been set up to avoid this as much as possible, but it still interferes with performance. For example, persons with phonetic deficits may be able to read *cat* from memory while missing other reading items, especially unfamiliar words or phonemes. Because of this, they may correctly answer items one would expect them to miss if they had the hypothesized deficit. The user must then evaluate whether any alternate functional system could be involved and must test such a hypothesis about brain integrity against other appropriate items that might use the same alternate skills.

A related problem is the assumption that a person missed an item because of a deficit in the major skill it measures. The scoring system has been set up to minimize this, since one may miss any item for a large number of reasons. Again, only pattern or syndrome analysis can reveal a true deficit.

With these cautions in mind, one can employ syndrome analysis (along with one's observations of the patient) as a powerful tool for analyzing the nature of behavioral deficits. This basic skill makes the Luria-Nebraska useful in planning rehabilitation and making prognostic decisions (along with such information as neurological course, age, education, family support, premorbid personality, financial strengths, timing of insurance settlements, and motivation). The information in the next chapters serves as the basis for these analyses.

2. The Motor Scale

The Motor scale of the Luria-Nebraska Neuropsychological Battery assesses the ability to organize, control, and carry out motor acts with the upper extremities and oral area. Movements of the hands are of utmost importance in human activity. Successful movement of the tongue, lips, and face is necessary for expressive speech. The organization of the Motor scale and the items utilized reflect Luria's (1966) thinking in regard to neuropsychological functioning. Motor activity is assessed as a complex functional system with both a sensory and a motor basis.

Luria considers any cortical function to be controlled by a complex functional system rather than by a discrete localized unit of the cortex. No one portion of the cortex is responsible for controlled movement. Rather, it requires the contributions of multiple cortical systems working together. Movement is made possible by the "organization of concertedly working zones, each of which performs its role" (Luria, 1973).

The initial requirement for the successful completion of any voluntary movement is adequate muscle tone and strength. The second requirement is an adequately functioning afferent (sensory) system that provides a precise, well-articulated, and defined destination for the movement impulses. Constant afferent-kinesthetic feedback from the musculature, mediated by the postcentral zones of the cortex, is necessary to maintain control over movement and to ensure accuracy of course and correct any mistakes.

Since most movement takes place within a spatial framework, adequate voluntary motion demands an intact optic-spatial system. In turn, integrity of the occipitoparietal division of the cortex is necessary to ensure adequate spatial organization.

Complex movements consisting of a chain of discrete movements require the progressive innervation and inhibition of different muscle groups. Small movements are not simply added to one another, they are joined to achieve smooth, coordinated, goal-directed motion. This requires flexible mobility of impulses over time to create "kinetic melodies'' (Luria, 1966), and it is mediated by the premotor areas of the cortex.

Finally, goal-directed movement entails maintaining intentionality throughout the activity and selecting the appropriate actions. The frontal lobes play a critical role in regulating, directing, and completing an intended action. Additionally, the goal of movement is often provided by, and mediated through, verbal directions. For this there must be integrity of the temporoparietal area of the left hemisphere.

Note that the entire cortical system is involved in the successful completion of voluntary movement. As a result, the Motor scale of the Luria-Nebraska is sensitive to a variety of dysfunctions. Though the scale primarily detects lesions of the posterior frontal lobe, lesions of the temporal, parietal, occipital, and anterior frontal lobe will also impair function. Though all items require all the elements necessary for movement, the weighting varies from item to item. Analyzing the requirements of each item and comparing performance among items by double discrimination will localize the part of the process that is impaired and add to our understanding of cortical function as a whole.

The items on the Motor scale of the Luria-Nebraska can be divided into eight sections to help us evaluate and understand motoric activity as a complex functional system. The items vary in terms of the weighting of the contributions of various elements of the functional system and in terms of the level of complexity and integration required for success. Both manual and oral functions are examined at each level of organization.

Simple Movement: Hands & Oral Motor Area

Simple motor movements of the hand are assessed by items 1–4 and simple movement of the oral motor area by items 28 and 29. Though, like all items on the Motor scale,

these tasks require multiple elements of the functional system for successful performance, they are most useful in evaluating pathological changes in muscle tone, power, and accuracy of movement. Patients may fail these items because they cannot complete the required motion or do not perform the sequential movements rapidly and repeatedly.

Changes in power of movement, in precision of movement, and in synkinesis (associated movements) occur secondary to lesions of the primary motor area of the cortex (area 4) or of its tracts. The severe end of this continuum would be evidenced in motor paralysis, whereas minor deficits appear on the Luria-Nebraska as an inability to reach criterion levels for normal performance.

In item 1 the patient is asked to touch each of the fingers of his/her right hand in turn with the thumb while counting them aloud. Item 2 is the same except that the left hand is used. For item 3 the patient is asked to alternately clench and extend the fingers of the right hand as quickly as possible. Item 4 examines the same movements of the left hand.

Successful and rapid performance of items 1–4 requires precise movement. The afferent basis of movement, as mediated by the postcentral area of the cortex, is evaluated according to the patient's ability to select the required impulses to complete the movement within a time limit. Subjects unable to utilize kinesthetic feedback to control and alter movement cannot retain the required topological pattern despite adequate motor strength. Motor impulses lose their selectivity, and there is a diffuse contraction of agonists and antagonists simultaneously. Luria terms such a deficit afferent (kinesthetic) apraxia and attributes this pathological process to lesions of the postcentral area of the cortical nucleus of the sensorimotor area (areas 1, 2, 3, 5).

Because these items are performed separately by both hands, comparisons of strength and accuracy between hands may reveal a significant unilateral disturbance defined by an idiopathic rather than a group norm. Such differences will also exert an effect on the Right and Left Hemisphere scales.

The need for persistent repetition of the simple motor movements in items 1 and 2 for 10 seconds renders this task sensitive to mild frontal lobe damage. Luria (1966) reports that such patients will have trouble sustaining the pattern of selective motions and will perseverate with movements that are even less complex (as in simply opening and closing the hand, or touching individual fingers without regard to the order requested). Such behavior is indicative of the failure of internal speech to regulate motor activity and the breakdown in goal-directed action observed in patients with frontal-lobe lesions.

Simple motor movements of the oral area are assessed by items 28 and 29. The patient is asked to puff out the cheeks for item 28, and on item 29 is told to stick out the tongue as far as possible. The requirements for successful performance of these items are similar to those of the simple manual movements, although repetition is not required and no visual model is provided. Impairment in muscle tone and defective innervation of the oral musculature will preclude successful performance and may occur secondary to damage to the primary motor area. Symmetrical movement is required for success on item 28, and failure to achieve this may indicate a paresis of the oral motor area. Elevated tension of the tongue muscles, and also spasms, which may develop during voluntary movements of the tongue, indicate disturbed muscle tone. The functional loading on both items 28 and 29 requires effective innervation of isolated muscles as mediated by the primary motor area of the cerebral cortex.

The items in the simple oral movement section of the Luria demand a somewhat different neuropsychological process than the simple manual movements because they are administered without a visual model: only verbal direction is provided. These items therefore demand a greater contribution from the left temporal area, which is involved in accurate discrimination and understanding of speech.

Though the tasks used to assess simple manual movement and those used to assess simple oral movement are designed to primarily evaluate the contribution of effective innervation and precision of movement, the somatotopic organization of the areas of the cortex that contribute to these skills makes it possible for simple manual movement to be unimpaired while simple oral movement is disturbed, or vice versa.

KINESTHETIC BASIS OF MOVEMENT

The afferent basis of motor movement is strongly emphasized in the next set of manual and oral motor tasks (items 5–8, 30–31).

For item 5 the patient is asked to close his/her eyes, and the examiner places the thumb of the patient's right hand against the fifth finger of that hand. The patient is then asked to reproduce that hand position. Item 6 is similar except that the left hand is used. In item 7 the right hand is placed in a specified position and the patient is asked to reproduce the position with the left hand. For item 8, the procedure is the same except it begins with the left hand. On item 30 the patient is told to stick out his/her tongue and roll it up. Item 31 requires the patient to place the tongue between the upper teeth and upper lip. Although these items require contributions from multiple elements of the functional system of motor movements, performance depends most heavily upon kinesthetic analysis. Kinesthetic stimuli, as mediated by the postcentral area of the cerebral cortex, contribute to adequate voluntary movement by aiding in selectivity of innervation and by preventing simultaneous stimulation of agonist and antagonist muscle groups. Interpretation of failures on these items, and on other items that place heavy emphasis on tactile feedback, may lead to an understanding of the integrity of the postcentral area of the cortex and may reveal which step in the motor process is leading to motor difficulties for the individual.

Visual cues are eliminated as a source of feedback in these tasks, and the patient must rely solely on correct information from deep sensation to perceive and precisely complete the required movement. These items, though using muscle systems organized in space, do not require the visual organization of external spatial coordinates.

Failure to complete items requiring kinesthetic-tactile feedback to the manual musculature, or the tendency for fatigue on such items (which will result in failure on items later in the series), may indicate afferent (kinesthetic) apraxia. It is expected that such patients will demonstrate difficulties on other items requiring that the kinesthetic bases of movement be intact. Disturbance of the postcentral area of the sensorimotor analyzer will concurrently produce imprecise, diffuse movement and tactile deficits.

The kinesthetic afferent system plays a larger role in oral praxis than in manual praxis (Luria, 1966), and deficits interfere with adequate, crisp articulation. Unsuccessful performance on items requiring that kinesthetic feedback be utilized to monitor oral movement (items 30, 31) is crucial to discerning expressive speech difficulty.

Damage to the postcentral area of the cortex may produce a deficit in the ability to use kinesthetic feedback, so that oral motor movements become diffuse and imprecise (Luria, 1966). Patients with such deficits have difficulty selecting the required movement, their responses become inadequately differentiated, and they need prolonged attempts to organize the appropriate movement.

Though the neuropsychological basis is the same for oral and manual motor movements that depend on kinesthetic feedback, the somatotopic organization of the postcentral sensory area makes it possible for one type to remain intact while there is apraxia in the other. Performance on tasks measuring the adequacy of the kinesthetic contribution to movement depends, to some degree, on motor tone and on adequate innervation of the muscles as measured by performance on the simple motor tasks. The quality of such underlying skills should be considered in interpreting performance on these higher-level motor tasks.

OPTIC-SPATIAL ORGANIZATION

Items 9–20 assess the patient's ability to organize motor movements in external space. The integrity of spatial or-

ganization of movement is more important in human manual motor activity than in oral motor activity. As with all the motor items, the tasks of this section require use of multiple elements of the functional system for movement, though they are designed so that the functional loading is heavily on visual-spatial organization. The need for corrective kinesthetic feedback is reduced in these items.

The tasks presented in this section require differing levels of organization. For items 9–18 the patient is asked to reproduce a variety of hand movements modeled by the examiner. On items 19 and 20 the patient is to follow the verbal commands "point to your left eye with your right hand" (19) and "touch your right ear with your left hand" (20). Items 13 and 14, which require simultaneous use of both hands in different spatial planes, are more complex tasks than those requiring reproduction in one spatial plane (items 9–12). Items 19 and 20 differ from the others in that no visual model is provided. The patient must complete motor tasks within a defined spatial scheme by following verbal directions.

The ability to construct motor activities within a system of spatial coordinates is mediated by the tertiary area that lies at the boundary of the occipital, parietal, and temporal areas (Luria, 1973). Disturbed functioning may occur secondary to either right or left hemisphere lesions. This area is unique in man and is slow to develop, not maturing fully until about the seventh year of life.

Disturbances in visual-spatial orientation can occur independent of more primary disturbances in a visual process, such as visual agnosia. But a lesion of the posterior portion of the inferoparietal region, which is contiguous with the occipital division, will inevitably be followed by a disturbance in the complex visual-spatial synthesis (Luria, 1966) required by the tasks in this section.

Disturbances in spatial orientation occurring secondary to lesions in the tertiary area of the posterior cortex may arise with lesions of either the right or the left hemisphere. Disturbances associated with left hemisphere damage tend to be more extreme. Patients with lesions affecting the inferior parieto-occipital area demonstrate a variety of disorders. This section of the Luria-Nebraska Neuropsychological Battery evaluates only the motor manifestations of the pattern of disabilities, spatial apractagnosia, in which defects in spatial perception are combined with deficits in spatially organized behavior (Luria, 1966).

Items 9–12, and items 15 and 16, require that the patient imitate a simple movement of one hand within one spatial plane. Any disturbances in visual-spatial orientation are apparent in failure to utilize external systems of spatial coordinates to orient the hand appropriately or in failure to use the correct hand. Because of the seating arrangement during testing, the patient must mentally reverse the visual picture so as not to produce a mirror image of the stimuli. This conscious transposition of spatial relationships is difficult for patients with lesions of the inferoparietal region, and such disturbances are especially marked on these tasks (Luria, 1966).

The level of spatial organization required by items 13, 14, 17, and 18 is greater than that required by earlier items. The subject must simultaneously reverse the visual image presented and organize both sides of the body in the correct spatial orientation. Mental recoding is necessary at two levels, along with adequate perception and integration of lateralized relationships. These tasks are more difficult and hence more sensitive to subtle disturbances in visual-spatial organization.

Items 19 and 20 provide a verbal stimulus for spatially oriented motor movements and exclude the visual model. Left temporal lobe function, necessary for perceiving and understanding verbal directions, attains a greater importance in these tasks. Rather than mentally rotating a visual image, the patient must use speech to spatially organize a motor act. Failure to successfully complete items 19 and 20, in conjunction with failures on the more visually mediated tasks given earlier in the test, emphasizes a spatial orientation deficit in the parieto-occipital area. Inadequate performance on these items, in contrast to success on earlier visual-spatial motor tasks, may be secondary to failures in receptive language. Success on items 19

and 20, in which external verbal directions support behavior, contrasted with failure on earlier items in which internal speech must be used to regulate behavior, suggests mild frontal lobe damage that produces echopraxia.

Patients with frontal lobe damage respond to the visual image in an echopractic manner. Without external verbal directions, the model provokes a direct imitation—a mirror-image response. Frontal lobe patients cannot analyze the problem to recode the visual image. They tend to perseverate and to lose the controlling influence of internal speech. With external verbal directions, patients with relatively mild frontal lobe deficits may perform adequately (Luria, 1966), for their primary deficit is not in visual-spatial organization, but in the ability to plan and carry out goal-directed behavior mediated by internal speech and to evaluate their own behavior.

Dynamic Organization: The following group of items assess the patient's ability to complete motor tasks requiring dynamic organization of complex movement. Items 21–24 assess ability to smoothly complete a series of manual motor movements, while items 32 and 33 assess the performance of complex oral movements. The items in this section emphasize not spatial and kinesthetic skills, but the ability to integrate multiple simple movements into a complex pattern. Luria (1966) notes that complex motor patterns are not merely simple movements attached to one another; they consist of a chain of movements organized in time to create smooth dynamic patterns. When the motor pattern becomes skilled and automatized, "kinetic melodies" are established; when the smooth transfer from one small movement to the next is disrupted, performance is disturbed. Each element then comes to require a special effort of will, and skilled motor tasks are not readily performed. The smooth, coordinated performance of motor behavior is mediated by the premotor zone of the cortex, Brodmann area 6 (Luria, 1973, 1966).

Item 21 assesses reciprocal coordination of the two hands. If the patient has adequate strength and muscle tone, as assessed in the first section of the motor scale, and has demonstrated adequate use of manual kinesthetic feedback (as evidenced in items 5–7), failure on this task may indicate a deficit in smooth coordination of motor skills. Failure on item 21 may be secondary to inability to persist at a task, inability to coordinate the two hands simultaneously, or failure to establish a smooth pattern of motion to meet the time criterion. Patients with lesions of the premotor zone of the cortex will be unable to perform the required reciprocal movements quickly and smoothly. Each movement will be completed separately, and coordinated performance is disrupted so that both hands perform the same action together or isolated movements are produced. Luria (1963) reports that with lesions of both the premotor and the postcentral areas one hand lags behind the other in completing this task. Patients with lesions of the anterior divisions of the corpus callosum, which connects the symmetrical points of the premotor and motor cortex, allowing mutually coordinated movements, will be unable to coordinate the two hands. Such patients will be able to complete tasks requiring smooth performance of complex movements in each hand independently, testifying to the integrity of the premotor zones (Luria, 1963, 1966, 1973).

Some patients have difficulty persisting for 10 seconds in the activity required in item 21. This is typical of patients with frontal lobe lesions. As previously noted, subjects with mild frontal lobe deficits will have trouble automatizing the required movements while maintaining their specificity, and simplified performance may result. Though the patient will begin performing the task correctly, he cannot continue throughout the 10-second period.

Item 22 requires that the patient tap out a specified rhythm using both hands. In item 23 the patient taps out the same rhythm but switches hands so that the order of performance is reversed. Both items are timed over 10 seconds, encouraging rapid performance. Patients with lesions of the premotor area are unable to create a smooth "kinetic melody," since each tap requires an exercise of will and they cannot perform the series rapidly. They may begin to add extra taps or to produce an incorrect and

equivalent performance with both hands.

Frontal lobe lesions may also produce deficient performance on items 22 and 23, and one may discriminate deficits due to premotor as opposed to frontal damage. Luria (1963) reports that when patients with premotor lesions begin to make errors on such items they are capable of recognizing and correcting them. When patients with frontal lobe lesions begin tapping a haphazard pattern, they are not critical enough of their performance to restructure it to meet task requirements. In addition, patients with lesions of the premotor zone can improve their performance by verbalizing directions. Patients with severe frontal lobe lesions cannot use speech to regulate behavior. External verbal reinforcement will have little effect on their performance of patients.

Item 24 is a drawing exercise that requires constant alteration of movement and thus is sensitive to a disturbance of the kinetic organization of movement. Patients with lesions of the premotor area of the cortex will be unable to make a smooth switch from one motion to another. They will attempt to create a simpler motor stereotype and will be unable to successfully copy the required figure; or, ignoring directions, they will lift the pencil from the paper, breaking the smooth copying task into unintegrated movements.

The dynamic organization of oral movement is assessed by items 32 and 33. Item 32 requires accurate kinesthetic feedback, a function mediated by the postcentral area of the motor cortex. Item 33 requires rapid, repeated, and skilled movement over time, so as to create a "kinetic melody." The ability to organize a complex system of oral motor movements and to switch quickly and rapidly from one to the other is necessary for crisp and clear articulation of language.

The skills assessed by the items in the dynamic organization section of the Motor scale depend most heavily on the capacity to convert individual motor acts into more complex movement over time. Inhibition of the original movement and smooth transfer to the next is necessary for complex manual and oral activities. Luria (1966) calls the failure to establish such smooth movement a defect in the kinetic aspect of motor activity, and he recognizes kinetic motor apraxia when manual movement is impaired and kinetic aphasia when there is a deficit of oral motor movement. Both syndromes represent a failure in the integration of simpler tasks into smooth kinetic melodies, which is associated with the premotor portion of the cortex.

COMPLEX FORMS OF PRAXIS

Complex manual praxis is assessed by items 25, 26, and 27. In item 26 the patient is asked to pretend to hold a teapot or a coffeepot and to show the examiner how to pour and stir tea or coffee. Next (item 27) he/she is asked to demonstrate how to thread a needle (no props are present). For item 28 the patient is to show how to cut with scissors. All three tasks require symbolic action unsupported by vision. The adequacy of performance of an imaginary act is a highly sensitive indicator of the extent to which integrative forms of praxis are preserved (Luria, 1966), but the level of integration and the multiplicity of skills required for accurate performance of these complex, multidetermined behaviors diminishes their significance for topical diagnosis. An accurate understanding of the factors necessary for success on these tasks is useful in assessing the pattern of strengths and deficits seen throughout the Motor scale.

Multiple elements of the functional unit for motor behavior are utilized in complex praxis. Motor tone and adequate innervation are, of course, basic requirements. The kinesthetic, afferent basis of movement is tapped as the patient rapidly selects the correct motions to fit the verbal directions. As we have been previously noted, patients with kinesthetic apraxia secondary to postcentral lesions cannot perform sufficiently differentiated movements as the motor impulses lose their selectivity. Luria (1966) notes that this deficit is exacerbated when, as in these items, no real object is present and the patient's actions are not supported by vision.

The optic-spatial system, as mediated by the parieto-temporo-occipital area, contributes to adequate performance on these items, since correct assessment of external coordinates is necessary. Integrity of the verbal receptive system and the efferent kinetic system are also prerequisites for success, but these items do not emphasize those components of motor behavior.

Integrative Oral Praxis: Integrative oral praxis is assessed by items 34 and 35. These oral tasks are similar to the manual tasks presented in the section on complex forms of praxis in that they represent a multifaceted skill and can demonstrate slight disturbances without allowing for an analysis of the conditions underlying the disability. Failure to complete these test items when the same actions can be performed in the environment indicates the general lowering of the level of organization of cortical activities characteristically seen in brain-damaged patients (Luria, 1966). These data in themselves have no localizing or analytical significance, though the information can be interpreted, in conjunction with that from other items in the neuropsychological battery, to establish a pattern of deficits.

Selectivity of Motor Acts: The six tasks presented in this section, items 36–47 (time to complete each figure is also scored), require the patient to draw geometrical figures from verbal directions and then to copy these same figures from a model. Performance is scored for both quality and time; specific scoring criteria are provided in the manual. Figure drawing tasks are frequently used to identify organic disorders because their complex nature makes them vulnerable to disruption by a variety of disorders. The sensitivity of these items to organic impairment is reflected in the Luria-Nebraska. Note that this section contributes five of the 33 items on the Pathognomonic scale. Luria (1966) reports that a disturbance in the selectivity of the motor act, for example, failure to respond to a verbal or visual command such as is required in the tasks in this section, may indicate a major disturbance in cerebral functioning.

The examiner must be sensitive to the range of deficits that can disrupt performance in drawing tasks. Though the items that require drawing a triangle from verbal directions and copying a triangle seem similar, each places different demands on the cortical system. Adequate interpretation of performance on these items demands that one attend to these differences as well as to the requirements of individual items and the subject's pattern of performance throughout the section.

The individual construction tasks may be disrupted by poor motor control, leading to scorable defects such as lack of closure in figures, overlaps in figures, and fine motor tremor. Such deficits may be secondary to inadequate afferent feedback leading to a disruption of the kinesthetic basis of movement. Such patients cannot select the appropriate movements, and specificity is lost. Lesions of the premotor zone, which disrupt smooth performance of skilled tasks by failing to inhibit the initial individual motor elements of fine movement, will also disrupt motor control on the construction tasks.

These construction tasks require frequent fine changes in the direction of movement, which makes them sensitive to defects in the optic-spatial system. Such deficits may reflect left or right hemisphere dysfunction. Construction difficulty is one of the most common disorders in individuals with right hemisphere lesions (Heimburger & Reitan, 1961). Such patients may have trouble changing directions when they come to corners and so produce rounded or dog-eared angles. Spatial dysfunctions are also exhibited in an inability to change directions when crossing the midline, so that impaired individuals draw a circle as two halves. Left-hemisphere lesions of the parieto-occipital area will also lead to defects in spatially organized activity.

Some patients demonstrate perseverative behavior on the construction tasks. This may limit their ability to inhibit individual and basic elements of the motor act, or it may be generalized, leading to failure in the inhibition of entire voluntary actions. Though both these dysfunctions indicate failure in the inhibitory system, they have differential significance in our understanding of the breakdown of the motor act and of the status of higher cortical functions. Perseveration on one part of the motor act is more indicative of premotor and deeper brain involvement and is consistent with the difficulty such patients encounter with smooth and successive excitation and inhibition of the muscle groups. More generalized perseveration is seen in patients with lesions of the frontal lobes and indicates inertia of the nervous process so that selective performance becomes impossible. The patient's intention loses its power to regulate behavior, and appropriate inhibition of the motor act does not occur.

The salient features of premotor versus frontal perseveration may be highlighted by the individual's performance over the entire construction section. The disintegration of selectivity associated with lesions of the frontal lobe may be observed in perseveration between figures as well as in the drawing of individual figures. Characteristically, patients with severe frontal lobe lesions can carry out the first in a series of actions, but they are unable to transfer to a second task upon verbal instruction. Retention of selective traces in such individuals is so difficult and the pathological inertia of the preceding instruction is so strong that there is a tendency to perseverate on the first task. Failure to adequately inhibit old associations disrupts the ability to create a new set of intentions in response to a new task.

The organization of motor acts by speech is the link most disrupted in lesions of the frontal lobe. A visual stimulus that provides the support of the optic afferent system may stabilize the intentions of individuals with frontal lobe lesions (Luria, 1966). With only verbal instructions they typically will not compare the results of their actions with the task or correct their perseverative repetition of an inert stereotype. When such an individual is asked to copy single figures, no perseveration may be noted, since the set is more clearly observable and comparable. The difference in functioning between oral and visual tasks is indicative of the weakness in retention and in the regulating influence of verbal traces in frontal lobe patients.

Failure in regulating motor behavior by speech and

difficulty in maintaining a stable set of intentions or verbal direction in frontal lobe patients have been previously noted. Problems in maintaining behavior for 10 seconds, as on items 1 and 2, and regression to simpler, more perseverative behavior, as on item 21, indicate the same deficit in higher cortical functioning.

Speech Regulation of Motor Acts: Items 48–51 of the Motor scale are similar to the construction tasks in that they assess how well the patient's motor act corresponds to a visual or verbal command. These tasks stress more seriously the stability of intentions and the regulatory function of verbal stimuli by requiring a series of responses and by presenting tasks in which the response is in conflict with the stimulus (e.g., in item 48, "If I knock once, you knock twice; if I knock twice, you knock once").

For item 49 the patient is asked to squeeze the examiner's hand if the examiner says "red" and to do nothing if he says "green." Item 50 requires the patient to raise the right hand if the examiner knocks once and to raise the left hand if he knocks twice. For the final item of the scale (51) the patient is to knock gently if the examiner knocks hard and to knock hard if the examiner knocks gently.

A prerequisite for success on these tasks is competent understanding of verbal directions. Lesions of the left temporal lobe will disrupt such performance. Additionally, these items require the subject to follow directions utilizing relational words. Understanding of complex grammatical structures is related to the integrity of the tertiary parietal areas of the left temporal lobe. Deficiencies in this function will be reflected in performance on the Receptive Speech section of the Luria-Nebraska.

The items in this section are most sensitive to disorders of the frontal lobe. The regulatory function of speech is emphasized. Patients with frontal lobe lesions demonstrate a dissociation between speech and movement. With complex instructions where the response must be the opposite of the stimulus the examiner provides, patients with lesions of the frontal lobe will exhibit disrupted performance and echopraxia. Rather than following the verbal directions, they will begin imitating the examiner's be-

havior, matching their response to the stimulus in direct contradiction of the instructions. Speech no longer creates a stable set of connections to organize, determine, and direct movement. Perseveration often occurs; for example, the patient will squeeze the examiner's hand three or four times rather than once, another indication of the failure of the regulatory function of speech in frontal lobe patients (Luria, 1966).

Echopraxia, as exhibited on these items, indicates the same pathological process frontal lobe patients evidence on the construction and optic-spatial organization tasks. Failure to regulate motor performance to conform with the verbal instructions on these tasks reflects their inability to inhibit responses to irrelevant stimuli. Just as perseveration between construction tasks resulted from the intrusion of a prior, now irrelevant stimulus, failure to follow verbal instructions on these later tasks indicates inability to inhibit responses to visual, auditory, or kinesthetic stimuli. Similarly, a failure in recoding visual stimuli on the optic-spatial organization tasks (items 10–18) so as to mirror rather than copy the action may indicate failure to inhibit a response to visual stimuli and to regulate activity by internal reorganization of the stimulus. Errors on these items reflect a dysfunction in the capacity to maintain a stable plan or to regulate activity by internal speech. Items 10–18 allow the patient a second chance to respond when errors reflect only problems in mirror-imaging. Continuing errors even after correction are seen as particularly severe, while normals may make initial errors of this kind due to lack of concentration or other factors.

Item Intercorrelations

Intercorrelation of the Motor scale items with all other Luria items reveals a number of significant correlations ($r > .35$; $p < .0001$), as is shown in Table 2.1 (Golden and Berg, 1980b, 1980c). As noted above, the Motor scale is one of the most complex scales on the Luria test, tapping a wide variety of motor skills involving both the right and left hemispheres.

Table 2.1: **Item Intercorrelations with Motor Scale**

Item	r*	Item	Description
1	.37	55	Listen to tones and hum
1	.37	134	Repeat *sp, th, pl, str, awk*
1	.37	185	Write words and phrases
1	.38	178	Copy *pa, an, pro, pre, sti*
1	.39	59	How many beeps in all groups together?
1	.39	71	Score #70, distance (mm) between two points (left hand)
1	.41	70	How many points do you feel? Two-point tactile stimulation—right hand
1	.41	84	Left hand stereognosis errors
1	.41	92	Number of errors on tasks from Raven's Matrices
1	.41	157	Name objects (guitar, can opener, table, candle, stapler)
1	.42	82	Right hand stereognosis errors
1	.42	187	Number of words written on specified subject in 60 seconds
1	.42	256	Analogies; e.g., good: ———::high: low
1	.43	62	Reproduce rhythm
1	.43	223	Memory for seven words scored for errors
1	.44	74	Identify shapes drawn on right wrist
1	.45	227	Draw geometric shapes from memory
2	.37	85	Left hand stereognosis—time
2	.37	178	Copy *pa, an, pro, pre, sti*
2	.37	187	Number of words written on specific subject in 60 seconds
2	.37	257	Which of these four does not belong in same group as other three?
2	.38	84	Left hand stereognosis errors
2	.38	218	What sign is missing? 10 ( ) 2 = 20; 10 ( ) 2 = 12
2	.40	92	Number of errors on tasks from Raven's Matrices
2	.41	70	Two-point tactile stimulation—right hand
2	.42	74	Determine what shape drawn on right wrist
2	.42	223	Memory for seven words scored for errors
2	.42	227	Draw geometric shapes from memory

*r = correlation

Table 2.1: **Item Intercorrelations with Motor Scale**   *Continued*

Item	r*	Item	Description
2	.43	256	Verbal analogies
2	.47	71	Two-point tactile stimulation left hand
3	.35	203	Write 17 and 71; 69 and 96
3	.36	84	Stereognosis—left hand errors
3	.36	223	Memory for seven words scored for errors
3	.37	86	Name visually presented objects
3	.38	256	Verbal analogies
3	.39	70	Two-point tactile stimulation—right hand
3	.39	71	Two-point tactile stimulation—left hand
3	.39	83	Stereognosis—right hand time
3	.39	92	Number of errors on tasks from Raven's Matrices
3	.39	157	Name objects from pictures
3	.39	205	Write 14, 17, 19, 109, 1023
3	.41	82	Stereognosis—right hand errors
4	.34	75	Determine shapes drawn on left wrist
4	.36	59	How many beeps in all groups together?
4	.36	84	Stereognosis—left hand errors
4	.40	85	Stereognosis—left hand time
4	.40	92	Number of errors on tasks from Raven's Matrices
4	.43	81	Muscle and joint sensation
4	.44	71	Two-point tactile stimulation—left hand
5	.34	84	Stereognosis—left hand errors
5	.34	210	Which is larger: 17 or 68; 23 or 56; 189 or 201?
5	.36	209	Read vertically printed numbers
5	.37	218	What sign is missing? e.g., 10 ( ) 2 = 20; 10 ( ) 2 = 12
5	.38	86	Name visually presented objects
5	.40	82	Stereognosis—right hand errors
6	.35	65	Cutaneous sensation—left side
6	.35	95	Draw hands on blank clockface at 12:50, 4:35, 11:10
6	.35	201	Write 7-9-3; 3-5-7
6	.37	81	Muscle and joint sensation—left arm
6	.37	178	Copy *pa, an, pro, pre, sti*

*r = correlation

Table 2.1: **Item Intercorrelations with Motor Scale** *Continued*

Item	r*		Item Description
6	.38	71	Two-point tactile stimulation—left hand
6	.38	84	Stereognosis—left hand errors
6	.39	69	Differentiation of hard and soft pin pressure—left hand
6	.40	177	Copy B, L, $\mathscr{L}$, $\mathscr{D}$, $\mathscr{B}$
6	.42	85	Stereognosis—left hand time
6	.43	77	What number is written on left wrist?
7	.35	71	Two-point tactile stimulation—left hand
8	.34	71	Two-point tactile stimulation—left hand
8	.34	82	Stereognosis—right hand error
8	.35	55	Listen to tones and hum them
8	.35	85	Stereognosis—left hand time
8	.35	201	Write 7-9-3; 3-5-7
8	.37	208	Read 27, 34, 158, 396, 9845
8	.38	65	Cutaneous sensation—left side
8	.39	69	Differentiation of hard and soft pin pressure—left hand
8	.39	108	Point to eye; nose; ear
8	.43	177	Copy B, L, $\mathscr{L}$, $\mathscr{D}$, $\mathscr{B}$
8	.44	178	Copy *pa, an, pro, pre, sti*
9	—		No correlations ≥.35 with items from other scales
10	.35	62	Reproduce rhythm
10	.35	65	Cutaneous sensation—left side
10	.35	71	Two-point tactile stimulation—left hand
10	.35	81	Joint and muscle sensation—left arm
10	.36	59	How many beeps in all groups together?
10	.36	95	Draw hands on blank clockface at 12:50, 4:35, 11:10
10	.36	217	Mental subtraction (24−18)
10	.37	204	Write 27, 34, 158, 396, 9845
10	.37	209	Read vertically printed numbers
10	.38	84	Stereognosis—left hand errors
10	.38	177	Copy B, L, $\mathscr{L}$, $\mathscr{D}$, $\mathscr{B}$
10	.43	205	Write 14, 17, 19, 109, 1023
11	.34	129	Logical grammatical structures—inverted grammatical constructions

Table 2.1: **Item Intercorrelations with Motor Scale** *Continued*

Item	r*		Item Description
11	.34	209	Read vertically printed numbers
11	.35	58	How many beeps do you hear?
11	.35	70	Two-point tactile stimulation—right hand
11	.35	210	Which is larger: 17 or 68; 23 or 56; 189 or 201?
11	.37	177	Copy B, L, $\mathscr{L}$, $\mathscr{D}$, $\mathscr{B}$
11	.37	205	Write 14, 17, 19, 109, 1023
11	.38	201	Write 7-9-3; 3-5-7
12	.36	75	Identify shapes drawn on left wrist
12	.36	94	Tell what time clocks tell
12	.37	59	How many beeps in all groups together?
12	.37	84	Stereognosis—right hand time
12	.37	95	Draw hands on blank clockface for 12:50, 4:35, 11:10
12	.38	208	Read 27, 34, 158, 396, 9845
12	.41	58	How many beeps do you hear?
12	.41	108	Point to eye, nose, ear
12	.41	204	Write 27, 34, 158, 396, 9845
12	.41	209	Read vertically printed numbers
12	.43	205	Write 14, 17, 19, 109, 1023
12	.44	177	Copy B, L, $\mathscr{L}$, $\mathscr{D}$, $\mathscr{B}$
12	.44	201	Write 7-9-3; 3-5-7
13	—		No correlations ≥.35 with items from other scales
14	.30	55	Listen to tones and reproduce them.
14	.30	130	If I had breakfast after I sawed wood, what did I do first?
15	.30	119	Point with key toward pencil; point with pencil toward key
15	.31	58	How many beeps do you hear?
15	.31	123	Draw a cross beneath a circle; draw a cross to the right of a circle
15	.31	251	Logical relationships; e.g., rose belongs to what group?
15	.32	159	Name objects from pictures
14	.35	54	Determine whether two groups of tones are different
15	.35	204	Write 27, 34, 158, 396, 9845
15	.35	205	Write 14, 17, 19, 109, 1023

*r = correlation

Table 2.1: **Item Intercorrelations with Motor Scale** *Continued*

Item	r*		Item Description
15	.35	209	Read vertically printed numbers
16	.35	213	How much is 3 + 4; 6 + 7?
16	.36	68	Discriminate between hard and soft pin pressure—right hand
16	.36	119	Point with key toward pencil; point with pencil toward key
16	.36	129	If Arnie hit Tom, which boy was the victim?
16	.37	209	Read vertically printed numbers
16	.39	58	How many beeps do you hear?
17	.34	109	Point to these in this order: eye-nose-ear-eye-nose
17	.36	55	Listen to tones and reproduce them
17	.36	157	Name objects from pictures
18	.35	95	Draw hands on blank clockface at 12:50, 4:35, 11:10
18	.35	97	Count all blocks in picture, including hidden ones
18	.37	157	Name objects from pictures
19	.40	64	Cutaneous sensation—right hand
19	.40	73	Determine whether stimulus is moving up or down left arm
19	.41	115	Whose watch is this? (examiner's); whose is this? (patient's)
19	.41	160	Count from 1 to 20
19	.41	201	Write 7-9-3; 3-5-7
19	.41	209	Read vertically printed numbers
19	.41	258	Discursive reasoning—elementary arithmetic
19	.45	72	Determine whether stimulus is moving up or down right arm
19	.46	210	Which is larger: 17 or 68; 23 or 56; 189 or 201?
19	.48	205	Write 14, 17, 19, 109, 1023
19	.48	206	Read 7-9-3; 3-5-7
20	.33	84	Stereognosis—left hand errors
20	.35	68	Determine whether pin pressure is hard or soft—right hand
20	.36	177	Copy *B, L, ℒ, 𝒟, ℬ*
20	.37	71	Two-point tactile stimulation—left hand
20	.37	206	Read 7-9-3; 3-5-7
20	.38	59	How many beeps in all groups together?
20	.38	113	Point to the picture that shows: typewriting; mealtime; summer
20	.39	158	What part of the body does picture represent?
20	.39	208	Read 27, 34, 158, 396, 9845
20	.40	73	Determine whether stimulus is moving up or down—left arm
20	.40	112	What do *cat, bat, pat* mean?
20	.42	124	Which is correct: Spring comes before summer, or Summer comes before spring?
21	.36	70	Two-point tactile stimulation—right hand
21	.36	87	What is picture supposed to be?
21	.36	84	Stereognosis—left hand errors
21	.36	92	Number of errors on tasks from Raven's Matrices
21	.36	106	Phonemic hearing—conditioned reflex
21	.36	144	Read *sp, th, pl, str, awk*
21	.36	202	Write IV and VI; IX and XI
21	.36	205	Write 14, 17, 19, 109, 1023
21	.37	55	Listen to tones and reproduce them
21	.38	59	How many beeps in all groups together?
21	.38	60	Count beeps in each group
21	.38	62	Reproduce rhythm
21	.38	71	Two-point tactile stimulation—left hand
21	.39	82	Stereognosis—right hand errors
21	.39	219	What number is missing? 12 − ( ) = 8; 12 + ( ) = 19
21	.41	256	Verbal analogies
22	.36	71	Two-point tactile stimulation—left hand
22	.36	106	Phonemic hearing—conditioned reflex
22	.36	257	Verbal analogies
22	.37	55	Listen to tones and reproduce them
22	.37	176	What is the second letter in *cat*? first letter in *match*?
22	.37	218	What sign is missing? 10 ( ) 2 = 20; 10 ( ) 2 = 12

*r = correlation

Table 2.1: **Item Intercorrelations with Motor Scale** *Continued*

Item	r*		Item Description
22	.38	60	Count beeps in each group
22	.38	70	Two-point tactile stimulation—left hand
22	.38	185	Write words and phrases
22	.38	187	Number of words written in 60 seconds on specified subject
22	.38	227	Draw geometric shapes from memory
22	.38	230	Write words from memory after visual presentation
22	.39	157	Name objects from pictures
22	.40	53	Which is higher, first or second tone?
22	.40	221	Serial seven subtraction from 100
22	.41	62	Reproduce rhythm
22	.41	223	Memory for seven words scored for errors
22	.41	256	Verbal analogies
22	.42	200	Time taken to read paragraph
22	.42	92	Number of errors on tasks from Raven's Matrices
23	.37	59	How many beeps in all groups together?
23	.37	185	Write words and phrases
23	.37	221	Serial seven subtraction from 100
23	.37	230	Write words from memory after visual presentation
23	.38	62	Reproduce rhythm
23	.38	123	Draw a circle beneath a cross; draw a circle to the right of a cross
23	.38	145	Read *see–seen; tree–trick*
23	.38	256	Verbal analogies
23	.39	60	Count beeps in each group
23	.39	223	Memory for seven words scored for errors
23	.40	55	Listen to tones and reproduce them
23	.40	106	Phonemic hearing—conditioned reflex
23	.41	71	Two-point tactile stimulation—left hand
23	.42	200	Time taken to read paragraph
24	.35	65	Cutaneous sensation—left side
24	.35	69	Determine whether pin pressure is hard or soft—left hand
24	.35	113	Point to picture that shows: typewriting; mealtime; summer
24	.35	208	Read 27, 34, 158, 396, 9845
24	.36	110	Point to picture of shoe; candle; stove
24	.37	177	Copy *B, L, ℒ, 𝒟, ℬ*
24	.38	81	Muscle and joint sensation
24	.38	95	Draw hands on blank clockface at: 12:50, 4:35, 11:10
24	.38	178	Copy *pa, an, pro, pre, sti*
24	.39	59	How many beeps in all groups together?
24	.39	205	Write 14, 17, 19, 109, 1023
24	.42	74	Identify shapes drawn on right wrist
25	.35	106	Phonemic hearing—conditioned reflex
25	.36	177	Copy *pa, an, pro, pre, sti*
25	.36	178	Copy *B, L, ℒ, 𝒟, ℬ*
25	.36	204	Write 27, 34, 158, 396, 9845
25	.36	209	Read vertically printed numbers
25	.36	259	Time to solve discursive arithmetic problem
25	.36	261	Time to solve discursive arithmetic problem
25	.39	59	How many beeps in all groups together?
25	.41	137	Repeat *hairbrush; screwdriver; laborious*
25	.42	129	If Arnie hit Tom, which boy was the victim?
26	.37	204	Write 27, 34, 158, 396, 9845
26	.35	160	Count from 1 to 20
27	—		No correlations ≥.35 with items from other scales
28	—		No correlations ≥.35 with items from other scales
29	.35	69	Determine whether pin pressure is hard or soft—left hand
30	—		No correlations ≥.35 with items from other scales
31	—		No correlations ≥.35 with items from other scales
32	.38	63	Make a series of taps
32	.37	230	Write words from memory after visual presentation
33	.44	157	Name objects from pictures
33	.44	227	Draw geometric shapes from memory

*r = correlation

Table 2.1: **Item Intercorrelations with Motor Scale** *Continued*

Item	r*		Item Description
33	.43	92	Number of errors on tasks from Raven's Matrices
33	.42	223	Memory for seven words scored for errors
33	.40	84	Stereognosis—left hand errors
33	.40	87	Visual identification of pictures of objects
33	.38	82	Stereognosis—right hand errors
33	.37	85	Stereognosis—left hand time
33	.37	109	Point to these, in this order: eye–nose–ear–eye–nose
33	.37	228	Tap the rhythm demonstrated
33	.37	235	Logical memorization—recall by visual aid
34	.46	115	Whose watch is this? (examiner's); whose is this? (patient's)
34	.41	108	Point to eye; nose; ear
34	.38	118	Point to specified objects
34	.36	112	What do *cat, bat, pat* mean?
34	.36	206	Read 7-9-3; 3-5-7
35	—		No correlations ⩾.35 with items from other scales
36	—		No correlations ⩾.35 with items from other scales
37	—		No correlations ⩾.35 with items from other scales
38	—		No correlations ⩾.35 with items from other scales
39	—		No correlations ⩾.35 with items from other scales
40	.42	118	Point to specified objects
40	.39	75	Identify shapes drawn on left wrist
40	.39	85	Stereognosis—left hand time
40	.38	71	Two-point tactile discrimination—left hand
40	.38	205	Write 27, 34, 158, 396, 9845
40	.37	83	Stereognosis—right hand time
40	.37	95	Draw hands on blank clockface at 12:50, 4:35, 11:10
40	.37	251	Logical relationships; e.g., rose belongs to what group?
40	.36	86	Name visually presented objects

*r = correlation

Table 2.1: **Item Intercorrelations with Motor Scale** *Continued*

Item	r*		Item Description
40	.35	92	Number of errors on tasks from Raven's Matrices
40	.35	99	Intellectual operations in space
40	.35	223	Memory for seven words scored for errors
41	.35	157	Name objects from pictures
42	—		No correlations ⩾.35 with items from other scales
43	—		No correlations ⩾.35 with items from other scales
44	—		No correlations ⩾.35 with items from other scales
45	—		No correlations ⩾.35 with items from other scales
46	.36	227	Draw geometric shapes from memory
46	.35	110	Point at picture of shoe, candle, stove
47	—		No correlations ⩾.35 with items from other scales
48	.42	205	Write 14, 17, 19, 109, 1023
48	.41	70	Two-point tactile discrimination—right hand
48	.41	71	Two-point tactile discrimination—left hand
48	.40	62	Reproduce rhythm
48	.39	177	Copy *B, L, ℒ, 𝒟, ℬ*
48	.38	59	How many beeps in all groups together?
48	.38	108	Point to eye, nose, ear
48	.38	201	Write 7-9-3; 3-5-7
48	.38	204	Write 27, 34, 158, 396, 9845
48	.38	210	Which is larger: 17 or 68; 23 or 56; 189 or 201?
48	.38	253	Concept formation—logical relationships
48	.37	52	Determine whether tone pairs are same or different
48	.37	252	Concept formation—logical relationships
49	.39	210	Which is larger: 17 or 68; 23 or 56; 189 or 201?
49	.38	58	How many beeps do you hear?
50	.40	59	How many beeps in all groups together?
50	.37	113	Point to picture that shows: typewriting; mealtime; summer

*r = correlation

Table 2.1: **Item Intercorrelations with Motor Scale**   *Continued*

Item	r*		Item Description
51	.47	59	How many beeps in all groups together?
51	.42	53	Determine which of two tones is higher
51	.41	113	Point to picture that shows: typewriting; mealtime; summer
51	.41	177	Copy *B, L, ℒ, 𝒟, ℬ*
51	.41	178	Copy *pa, an, pro, pre, sti*
51	.40	62	Reproduce rhythm
51	.40	208	Read 27, 34, 158, 396, 9845
51	.40	234	Repeat story
51	.39	230	Write words from memory after visual presentation
51	.38	58	How many beeps do you hear?
51	.38	68	Determine whether pin pressure on right hand is soft or hard
51	.38	71	Two-point tactile discrimination—left hand
51	.38	84	Stereognosis—left hand errors
51	.38	99	Intellectual operations in space
51	.37	108	Point to eye; nose; ear
51	.37	140	Repeat *streptomycin; Massachusetts Episcopal*

*r = correlation

The first four items on the scale involve simple hand movements and are especially sensitive to disorders in or near the posterior frontal lobe (Golden, Purisch, and Hammeke, 1979). These items (1–4) are highly correlated with items tapping tactile and kinesthetic functions, suggesting sensitivity to anteriorparietal injury. Simple hand movements also appear to be related to memory for words and designs as well as to visual-spatial functions. Memory, especially for verbal material, and visual-spatial disorders have been associated with frontal lobe injury (Luria, 1966; Teuber, 1963; Milner, 1971). Not surprisingly, these items also correlate highly with several tasks involving writing and motor reproduction of rhythmic sequences, reflecting the importance of the motor component in these tasks.

Items 5–8 require kinesthetic and tactile feedback for proper performance, thus implicating parietal lobe dysfunction. The items in this section demonstrate an expected correlation with a number of other items that require intact kinesthetic and tactile feedback systems. These items (5–8) also appear to be influenced by deficient spatial, writing, and, to a lesser extent, arithmetic abilities. Deficiencies in the functions mentioned here often can be localized to the temporoparietooccipital areas of the contralateral hemisphere. Items 9–20 are again simple motor movements, but these items require intact spatial organization. As noted earlier in the chapter, these items are thought to be sensitive to both frontal lobe disorders and disorders of the right hemisphere. With the exception of items 9 and 13, they demonstrate a significant relationship with arithmetic, reading, and writing abilities and also appear to require tactile and kinesthetic feedback, a notion that seems reasonable given the nature of this section of the scale. In addition, the ability to process pitch and rhythm relationships, a right hemisphere function (McFie, 1970), is associated with these items.

Several of the Motor scale items in this section (items 12, 14, 15, 16, 17, 19, 20) are also significantly correlated with items assessing ability both to understand verbal instructions and to perform or answer as directed. Such abilities can be affected by left hemisphere injury. Significant correlations are also found relating these items to those that require comparisons and are theoretically sensitive to damage in the parieto-occipital areas of the left hemisphere (Golden, Purisch, & Hammeke, 1979).

Only items 9 and 13 of the first 24 items on the scale did not demonstrate significant correlations with other test items. It may be, therefore, that these items are unique in the abilities they tap. An inspection of the correlations, however, shows that items 9 and 13 show attenuated correlations with many of the same items of the Luria-Nebraska battery as the rest of the items in this section (items 9–20). Both items 9 and 13 require optic-spatial organization and use the right hand, the motor aspects of which are controlled by the left hemisphere. Luria (1973) has noted that a local focus in the parieto-occipital region disturbs the spatial organization of perception and movement.

Items 21–24, requiring complex movements of various kinds, are very sensitive to injury in both the motor area of the frontal lobe and the prefrontal areas that are involved in the organization of behavior. The item intercorrelations suggest that these items are influenced by tactile and kinesthetic feedback, anterior parietal lobe functions. Owing to the proximity of the motor areas, motor difficulties may be associated with verbal-expressive deficiencies. Such verbal-expressive disorders may result from lesions in the primary area of the frontal lobe. Luria (1966) has also suggested that such injuries lead to thinking disorders because they interfere with the execution of internal speech, which he feels is the basis for thought. The items in this section (21–24) are also closely associated with writing, reading, and memory skills, all of which can be affected by frontal lobe dysfunction.

Items 25–27 require complex movements and are sensitive to injury both in the motor area of the frontal lobes and in prefrontal areas that are concerned with the organization of behavior. Since these items are sensitive to frontal lobe damage, it is no surprise that they correlate highly with other items sensitive to frontal injury. Items 25 and 26 are related to items that involve speech and writing as well as to items requiring comparisons and word fluency. Additionally, there appears to be a relationship between these items and spatial functions. Consequently, poor performance of these items (25–27) may also reflect injury in the temporoparietooccipital areas.

Items 28–35 involve oral movements. Items 28 and 29 reflect simple oral movements and appear to require kinesthetic feedback, as do items 30 and 31 as reflected by the item intercorrelations. Items 32 and 33 measure complex oral skills and are also strongly influenced by kinesthetic feedback, memory, and visual-spatial organization. These functions are sensitive to disruption of the frontal lobe areas and also to parietal disorders (Warrington, Logue, & Pratt, 1971; Luria, 1966, 1973). Disorders of the left parietal areas may lead to a loss of the

ability to associate names and objects (Butters & Brody, 1969), an ability that also is significantly correlated with this section of the Motor scale.

Several items (items 28, 30, 31) in this section do not correlate highly with other Luria items. All these items measure praxis at varying levels of complexity and may reflect either inability to carry out intentional behaviors owing to frontal lobe dysfunction or dyspraxia owing to parietal lobe injury (Luria, 1973).

Items 34 and 35 tap an individual's ability to perform simple oral movements on the basis of verbal instructions. These items obviously can be affected by an impairment of the motor area. They also appear susceptible to temporoparietal dysfunction, as suggested by correlations with tasks involved with receptive language and comprehension.

Items 36–47 are concerned with construction difficulty, as is readily confirmed by significant correlations with other Luria-Nebraska items requiring spatial organization skills. Poor performance on these items often reflects severe spatial disorganization characteristic of injuries to the right hemisphere (Klove & Reitan, 1958; Wheeler, 1963; Wheeler & Reitan, 1962) or to the left parietal area (Luria, 1966, 1973; DeRenzi, Faglioni, & Scotti, 1968). However, slow performance on these items may simply reflect motor dysfunction of the dominant hand and the contralateral cerebral hemisphere, since items in this section are not significantly correlated with items from other scales.

Items 48–51 involve the ability to respond to speech regulation of a motor act. In each of these final items, the patient must keep instructions in mind, interpret them, then respond appropriately. These items involve the temporoparietal areas of the left hemisphere, basic to the understanding of what is required, as well as frontal lobes, which are responsible for the verbal command of motor movements (Golden, Purisch, & Hammeke, 1979). Individuals with frontal lobe dysfunction frequently understand what is to be done but are unable to direct the proper motor movements to respond. The items of this final section of the scale are also correlated with tasks requiring spatial organization as well as cutaneous sensation and kinesthetic feedback, all of which are considered parietal lobe functions. Items that demand following directions and understanding both relational words and arithmetic relations are similarly correlated with items 48–51. Performance on these and similar tasks can be disrupted by disorders of tertiary parietal areas (Golden, 1978). Finally, nonverbal visual memory tasks, a right frontal lobe function (Milner, 1971), are also related to those final Motor scale items.

Factor Analysis

Factor analysis of the Motor scale yields several factors, as can be seen in Table 2.2 (Golden, Sweet, Hammeke, Purisch, Graber, & Osmon, 1980). The majority of items (5, 6, 7, 8) contributing to the first factor (Table 2.3) involve hand movements that are highly dependent on kinesthetic feedback. The last two involve a test for perseveration (copying geometric figures with alternating peaks and plateaus) and the use of language in acoustic-visual cues to control motor acts. Why these last two items contribute to the factor is not altogether clear. Perhaps cerebral dysfunction in the postcentral region is likely to be related to the kinesthetic element in the first four items loading on this factor as well as affecting the subcortical connecting pathways responsible for acts dependent on visual-auditory cues. Other items dependent only on auditory or only on visual cues did not load on this factor.

The perseveration items are more explainable. Specific drawing tasks with alternating plateaus and points require extensive kinesthetic feedback from the hand, since they must be done quickly and somewhat automatically. The loading suggests that not only will damage to the premotor area interfere with this item, but apparently so will damage to the kinesthetic area of the brain. This is important in interpretation because the two causes have distinct etiologies and different implications for brain localization. This is supported by the item intercorrelations (see previous section).

The second motor factor (Table 2.4) involves the quality of drawing where simple figures are drawn by copying or on command. Each of the items, except item 36, represents the time it took to draw the required figure. Thus motor speed seems to emerge as a separate factor with diagnostic significance independent of quality, the dimension most often used in interpreting drawing items. These items need to be compared with those appearing on factor 7 (Table 2.5), the quality of the drawings, which is generally independent of motor factor 2, and overall accounted for less variance on the scale than did the time needed to do the drawing.

One possible reason for this is that the figures to be drawn on the Luria-Nebraska are rather simple. Individuals with mild construction difficulty often show their deficit not in quality but in time. Those with quality deficits as well generally have fairly severe construction difficulty. This localizes more clearly to the right hemisphere than does the drawing of complex figures such as Greek crosses or items similar to those on the Bender or the Benton Visual Retention Test.

Eight items contributed to motor factor 3 (Table 2.6). In general, this appears to represent a simple hand movement factor dependent upon visual feedback or visual-spatial analysis of complex coordinated activities.

Seven items contribute to motor factor 2 (Table 2.7), all measuring speed in repeating serial motor acts. The set of movements represented by the items loading on this factor correspond to Luria's (1966) concept of dynamic organization of movement.

The contribution of visual feedback to motor skills appears to be reflected in factor 5 (Table 2.8). These items require imitation of hand movements demonstrated by the examiner. They are simple and unilateral and generally do not involve crossing the midline of the body field. These items are successful as optic-spatial organization of motor acts (Luria, 1966). In many respects, motor factor 5 appears to be closely related to motor factor 3, which appears

Table 2.2: **Motor Factor Structure**

Item	Factor 1	Factor 2	Factor 3	Factor 4	Factor 5	Factor 6	Factor 7
1	37	22	36	−74	−20	31	38
2	38	28	37	−73	−19	30	30
3	27	17	10	−78	−32	18	41
4	23	14	11	−74	−24	17	35
5	61	16	26	−40	−21	20	38
6	58	16	22	−32	−15	17	29
7	59	23	23	−23	−20	15	18
8	57	20	22	−33	−27	28	27
9	25	22	20	−21	−55	17	27
10	32	16	27	−34	−64	40	34
11	34	16	30	−34	−62	29	34
12	33	21	27	−39	−69	36	46
13	19	11	56	−14	−23	16	14
14	22	12	61	−29	−35	22	14
15	19	13	50	−28	−69	02	11
16	25	13	53	−31	−65	11	14
17	35	19	74	−44	−27	13	21
18	29	19	76	−38	−24	15	22
19	38	13	15	−26	−40	31	24
20	37	33	19	−26	−31	36	11
21	31	20	34	−75	−20	24	26
22	27	19	45	−67	−16	25	41
23	27	21	41	−66	−17	29	36
24	42	23	22	−32	−24	32	38
25	30	17	16	−36	−24	36	26
26	29	06	16	−23	−26	42	20
27	25	19	16	−25	−18	29	20
28	32	15	10	−13	−21	21	−04
29	36	07	15	−14	−03	54	12
30	40	25	15	−26	−16	23	09
31	40	05	27	−14	01	32	04
32	35	12	32	−24	−10	49	09
33	37	25	38	−43	−08	35	20
34	10	08	02	−11	−08	44	03
35	11	06	09	−17	−12	56	13
36	27	59	16	−29	−17	21	70
37	15	63	00	−08	−02	12	03
38	26	00	13	−36	−13	12	53
39	24	79	13	−16	−08	08	04
40	32	26	15	−41	−33	25	63
41	25	71	18	−29	−25	08	17
42	12	23	08	−30	−22	16	66
43	18	78	14	−12	−14	01	08
44	15	06	14	−35	−21	06	65
45	03	81	10	−18	−11	08	04
46	29	14	24	−38	−25	14	68
47	19	75	16	−28	−15	14	23
48	45	20	27	−41	−30	26	35
49	20	14	14	−22	−20	40	14
50	59	16	26	−31	−30	35	31
51	41	19	32	−36	−37	39	33

to be an extension of motor factor 5 in that it involves relatively more complex items.

Motor factor 4 appears to identify simple movements of the mouth and tongue. Its emergence as a separate factor establishes that motor activity of the hands is not necessarily related to motor activity of the mouth and tongue. Two items show significant loading on this factor: items 29 and 35.

The factors emerging on this scale generally support Luria's formulation of motor acts. Separate factors emerge for motor functions that are highly dependent on the integrity of alternate sensory systems (kinesthetic and visual). Also, separate factors were found for repetitive serial movements of the hand or movements in construction abilities, all of which require a separate set of component skills, according to Luria (1966).

On the other hand, several items in the Motor scale do not contribute to any of the factors. Some of these involve simple and complex oral movements. There are also several items in the production of complex motor activity that do not form a factor. This might be expected on the basis of Luria's theory, however. Since these acts are relatively complex, they can be disrupted for a variety of reasons and can also be completed through a variety of channels. In addition, Luria's hypothesis regarding the verbal control of motor acts did not clearly show itself in the factor structure. Again, this may be because verbal processes are used, almost by necessity, in all items. Alternatively, however, it may be that the use of verbal skills in controlling motor acts depends upon the specific nature of the item, thus tending to make the items generally independent of one another.

Summary

The Motor scale of the Luria-Nebraska Neuropsychological Battery assesses motor function as a complex functional unit. Motor behavior may be disrupted by dysfunctions at different junctures and by deficits in the optic-spatial, verbal, kinesthetic, kinetic, or inhibitory processes. To adequately interpret motor defects, we must determine what features of the motor process are disturbed. We can do this by thoroughly analyzing the cortical requirements of the items an individual misses, so as to establish a pattern of deficits within each scale and over the test as a whole.

Table 2.3: **Items on Motor Factor 1**

Loading	Item	Description
.61	5	With your eyes closed, place your right hand in the same position I place it in. (Press patient's thumb against fifth finger for 2 seconds.)
.58	6	Left hand
.59	7	With your eyes closed, place your right hand in the same position I place your left hand in. (Thumb and middle finger are placed against each other for 2 seconds.)
.57	8	Left hand
.42	24	Draw this pattern without lifting your pencil from the paper.
.59	50	If I knock once, raise your right hand; if I knock twice, raise your left hand.

Table 2.4: **Items on Motor Factor 2**

Loading	Item	Description
.59	36	Without lifting your pencil from the paper, I want you to draw the best circle you can.
.63	37	Scoring (circle, time)
.79	39	Scoring (square, time)
.71	41	Scoring (triangle, time)
.78	43	Scoring (copy circle, time)
.81	45	Scoring (copy square, time)
.75	47	Scoring (copy triangle, time)

Table 2.5: **Items on Motor Factor 7**

Correlation	Item	Description
.46	12	Left hand
.70	36	Without lifting your pencil from the paper, I want you to draw the best circle you can.
.53	38	Without lifting your pencil from the paper, I want you to draw the best square you can.
.63	40	Without lifting your pencil from the paper, I want you to draw the best triangle you can, and make all three sides equal.
.66	42	Copy this figure as best you can without lifting your pencil from the paper (circle).
.65	44	Copy square, quality
.68	46	Copy triangle, quality

Table 2.6: **Items on Motor Factor 3**

Correlation	Item	Description
.56	13	Right hand held horizontal to vertical left.
.61	14	Left hand held horizontal to vertical right.
.50·	15	Raise the right hand.
.53	16	Raise the left hand.
.74	17	Right hand points to left eye.
.76	18	Left hand points to right eye.
.45	22	With your hands in front of you, tap your right hand twice and your left hand once, changing smoothly from one hand to the other. Do it as fast as you can until I tell you to stop.
.41	23	Same as #22, but reverse order of hands.

Table 2.7: **Items on Motor Factor 4**

Correlation	Item	Description
.74	1	Using your right hand, touch your fingers in turn with your thumb as quickly as you can while you count them.
.73	2	Left hand.
.78	3	Do as I do. Clench your right hand and then repeatedly stretch your fingers until I ask you to stop. Make sure you extend your fingers all the way and then completely close your hand. Do it as quickly as you can.
.74	4	Left hand.
.75	21	Do as I do. Change the position of your two hands at the same time. First you are to clench your right hand and at the same time extend the fingers of your left hand. Then I want you to reverse the position of your two hands. That is, I want you to then clench the fingers of your left hand and extend the fingers of your right hand at the same time.
.67	22	With your hands in front of you, tap your right hand twice and your left once, changing smoothly from one to the other. Do it as fast as you can until I tell you to stop.
.66	23	Same as #22, but reverse order of hands.

Table 2.8: **Items on Motor Factor 5**

Correlation	Item	Description
.55	9	Do as I do. (Place right hand under chin with bent fingers.) Be sure to use the same hand I do.
.64	10	Left hand.
.62	11	Right hand fingers extended in sagittal plane touching chin.
.69	12	Left hand.
.69	15	Raise the right hand.
.65	16	Raise left hand.
.40	19	Point to your left eye with your right hand.

3. Rhythm (Acoustic-Motor) Functions

The assessment of memory, spatial, and verbal functions in brain-injured individuals is a long-standing tradition. In contrast, the investigation of acoustic-motor functions has only recently gained currency in describing deficits stemming from brain injury (Luria, 1970). Acoustic-motor functions refer to the formation and coordination of motor acts based on nonverbal properties of auditory input (e.g., pitch, intensity, rhythm). The efficiency of this process ultimately depends on the integrity of the auditory afferent system.

The auditory afferent system performs perceptual functions similar to those of the tactile and visual systems. It selects and analyzes critical stimulus characteristics while simultaneously suppressing nonessential features. However, there appear to be fundamental differences in the way stimulus features are integrated in these modalities. The tactile and visual systems appear to rely heavily on a simultaneous, spatially organized synthesis of input elements. For example, many pictorial details are simultaneously integrated in recognizing a familiar face. The auditory system appears to rely more on a sequential, temporally organized synthesis of information. A series of acoustic signals are integrated into a single sequential perception (e.g., a melody or a rhythm), the pattern of which may underlie and afford a starting point for a motor sequence.

The ability to recognize and recall sequential patterns must be evaluated in any comprehensive examination of adaptive abilities. The importance of this is further enhanced by the observation that completely different sets of cortical zones are responsible for the synthesis of spatial and sequential information. Whereas spatial information is processed in the parieto-occipital region, sequential information is mediated in the temporal and frontotemporal regions (Luria, 1970).

Luria (1966) says that motor acts have "a precise serial organization, and, in their purest form, consist of 'motor melodies' in which the sequence is based on time intervals" (p. 341). In other words, each of our actions (e.g., brushing teeth, eating, conversing) requires a sequential integration of component muscle movements. Luria proposes that many motor sequences have their origin in rhythms provided through acoustic signals. In time these motor sequences may become automated so that the individual no longer needs the acoustic signals as cues. The adequacy of a behavior depends in part on the precision with which the component movements are temporally organized in the motor sequence.

Some behaviors demand precise timing of component movements. In others timing is less important. Also, tasks vary in the degree to which they depend on acoustic signals. Obviously the performance of a musician in an orchestra is heavily dependent on the ability to arrange actions in concert with the tempo and rhythmic cues of the music. In oral speech, considerable information is conveyed by the voice tempo, intensity, and inflection, which depend in part on the adequacy of acoustic analyzers. Most athletic activities require relatively precise timing of responses (e.g., tennis, ping pong, basketball), but the role of acoustic cues is less important. Many kinds of work, such as assembly lines, require a rhythmic sequence of actions for efficient production, often subject to acoustic signals. Thus the consequences of poor acoustic-motor skills depend on the severity of the impairment and on the activities in which the individual engages.

Evaluating acoustic-motor functions involves two types of task materials, melodic and rhythmic, of varying complexity. First one examines the patient's perceptual skills by requiring discrimination among increasingly complex stimuli. Next one examines the ability to motorically reproduce melodic and rhythmic sequences following model stimulus patterns. Finally, one evaluates the ability to spontaneously produce melodic and rhythmic sequences without the aid of a stimulus pattern.

Assessment of Acoustic-Motor Functions

GENERAL DESCRIPTION OF THE TEST SECTION
The test of acoustic-motor functioning contains 12 items

(items 52 through 63). This section is broken down into four subtests: perception of pitch relationships (3 items); reproduction of pitch relationships and musical melodies (3 items); perception and evaluation of acoustic signals (4 items); and motor performance of rhythmic patterns (2 items).

Most of the stimulus materials in this section are presented on tape. Because many of the tasks require rather subtle discriminations in the taped material, ambient noise levels and other distractions should be kept to an absolute minimum. The volume of the tape player should be adjusted to the comfort and needs of the patient. If the patient requests volume changes, adjustments should be made before beginning a trial or between trials so as not to confound the task administration. It is best to let the patient listen to the announcement of the item on the tape and to make volume adjustments accordingly.

Only the beginning of each item is announced on the tape. There are no warning signals for each trial within the item. Consequently, the patient should be warned that the next stimulus will be presented immediately and encouraged to keep listening to the tape material. Enough time should be allowed for the player to reach normal operating speed before each stimulus begins. In our practice the player is routinely stopped about 4 seconds after the stimulus presentation if no response has been made. This gives the patient more time to consider the response or allows time for the examiner to regain the patient's attention with adequate lead time on the tape before the next stimulus presentation.

Only when there is an obvious distraction, such as someone's coming into the room, should a trial be replayed. Patients are discouraged from requesting a replay of the trial stimulus by warning them before the task is started that they will have only one chance to listen, and the examiner should be reasonably sure that the patient's attention is on the task before beginning each trial. Of course, after completion of the standardized administration, the examiner is encouraged to readminister any items with any desired modifications in procedures or materials. The performance ratings of the standardized administration are used in computing summary indexes, but any significant observation with modified or repeated administrations should be incorporated in the clinician's interpretation of the results.

The items in this section of the battery require sustained concentration. Because of this, and because the examiner has somewhat limited control over the exact time of stimulus presentations, this section is particularly sensitive to attentional difficulties. To interpret whether a poor performance on these items is primarily due to deficits in particular acoustic-motor abilities, the examiner should note any signs of poor attention (e.g., drowsiness, lethargy, instability, restlessness, excitability, distractibility). If many such signs occur one may interpret a poor performance as at least partially due to attentional deficits, which precludes a valid evaluation of acoustic-motor skills.

PERCEPTION OF PITCH RELATIONSHIPS
These items are intended to assess the patient's ability to discriminate differences in both simple and more complex musical stimuli. All the test stimuli are presented on tape. Item 52 poses the simplest and most basic pitch discrimination problem. Five pairs of tones are presented, and the task is to identify whether the two tones in each pair are the same pitch or different. All the tones are one of three pitches (approximately 500, 540, or 600 Hz).

Item 53 requires the patient not only to be sensitive to differences in pitch, but also to report the directional relationship of the differences. Again five pairs of tones are presented on tape. The approximate frequencies (Hz) presented in the five trials are as follows: 600/500, 500/540, 500/600, 600/540, and 540/600. On each trial the patient is asked to state which tone in the pair is higher, the first or the second.

Item 54 increases the complexity of the pitch discrimination task. Six pairs of tone groups (each group involving four or five individual tones at either 540 or 600 Hz) are presented, and the patient is to state whether the tone

groups (or melodies) in each pair are the same or different. The complexity of this task is greater not only in the number of tones to be processed, but also in the memory requirement. The patient has to retain the melody of the first group of tones to compare it with the melody of the second group. A few patients may answer after the first melody of the pair, and it is obvious that they have failed to understand the task. In such situations it will be necessary to stop the tape, repeat the instructions, and ask the patient to withhold the response until both groups of tones are presented.

Patients with scores in the impaired ranges on these items may have difficulty analyzing pitch differences. This inability to discriminate pitch relationships in severe form is referred to as *sensory amusia*. Luria (1966, 1973) proposes that the temporal lobes are involved in the analysis and synthesis of acoustic information. Severe impairment on tasks requiring pitch discrimination and retention of melodic patterns suggests temporal lobe dysfunction. While both temporal lobes appear to be heavily involved in acoustic analysis of pitch, the right hemisphere appears to play a greater role (Luria, 1966; Milner, 1958). Where the patient's performance is impaired on all these items, one might expect difficulties on any task that depends on adequate discrimination of pitch—for example, appreciation of music, vocal reproductions of melodies, and, to a somewhat lesser extent, the communication conveyed by voice inflections in speech.

When items 52 and 53 are performed within the normal range but the performance on item 54 is impaired, the basic ability to discriminate pitch differences is intact but the ability to process and retain melodic information is compromised.

Apart from the ability to discriminate differences in pitch, these items also demand sustained concentration, particularly item 54. Consequently, poor scores may reflect attentional problems. Ways to discern whether an attentional problem or a problem in pitch discrimination is primary were suggested earlier. Poor performance from patients who appear to be attending to the task, making comments about its difficulty, or who seem somewhat unsure of their responses suggest pitch perception difficulties. Many patients appear confident in their responses and seemingly are unaware of any mistakes they have made. This observation in itself does not necessarily suggest either attentional or perceptual difficulties, but it may be diagnostically useful and should be noted, particularly if it characterizes much of the patient's test behavior.

REPRODUCTION OF PITCH RELATIONSHIPS
AND MUSICAL MELODIES

The ability to vocalize perceived pitch patterns of both familiar and unfamiliar stimuli is evaluated next. Many patients are apprehensive about displaying their vocal abilities, and some may require considerable encouragement. In such cases patients should be informed that no one is expected to be a professional singer and that all that is required is their best effort.

If the examiner has difficulty distinguishing pitch relationships reliably, scoring this subsection will pose problems. Generally, if the examiner can respond correctly to all the pitch perception trials in items 52–54, he or she has adequate musical skill for scoring the items in this subsection. If the examiner makes errors, it is recommended that someone who is reliable in discriminating pitch relationships be called in for scoring the items, or that the patient's reproductions be tape-recorded for later scoring.

Item 55 involves the simplest pitch vocalization. Four trials require the patient to reproduce tones either by singing (e.g., "la, la, la") or humming them. Each of the first two trials contains only two notes; the last two involve three notes. So that the patient does not begin responding before the end of the stimulus sequence on trial 3, one should mention just before the trial that the stimulus has three tones. For each trial the patient's response is scored as correct if it accurately reflects the *directional sequential relationship* of the pitches presented in the stimulus. Responses that are sung in a different key or fail to maintain the musical intervals presented in the stimulus should

be scored correct provided the directional relationship of the tones is accurate. However, reproductions are scored incorrect if the patient adds to or subtracts from the stimulus or if the response has so little pitch separation that it is difficult to discern the directional relationship. This is not a frequent problem. Most patients exaggerate rather than minimize pitch differences.

In contrast to the novel musical stimuli presented in item 55, items 56 and 57 involve familiar melodies. In item 56 the patient listens to a melody ("My Bonnie Lies over the Ocean"), then is asked to sing it. Regardless of how familiar the patient is with this melody, the stimulus alone allows most people to perform adequately. Item 57 assesses the patient's ability to spontaneously sing a familiar song, the first line of "Home on the Range." The patient may sing either the first line of the chorus ("Home, home on the range") or the first line of the verse ("Oh, give me a home"). While it is highly unlikely that this tune will be unfamiliar to the patient (a denial most likely reflects apprehension and possibly an attempt to avoid singing), the examiner may choose an alternate melody, such as "Jingle Bells" or "Mary Had a Little Lamb" or may ask the patient to suggest a song they both know. The same scoring criteria used for the test melody can be applied to the alternate song.

Scoring for items 56 and 57 is the same. The patient's reproduction is considered incorrect if it does not maintain the proper melody of the tune, that is, if any alterations are made in the sequential relationship of tones. In contrast to the scoring of item 55, the patient is required to maintain the proper musical intervals in the melody (both in pitch and in temporal arrangement) to receive a correct score; however, the melody may be sung in a different key from that presented on the tape. Thus, responses that include unstable intonations, irregular melodic patterns, or monotonic reproductions are scored as incorrect.

Provided the patient is giving maximum performance, impairment on these items reflects either a perceptual or a kinetic difficulty. Of the three items, item 55 depends most upon adequate perceptual skills. When item 55 is performed poorly but there is no difficulty with items 56 and 57, the patient may be having difficulty not with vocalization itself but with perceiving the task stimuli. Poor performance on all items in the previous subsection (52, 53, 54) would corroborate this.

When sensory amusia is implied by poor performance on items 52, 53, and 54, one would expect the ability to retain memory traces for novel stimuli to be unstable (Luria, 1966). Indeed, it is possible that the amusia may be primarily due to a defect in sensory memory that precludes pitch discrimination. The patient may be able to improve intonation when familiar tunes are used that afford more stable, long-term traces as the reproduction stimulus. Consequently the clinician should contrast the performance on item 55 with performance on items 56 and 57.

When the examination suggests that pitch discrimination is adequate, yet the patient has difficulty producing smooth, stable individual tones, one may suspect dysfunction in the neural mediation of intonation (*motor amusia*). Lesions in the inferior portions of the motor strip (those divisions responsible for primary motor innervation of the mouth, tongue, larynx, and pharynx), particularly in the right hemisphere, are associated with this disability (Luria, 1966). The patient has trouble switching from one tone to another, creating a halting, unstable, and perhaps somewhat perseverative reproduction of the same tone.

Conversely, difficulty in switching from one tone to another may be due to a lesion in the inferior premotor region, where the organization of the motor sequence is disrupted. In this case the production of individual tones is not seriously impaired, but the response may take the form of a series of isolated vocal impulses whose temporal pattern is disarranged and choppy. Difficulties in tone switching may also be symptomatic of disruption in kinesthetic feedback (lesions in the inferior sensory strip) from the lips, tongue, and vocal cords, causing kinesthetic apraxia. In this case the individual is receiving diminished and perhaps inaccurate feedback on the position of the vocal musculature.

In practice it is often difficult to distinguish motor amusias that have their primary origin in lesions of the sensorimotor strips from those resulting from premotor lesions. The problem of differential diagnosis is partially related to the anatomical proximity of these regions in the cerebral cortex as well as to some overlap of neural function in all the regions (motor, premotor, kinesthetic). The examiner should look at results on other portions of the battery for a pattern consistent with any hypothesized location of the dysfunction. For example, if one sees premotor perseveration of vocal intonation, one may look for similar perseverative features in other motor responses (e.g., sequential organization of mouth movements or drawings and disruption of responses requiring integration of right and left hand movements, as in dynamic organization of hand movements). Perseverative vocal responses originating from kinesthetic apraxia may be corroborated by impairments of tactile sensation, particularly on the left side. On occasion a similar kinesthetic switching problem may be observed in expressive speech, whereby sounds involving similar articulatory movements (e.g., d–t, g–k) are used interchangeably.

In contrast to items 55 and 56, item 57 requires spontaneous reproduction of a melody from remote memory. Poor performance on 57, when pitch perception and intonation are adequate, suggests difficulty in recalling information from long-term storage. One should look for similar memory deficits in other modalities (auditory-verbal, visual-verbal, visual-spatial, and tactile).

PERCEPTION AND EVALUATION OF ACOUSTIC SIGNALS
Analyzing acoustic information requires more than accurate recognition of pitch relationships. It also requires appreciation of the temporal sequence of the information and of the intensity of various components of the signal. Items in this subsection assess the ability to analyze these properties of acoustic signals. Test stimuli of varying complexity are presented on tape. A uniform pitch is used to control for the effects of poor pitch perception. Item 58 involves four trials on which the patient must simply count the beeps (tones are of equal intensity) presented on tape.

On the first two trials the beeps are presented at approximately .20-second intervals. The complexity of the task is increased on the last two trials, which use interstimulus intervals of approximately .12 second. The first two trials are presented slowly enough to allow the patient to vocally or subvocally count the beeps as they are presented. The more rapid presentation of the last two trials most likely requires the patient to mentally or motorically rehearse the trial to count the beeps.

Errors on the first two trials are usually seen only where there is severe dysfunction of attentional skills, such as in cases of extensive frontal lobe injuries or elevated intracranial pressure (e.g., hydrocephalus). Errors on the last two trials are most often overestimation. Again, one may suspect attentional deficits or a defect in the synthesis of sequential rhythmic stimuli (temporal lobes).

Item 59 involves two stimulus patterns presented on tape in which the patient is to count the *total* number of beeps. In each trial the beeps are temporally arranged in groups of two or three. In the first trial, eight tones are presented in four groups (" " " "); the second trial has 12 tones presented in four groups (‴ ‴ ‴ ‴).

Most patients appear to adopt one of two strategies on the task. Some can be seen to count each individual tone aloud or in a whisper as it is presented. Others count individual tones in the first group and, upon realizing that the second group is identical, begin to count groups of tones and then multiply for the final answer. The latter strategy appears to be more efficient and affords less chance for error. Item 59 requires sustained concentration and the ability to process and store acoustic information at least for short periods. The more the patient externalizes the task (i.e., counts aloud or with fingers), the less are the memory demands.

Item 60 is designed to evaluate acoustic processing of signals that contain tones of varying intensity. Four trials with series of tones of unequal intensity are presented, and the patient is to count the beeps in each series. The same pitch is used for all the tones in each series. Incorrect responses are summed across trials.

Processing acoustic signals of variable intensity is further evaluated in item 61, with more complex stimuli. The patient is given two trials. As in the previous item, each trial contains a series of tones representing two intensity levels, and the patient is to count the total number of beeps in each series. On the first trial three tones of low intensity (soft) are followed by three tones of high intensity (loud). The second trial mixes the temporal sequence of high- and low-intensity tones (H H L L H L H H). In the original standardization samples (Golden, Hammeke, & Purisch, 1978) subjects were asked to identify the exact number of loud and of soft tones in each series, a task of considerable difficulty even for normal subjects. Subsequently the task was simplified to merely counting the total number of beeps without regard for intensity.

Items 58 through 61 are particularly susceptible to attentional difficulties, whether secondary to neuropathological processes (often seen in frontal lobe disorders) or to emotional disturbances. Schizophrenic and neurological patients were found to perform equally poorly on these items (Purisch, Golden, & Hammeke, 1978). While we suspect that the poor performance of schizophrenics on these items is primarily related to attentional deficits, it is possible that there is dysfunction in acoustic perception.

If attentional problems can be ruled out, poor performance indicates a defective cortical analysis of rhythmic stimuli. Normal performance on item 58 with impaired performance on the following three items suggests that the fundamental process of acoustic analysis is intact but that difficulties arise when mnemonic requirements and intensity discriminations are added. Poor performance on item 58 accompanied by normal scores on the following three items is most likely due to lack of attention.

Defective analysis of rhythmic stimuli is most commonly associated with lesions in the temporal lobes (Luria, 1966, 1973). Some authors propose that such deficits are more often associated with left temporal lesions (Luria, 1966; Christensen, 1975); others argue for more right temporal mediation (Kimura, 1961; Milner, 1962, 1971). Although research is inconclusive, most findings support the notion that the right temporal lobe is dominant for nonverbal auditory perception (Hecaen & Albert, 1978). In our own experience with the Luria battery, rhythm perception deficits are more common in right hemisphere lesions, particularly in the absence of any language deficits.

When the items of this subsection are performed poorly, it may be useful to readminister them, replacing the taped stimuli with pencil taps made by the examiner. In this way one may examine whether adding a visual display to the nonverbal acoustic signals enhances performance. When this happens, the combination of the visual and acoustic presentation readily can be incorporated in the rehabilitation of the rhythm deficit. We recommend that such an expanded evaluation of skills be done only after the rhythm section is completed, so as not to confound the interpretation of test data obtained in the standardized administration.

MOTOR PERFORMANCE OF RHYTHMIC GROUPS

The set of component brain functions that enables motor production of rhythmic patterns differs when the pattern is produced (matched) to a rhythm presented auditorily and when it is produced to a verbal description. In the first case the auditory analyzers permit an internal representation of the rhythm that is conveyed to premotor regions for formation of the motor program. The integrity of the auditory analyzer is crucial to adequate performance. In the second case the production of a motor program is subordinated to higher cognitive centers. While the auditory analyzer is necessary to comprehending task instructions, the role of language centers (left frontal and parietotemporal regions) in guiding and directing the formation and execution of the motor program is more prominent. This section evaluates motoric production of rhythmic patterns under both auditory and verbal conditions.

The section is not intended to assess general motor functions. In cases of hemiparesis or other lateralized disorders, the patient should be allowed to use the hand whose function is least impaired. When no obvious impairment is noted, the patient should use the preferred hand.

Item 62 requires the patient to listen to a rhythmic pattern on tape and then tap the pattern on a table or lap board. The patient may use a finger (or fingers) or knuckles and can use one hand or both. When both hands are restricted by medical procedures (e.g., intravenous feeding) or by peripheral disorders, the patient may be given a pencil to tap with so the examiner can more clearly evaluate the productions. The examiner should note which hand is used, or whether both hands are used, since this may have lateralizing significance. Five trials are given. The first three involve rhythmic patterns where all beats are of equal intensity and the beats are arranged in groups of two or three (e.g., " " ", " ' " ' " '). Before the last two trials are administered, the tape is stopped and the patient is informed that the following trials contain loud and soft beats (e.g., "uuu"uuu"uuu", "'u"'u, where ' refers to loud beats and u refers to soft beats). The patient is then instructed to tap hard for loud beats and gently for soft beats.

Responses for item 62 are scored as incorrect when the wrong number of taps is included in the rhythm groupings, when the tap groupings are not clearly discernible by the examiner, or when the taps do not clearly reflect the intensity differences in the stimulus series. The exact number of beats on the tape need not be reproduced, just the rhythm. In general the patient is not required to reproduce the rhythm at the same speed as on the tape, but reproductions performed so slowly that they lose their rhythmic properties should be scored as incorrect. By these scoring criteria, many normal patients were found to have some difficulty with this task, particularly with trials 4 and 5, where the intensity component is present and the pattern is presented at a relatively rapid pace.

Item 63 evaluates the ability to produce rhythmic patterns under verbal control. The patient is to produce a pattern that is verbally described—for example, ''Make a series of two taps.'' A few patients repond to this request by just tapping twice. On these occasions the patient should be reminded to produce a *series* of two taps, to ''do the rhythm more than once.'' The patient is given six trials. In the first three the requested rhythms are comparable to the patterns presented auditorily in the first three trials of item 62. The rhythms requested in the last three trials are somewhat more complex, including variations in grouping and in intensity—for example, ''Make a series of two strong and three weak taps.'' On the first three trials the patient should be allowed to complete at least three tap groupings before the response is scored. On the last three trials the requested sequences should be completed at least twice before the performance is scored. If the patient fails to produce a series of taps as instructed after the second request for a ''series,'' the response is considered incorrect. Otherwise the scoring criteria for item 63 are the same as those for item 62.

One would expect poor performance on item 62 when impaired rhythm analysis skills have been demonstrated on items 58 through 61. If the patient has difficulty evaluating and recalling the stimulus pattern, attempts to reproduce the patterns motorically may appear to be a conglomeration of taps with no appreciation for groupings. When intensity requirements are added, performance suffers even more. Lesions in either of the temporal lobes may be suspected. With right temporal and frontal injuries, patients frequently appear totally unaware of mistakes. When questioned about the difficulty of the task, they may deny having any difficulty or may acknowledge problems but appear unconcerned.

When the disruption of rhythm productions is based on deficits in acoustic analysis, one would expect performance on item 62 to be more greatly impaired than performance on item 63 (except in cases of extensive left temporal lesions, which create severe impairment in comprehension of verbal instructions). The patient's difficulty in producing rhythmic patterns is minimized when a verbal description is the basis of formation of the motor program. Such patients also show improvement when they are allowed to organize the rhythm along spatial dimensions. For example, asking the patient to make the hard taps in a different place on the table from the gentle taps, or to use knuckles (or right hand) for hard taps and finger (or left hand) for gentle taps may enhance performance. Many patients spontaneously use one or more of these strategies to improve their performance. In these cases the examiner may have the patient perform the task without such response strategies to see if performance breaks down.

When item 63 is performed more poorly than item 62, impairment in the controlling function of speech is implied. This type of disturbance is frequently seen in extensive injuries to the dominant hemisphere and is most striking in frontal lobe injuries. The patient perseverates in forming rhythms, particularly when a verbal description is the sole stimulus. Often such patients perform better when their formation of the rhythm is based on an immediate sensory trace of the acoustic pattern, as in item 62. Additional evidence for impairment in the regulatory function of speech may be found on items 49, 50, and 51, where this aspect is evaluated using simpler motor responses.

When both items 62 and 63 are performed poorly although rhythm perceptual skills appear normal, dysfunction in motor output is suggested. Like dysfunction in the reproduction of musical melodies, impairment in the motor response may be symptomatic of lesions in the motor, sensory (kinesthetic), or premotor regions. The same problem in differential diagnosis is presented. However, impairment in primary motor functions may be more obvious in the investigation of rhythm skills than in melodic intonation. Lesions in the motor strip are reflected in paresis of the contralateral limb, whereas lesions restricted to premotor or kinesthetic divisions are not accompanied by obvious paresis.

Luria (1966) proposes that in severe premotor lesions motor responses are reduced to isolated impulses that prevent automatic renditions of complete sequences. Perseveration in both simple and complex motor sequences is often observed. In milder cases simple motor programs may remain operative, but more complex programs requiring precise synchronization of muscle systems and sophisticated temporal arrangement of component movements

Table 3.1: **Item Intercorrelations with Rhythm Scale**

Item	r*	Item	Description
52	.37	48	If I knock once you knock twice; if I knock twice, you knock once
52	.36	99	Intellectual operations in space
52	.36	247	Understanding of thematic text—proverbs
53	.40	22	Tap your right hand twice and your left hand once as quickly as you can
53	.42	51	If I knock hard, you knock gently; if I knock gently, you knock hard
53	.38	92	Number of errors on tasks from Raven's Matrices
53	.35	189	What word is made by these letters: s–t–o–n–e; k–n–i–g–h–t?
53	.38	207	Read IV, VI, IX, XI; 17, 71, 69, 96
53	.36	213	How much is: 3 + 4; 6 + 7?
53	.36	230	Write words from memory after visual presentation
53	.38	247	Understanding of thematic text—proverbs
53	.35	252	Concept formation—logical relationships
54	.36	2	Using your left hand, touch your fingers in turn with your thumb while you count them
54	.35	14	Left hand held horizontal to vertical right
54	.41	92	Number of errors on tasks from Raven's Matrices
54	.35	109	Point to these, in this order: eye-nose-ear-eye-nose
54	.36	144	Read sp, th, pl, str, awk
54	.37	223	Memory for seven words scored for errors
54	.39	232	Homogeneous interference—memory for words
55	.38	1	Using your right hand, touch your fingers in turn with your thumb as you count them
55	.36	2	Same as #1 with left hand
55	.36	17	Right hand points to left eye
55	.37	21	Clench right hand and extend fingers of left, then reverse
55	.37	22	Tap your right hand twice and left hand once as quickly as you can
55	.40	23	Same as #22 but reverse order of hands

Table 3.1: **Item Intercorrelations with Rhythm Scale**   *Continued*

Item	r*	Item	Description
55	.36	92	Number of errors on tasks from Raven's Matrices
56	—		No correlations ≥.35 with items from other scales
57	—		No correlations ≥.35 with items from other scales
58	.36	2	Using your left hand, touch your fingers in turn with your thumb while you count them
58	.41	12	Left hand fingers extended in sagittal plane touching chin
58	.36	48	If I knock once, you knock twice; if I knock twice, you knock once
58	.38	49	If I say red, squeeze my hand; if I say green, do nothing
58	.36	51	If I knock hard, you knock gently; if I knock gently, you knock hard
58	.42	129	If Arnie hit Tom, which boy was the victim?
58	.39	160	Count from 1 to 20
58	.37	185	Write words and phrases from dictation
58	.43	205	Write 14, 17, 19, 109, 1023
58	.36	207	Read IV, VI, IX, XI; 17, 71, 69, 96
58	.36	223	Memory for seven words scored for errors
58	.37	230	Write words from memory after visual presentation
58	.39	251	Concept formation—logical relationships
58	.36	253	Concept formation—logical relationships
58	.35	268	Discursive reasoning—complex arithmetic problems
59	.39	1	Using your right hand, touch your fingers in turn with your thumb while you count them
59	.39	24	Draw this pattern without lifting your pencil from the paper
59	.40	50	If I knock once, raise your right hand; if I knock twice, raise your left hand
59	.47	51	If I knock hard, you knock gently; if I knock gently, you knock hard
59	.39	82	Stereognosis—right hand errors
59	.42	92	Number of errors on tasks from Raven's Matrices

*r = correlation

Table 3.1: **Item Intercorrelations with Rhythm Scale**   *Continued*

Item	r*	Item	Description
59	.40	94	Tell me exactly what time these clocks tell
59	.39	97	Determine number of blocks in a stack, including hidden ones
59	.42	129	If Arnie hit Tom, which boy was the victim?
59	.40	150	Read *cat–hat–bat*
59	.39	176	Phonetic analysis; e.g., what is the second letter in *cat*, first letter in *match*?
59	.41	178	Copy *pa, an, pro, pre, sti*
59	.45	205	Write 14, 17, 19, 109, 1023
59	.41	207	Read IV, VI, IX, XI; 17, 71, 69, 96
59	.39	208	Read 27, 34, 158, 396, 9845
59	.46	219	What is the missing number? 12 − ( ) = 8; 12 + ( ) = 19
59	.40	222	Serial 13 subtraction from 100
59	.41	256	Verbal analogies
59	.40	257	Which word of these four does not belong to the same group as the other three?
60	.37	21	Clench right hand and extend fingers of left hand, then reverse
60	.37	22	Tap your right hand twice and your left hand once as quickly as you can
60	.39	23	Same as #22, but reverse order of hands
60	.41	257	Which word of these four does not belong to the same group as the other three?
61	—		No correlations ≥.35 with items from other scales
62	.43	1	Using your right hand, touch your fingers in turn with your thumb while you count them
62	.36	2	Same as #1 with left hand
62	.36	21	Clench right hand and extend fingers of left hand, then reverse
62	.41	22	Tap your right hand twice and your left hand once as quickly as you can

r = *correlation*

Table 3.1: **Item Intercorrelations with Rhythm Scale**   *Continued*

Item	r*	Item	Description
62	.38	23	Same as #22 with left hand
62	.35	24	Draw this pattern without lifting your pencil from the paper
62	.41	33	Do three oral movements repeatedly and in sequence
62	.39	48	If I knock once, you knock twice; if I knock twice, you knock once
62	.40	51	If I knock hard, you knock gently; if I knock gently, you knock hard
62	.39	92	Number of errors on tasks from Raven's Matrices
62	.39	106	If you hear *ba*, raise your right hand; if *pa*, raise your left hand
62	.37	129	If Arnie hit Tom, which boy was the victim?
62	.37	178	Copy *pa, an, pro, pre, sti*
62	.37	221	Serial seven subtraction from 100
62	.39	228	Motorically reproduce rhythm sequence
62	.37	233	Memory for sentences
62	.40	256	Verbal analogies
62	.38	257	Which word of these four does not belong to the same group as the other three?
63	.36	32	Perform three oral movements in sequence
63	.35	90	What objects can you make out in this picture?
63	.37	156	Repeat sentence
63	.37	215	How much is: 27 + 8; 44 + 57; 31 − 7; 44 − 14?
63	.38	219	What is the missing number? 12 − ( ) = 8; 12 + ( ) = 19
63	.40	220	Mental arithmetic
63	.35	223	Memory for seven words scored for errors
63	.37	253	Concept formation—logical relationships
63	.39	256	Verbal analogies

r = *correlation*

are disrupted. With kinesthetic apraxia the motor program may be slowed and perhaps more spatially than temporally disrupted. Again, examining performance on other portions of the battery may clarify the primary dysfunction in performance of rhythms.

Besides being symptomatic of many cortical lesions, marked lack of coordination is often seen in disorders of subcortical extrapyramidal structures such as the cerebellum and basal ganglia (Chusid, 1973; Curtis, Jacobsen, & Marcus, 1972). With focal cerebellar disorders, no accompanying cognitive disturbances are usually encountered (Golden, 1978), so localization of disturbance is not a problem. For a more detailed description of the effects of extrapyramidal disturbances on test performance, see the chapter on assessment of motor functions. Gross disruption on all tests of acoustic-motor skills is observed with extensive frontotemporal injuries.

Item Intercorrelations

Intercorrelations between the Rhythm scale and other Luria scales have revealed several significant correlations ($r > .35$; $p < .0001$), as seen in Table 3.1 (Golden & Berg, 1980d). As we noted earlier in this chapter, the 12 items that compose the Rhythm scale share the requirement of acoustic analysis, usually localized in the right or left temporal area (e.g., Lackner & Teuber, 1973; Luria, 1966).

Items 52–57 assess capacity to analyze differences in both simple and complex groups of tones as well as to reproduce groups of tones. Whereas the initial items (52–54) involve the perception of tonal qualities, the latter items involve the expression of tonal relationships, a task theoretically assigned to the right frontal lobe (Botez & Wertheim, 1959). Golden, Purisch, and Hammeke (1979) have noted that individuals with disorders of the right frontal lobe demonstrate deficits on these expressive items. In light of the apparent frontal lobe involvement with performance of these tasks, it is not surprising that

items evaluating motor skills, visual-spatial organization, nonverbal memory, the regulatory role of speech, and concept-formation skills are highly correlated with this section of the scale (Golden & Berg, 1980d). Patients with frontal lobe injury may show extreme memory deficits for verbal (Luria, 1966) and nonverbal visual material (Milner, 1971). Additionally, individuals with disorders of the tertiary right frontal areas demonstrate impairment on spatial tasks, especially complex ones (Golden, 1978).

Items 58–61 involve the evaluation of acoustic signals. This series of items demonstrated a relationship with motor skills, writing skills, and visual memory, indicating that deficiencies on these tasks may reflect disorders in or near the frontal lobes. A number of items demanding intact visual-spatial integration and stereognostic abilities also correlated highly with this section of the Rhythm scale, suggesting that these items are sensitive to generalized right hemisphere dysfunction. Impairment of receptive language functioning will also apparently hinder performance on items 58–61, further confirming the involvement of the left temporal region.

The left temporal lobe has been implicated in the decoding of speech (Kimura, 1961; Lansdell, 1970; Neff & Goldberg, 1960; Zurif & Ramier, 1972). The secondary temporal regions are responsible for the analyzing and integrating speech and decoding language phonemes (Luria, 1966, 1973; Zurif & Ramier, 1972). Lesions of this area cause an inability to understand or decode spoken words. This area also plays a role in the phonemic analysis necessary for writing, reading, and speaking (Golden, 1978), so lesions there may lead to deficits in these skills as well, as is demonstrated by Luria-Nebraska items that correlate highly with the Rhythm scale.

The last two items in the Rhythm scale deal with the perception and reproduction of rhythm. Item 62, which measures the ability to reproduce rhythmic patterns, requires both the perception of rhythmic patterns in the right temporal area and the reproduction of sounds, usually using the dominant hand. Item 63 requires the production of a series of rhythms from verbal commands and, as it

Table 3.2: **Rhythm: Rotated Factor Matrix**

Item	Factor 1	Factor 2
52	52	23
53	56	28
54	57	26
55	51	49
56	07	64
57	10	66
58	59	08
59	66	07
60	58	10
61	33	16
62	65	08
63	61	04

Table 3.3: **Items on Rhythm Factor 1**

Loading	Item	Description
.52	52	Now you are going to hear two tones on a tape recording. Tell me whether the tones you hear are the same or different.
.56	53	Again, you will hear two tones. Tell me which is higher, the first tone or the second tone.
.57	54	Now you will hear two groups of sounds. There will be about four tones in each group. You will hear the first group of four tones, then there will be a pause, then the second group of four tones. I want you to tell me whether the two groups of tones you hear sound the same or different.
.51	55	Listen to these tones, then hum them.
.59	58	Tell me how many beeps you hear (tape).
.66	59	How many beeps are there all together in these groups?
.58	60	How many beeps are there in each of these groups?
.65	62	You will now hear a rhythm on the tape. When I tell you that rhythm is over, I want you to tap with your hand the rhythm you heard on the tape.
.61	63	Please make a series of: two taps; three taps; two taps; two strong and three weak taps; three weak and two strong taps; a series of two taps followed by three taps.

requires a combination of rhythmic and verbal material, is sensitive to injuries in either hemisphere. Item intercorrelations demonstrate that a variety of abilities are closely allied with these two items, including motor skills, writing, written and mental arithmetic, memory, visual-spatial integration, and concept formation. This suggests the involvement of the frontal, parietal, and, to a somewhat lesser extent, occipital regions of the brain.

Factor Analysis

Factor analyses of the Luria-Nebraska Neuropsychological Battery demonstrated clear factors for the Rhythm scale (Golden, Sweet, Hammeke, Purisch, Graber, & Osmon, 1980). Analysis of the Rhythm section of the battery yielded two principal factors. The main items in this section that contribute to the first factor are listed in Table 3.3. The stimuli for each of these items are quantitative; however, each item requires attention and concentration. It is likely, therefore, that rhythm factor 1 represents an attention/concentration functional system rather than acoustic perceptual analysis.

The second factor on the rhythm scale consisted of two items listed in Table 3.4. Both items consider the ability to sing a familiar melody. That these two items produce a factor by themselves suggests that the ability to accurately perceive melodic information does not always coexist with the ability to carry a tune (Golden, Sweet, Hammeke, Purisch, Graber, & Osmon, 1980).

Table 3.4: **Items on Rhythm Factor 2**

Loading	Item	Description
.64	56	Listen to this melody (tape). Will you please sing it? ("My Bonnie Lies over the Ocean.")
.66	57	Please sing the first line of "Home on the Range."

Summary

It is important to evaluate acoustic-motor skills not only because analysis and synthesis of acoustic information is fundamentally different from tactile and visual processes, but also because different anatomical zones are responsible for these perceptual activities. Whereas tactile and visual perceptual processing occurs in the posterior cortical divisions, analysis of acoustic properties in auditory input is performed in the temporal and frontotemporal regions. Impairment of acoustic-motor skills may have important consequences depending on the severity of the deficit and the extent to which the individual is required to use these skills. With any impairment in perception and reproduction of pitch relationships, musical melodies, and rhythmic patterns, the examiner should carefully analyze the nature of the deficit to ascertain its implications for disturbances in other cognitive functions as well for rehabilitation.

Perhaps more than any other section of the battery, the Rhythm scale is sensitive to difficulties in attention and concentration. Brain-injured and emotionally disturbed patients perform equally poorly on these items. Consequently the examiner should be careful to elicit maximum performance from the patient and should be sensitive to indications of diminished attention to the test procedures. Finally, the interpretation of scores in this section can depend as much on conscientious observation of the patient's behavior as on the objective performance ratings.

4. Tactile Functions

The movement involved in all our daily activities requires a smooth and continuous flow of afferent impulses from the skin's surface as well as from muscles and joints. Without such cutaneous and proprioceptive feedback, simply tying one's shoelace would be exceedingly difficult. Cutaneous receptors provide impulses that let us recognize an object in contact with the skin's surface, noting its location, its temperature, its texture, and its shape as well as other attributes such as vibration and sharpness. Kinesthetic receptors in muscles and joints provide information that lets us determine the relative positions of our limbs in space. This positional awareness provides for direction and for destination in our movement, as well as for other functions such as estimating the weight of an object. Thus assessment of cutaneous and kinesthetic functions is essential to a thorough neuropsychological evaluation. Indeed, many of the items of this section overlap with procedures in routine neurological examinations.

While perception of the most elementary tactile sensations (gross touch, temperature, pain, vibration, pressure) is thought to occur at the level of the thalamus, somatosensory information is primarily processed in the sensorimotor, postcentral, and posterior parietal regions. The primary projection area is in the anterior portion of the postcentral gyrus (Broadmann's area 3). This sensory strip, from the medial and superior sagittal surface across the lateral and inferior region of the postcentral gyrus, maintains a somatotopical organization of somatosensory projection. Generally, sensory information from the lower extremities is projected to the medial and parasagittal portion of the strip, while sensory information from the arms and head are received in the lateral and inferior regions of the strip, respectively. The amount of cortical space allotted to various portions of the body reflects their functional importance. Thus projections from the vocalizing musculature (lips, tongue, larynx, and pharynx) and the hands occupy the most cortical space on the strip. The secondary parietal areas lie posterior to the primary projection area in Broadmann's areas 1, 5, 7, and 40. These areas are responsible for more complex forms of somatosensory processing, those involving integration of tactile input data, such as the ability to recognize an object by touch. A few primary sensory functions are indirectly evaluated in this section (gross touch, pain, pressure). Most test items are geared to assess higher integrative tactile abilities.

In contrast to the sequential integration (temporal synthesis) in sensory inputs of the auditory modality, tactile information appears to primarily involve a simultaneous spatial synthesis of information. Successive somatosensory impulses are converted into simultaneously processed groups or patterns of information from which the individual draws meaning.

Assessment of Cutaneous and Kinesthetic Functions

Three areas of tactile function are examined: cutaneous sensation, muscle and joint sensation, and stereognosis. Assessment and interpretive procedures for each of these areas are described separately.

Because this section is intended to assess abilities that depend on tactile functions, it is important that the examiner reduce the chance that other abilities (e.g., those dependent on visual and auditory skills, or kinesthetic functions when they are not the intended focus of the item) will be used to perform the task. Although a few patients can be trusted to keep their eyes closed, we have found it better to routinely use a blindfold to ensure that the measures obtained are related to tactile functions alone. Ski goggles opaqued with black paint or tape or such are useful because they are easy to slip on the patient and there is no contact with the eyelids to transmit infection. Some patients may become particularly apprehensive about being deprived of vision, and frequent breaks during the section may be required to reduce anxiety.

For the items of the cutaneous section, it is best if the arm, hand, or finger tested is held immobile to prevent kinesthetic cues from aiding the patient's performance. It is also important that the instruments used produce no

sounds, since these too can provide cues. In the description of each item, procedures will be elaborated to reduce the influence of undesired factors.

CUTANEOUS SENSATIONS
Assessment: These items (64–79) are intended to provide a cursory assessment of the elementary tactile skills of localizing touch, discriminating differences in sharpness and pressure, making two-point discriminations, and perceiving the direction of a moving stimulus, as well as more complex tactile skills involving recognition of geometric, alphabetic, and numeric configurations on both right and left sides of the body. Poor performance on these items may result from a variety of causes. Gross attentional deficits, injury to cortical and subcortical structures, and injuries to the spinal cord or peripheral nerves may be sources of difficulty. The characteristics of cortical and subcortical dysfunctions on task performance will be described after we describe administration and scoring procedures.

Items 64 and 65 assess the ability to localize a source of tactile stimulation on right and on left body sides. While in a sitting position, the patient is asked to place the hands in front, on table or bed, with the palms facing up. The hands should be placed as flat as possible. The examiner then tells the patient that she or he will be touched on various parts of the body. The task is to identify the location of the stimulation. Before beginning, the examiner must establish a finger labeling system with the patient. Either a numbering system (1 through 5 for thumb through little finger) or a verbal system (thumb, index, middle, ring, little) may be used. The patient should be checked on the labeling procedures with eyes open before placing the blindfold and beginning the task. If the patient appears to have any difficulty labeling the fingers (e.g., consistently calls the index finger number 1 or has difficulty recalling the names of the fingers), the examiner should have the patient point to the locus of stimulation with the opposite hand. In such cases the patient may remove the blindfold to point.

Once the labeling system has been established, the examiner touches with the eraser end of a pencil the sequence of loci specified on the protocol, alternating between right and left body sides. Each locus should be touched with enough pressure for the patient to recognize that contact has been made. Any fluctuations in thresholds needed at the various loci should be noted. Care should be taken not to apply so much pressure that the joint in the finger or limb is moved, so as to prevent kinesthetic feedback from aiding the cutaneous localization process. Having the patient's hand as flat as possible on the bed or table allows a greater amount of cutaneous pressure while keeping kinesthetic feedback to a minimum. Errors in identification of locus of stimulation are recorded for the right (item 64) and left (item 65) sides.

Items 66 and 67 are intended to assess the ability to make sharpness discriminations. The patient's hands are turned palms down against the table or bed and the backs are then touched with either the point or the head of a pin. The examiner should be careful to touch the patient between the tendons on the back of the hand to minimize lateral displacement of the skin surface on either side of the tendon, thereby keeping the item a measure of sharpness discrimination rather than skin displacement.

The pressure applied to the surface of the patient's hand should remain constant for both the sharp point and the dull head. A useful way to control the pressure applied is to stick the pin through a short piece of wood, such as a tongue depressor, and hold the opposite end while proceeding with the task. Again, a uniform pressure should be used throughout the trials. The amount of pressure should be established on the first trial on each hand. If the patient fails to respond to this same amount of pressure on subsequent trials, an error of omission is recorded. To prevent infection, however, the examiner should not apply enough pressure to break the skin. For interpretation, errors of omission should be differentiated from errors of commission.

Items 68 and 69 are intended to provide a relatively gross measure of the ability to discriminate differences in pressure applied to the skin surface for the right and the left body sides. Touching the head of the pin to the back of the patient's wrist, the examiner depresses the skin approximately 3 mm, saying "This is strong," then depresses the skin approximately 1 mm, saying "This is weak." In cases of hemiplegia, the training task should be done on the side not affected.

The patient is touched with either a strong or a weak stimulus and asked to identify the intensity. The relative pressure applied on each trial should remain as close as possible to the training stimuli across all trials for both hands. Again, the examiner should be careful not to apply the stimulus directly above the tendon, since with the strong stimulus the surface tissue may be displaced to one side, providing an additional cue for the patient to discriminate differences in the trials.

Items 70 and 71 provide a measure of two-point discrimination on the inner surface of the middle fingers of the right and the left hands. Using a compass or caliper, the examiner begins by simultaneously touching the two points of the instrument, separated by 5 mm, to the right middle finger and asking the patient "How many points do you feel?" The same trial is then given to the left middle finger. All subsequent trials alternate between right and left hands. With each trial on a given hand, the examiner increases the separation of the two points of the compass by 5 mm. Thus, on the second round of trials for each hand the two points should be separated by 10 mm, on the third trial point separation should be 15 mm, and so on. The 5 mm increment between each two trials for each hand is continued until the patient accurately reports two points.

When a correct report occurs, to ensure the reliability of the discrimination, the examiner follows with a one-point check, then another two-point check at the same distance. When the report is accurate on these two subsequent checks, two-point discrimination is considered reliable for that distance. If the patient makes an error on either of the two subsequent checks for discrimination, the examiner increases the distance by 5 mm and continues the task until accurate and reliable discrimination is obtained.

Each check is held for about two seconds. At least five seconds should be allowed between any point check on the same hand so as to avoid confounding the task by stimulus aftereffects. If at any time the patient reports more than two points, the trial is considered incorrect and the distance is increased.

For all two-point discrimination trials, the points must be aligned parallel to the fingers. Care should be taken to make simultaneous contact of both points on the skin surface, so that different stimulus onset times cannot contribute to a correct response. As the distance between the two points is increased, it will become necessary to span the finger creases. The patient is not allowed to move the finger in any fashion during each check. To help ensure that the two points make skin contact at the same time and that equal pressure is applied to each point, we recommend that the patient's finger be held immobile for each trial. Also, it is easier to control contact and pressure if the examiner rotates the points downward onto the fingers for each trial rather than lowering the points from directly above the fingers.

When tactile sensation on the middle finger is impaired owing to peripheral neuropathy or lesions of the spinal cord (e.g., quadriplegia), two-point discrimination may be checked on areas of the body that are spared. For example, in quadriplegics the two-point discrimination may be tried on the tongue or on the right and left cheeks. (Caution: the upper portion of the face has bilateral cortical representation, and impaired performances cannot readily be used as lateralizing indicators.) However, the distribution of cutaneous sensitivity varies considerably throughout the body. Thresholds of two-point discrimination are about 1 mm on the tip of the tongue, 2–5 mm on the fingertips, 4–6 mm on the dorsum of the fingers, 8–12 mm on the palm, and 20–30 mm on the dorsum of the hand. Greater distances are required for the forearm and upper arm, torso, thigh, and leg.

The general procedure for assessing two-point discrimination can be used on any body part. However, such assessment on various body parts may differ in reliability of measurement. For example, initial validity studies (Hammeke, Golden, & Purisch, 1978; Golden, Hammeke, & Purisch, 1978; Purisch, Golden, & Hammeke, 1978) on the Luria-Nebraska battery included an assessment of two-point discrimination on the palms as well as on the middle fingers, but the measurement on the palms was found to be considerably less reliable than that on the fingers. It is suspected that the uneven surface of the palm made it difficult to control pressure between the two points and to make simultaneous contact of the two points with the skin.

Items 72 and 73 assess the ability to discriminate direction of movement across the skin. The handle of a compass is moved approximately 150 mm (about 6 inches) up or down the lateral surface of the arm. The patient is asked to report which direction (up or down the arm) the stimulus is moving. Two trials are given on each arm, alternating between right and left sides. For this task, the patient's sleeve should be removed or rolled up so the stimulus object has direct contact with the skin. For quadriplegic patients the cheeks may be used as a site of stimulation.

Items 74 through 79 assess the ability to recognize symbols traced on the skin (graphesthesia). Items 74 and 75 involve tracing geometric symbols (cross, triangle, and circle) on the back of the right and the left wrists. In tracing the geometric symbols, a roughly sharpened pencil is used and the figures are made approximately 30 mm in diameter. The tracings should be made with smooth movements, and equal pressure and time should be given per hand so that each design is administered once to each hand and order is counterbalanced, as indicated on the protocol.

Items 76 and 77 involve tracing numerals on the backs of the wrists. A number (3) is drawn first on the right hand, then on the left, and with each trial the patient is asked to indicate what number has been traced. Items 78 and 79 involve tracing a letter (S) the back of the patient's wrists as in the previous items. In cases of quadriplegia, these symbols may be drawn on the right and left cheeks.

Interpretation of Cutaneous Performance: Experimental research on animals and humans indicates that the functional relations between various tactile skills are not well defined (for review, see Hecaen & Albert, 1978). For example, reduced tactile localization does not mean that two-point discrimination will be similarly impaired. Complex tactile tasks can be impaired when more elementary sensations are intact and vice versa. Moreover, the relationship between cortical locus of injury and type of cutaneous deficit is somewhat unclear. Semmes, Weinstein, Ghent, and Teuber (1960) found impairment in two-point discrimination and cutaneous sensation of directionality with both postcentral and posterior parietal lesions. In addition, these authors obtained evidence suggesting hemispheric differences in the way somatosensory information is represented. In the left (dominant) hemisphere, impairment in tactile functions was observed only following lesions to the sensorimotor, postcentral, and posterior parietal regions. In contrast, tactile deficits were observed with lesions to the right hemisphere that were outside the borders of these divisions. These data suggest that tactile functions are represented more focally in the left hemisphere and more diffusely in the right hemisphere (Semmes, 1968).

Research also indicates that bilateral as well as isolated ipsilateral tactile deficits can occur with unilateral lesions (Hecaen & Albert, 1978). A few studies suggest that the left hemisphere has a predominant bilateral influence; others suggest that the right hemisphere is predominant. The problem of cerebral dominance further complicates the picture. To some extent, the occurrence of bilateral deficits with unilateral lesions appears to be task-related. For example, if the task involves a spatial discrimination component, bilateral deficits may be seen with lesions restricted to the right hemisphere (Carmon & Benton, 1969; Fontenot & Benton, 1971). While these findings draw into question previous notions of strict contralateral representation of function, it must be recognized that results of tactile evaluations still remain one of the most powerful indicators of lesion lateralization.

Thus the structural and functional representation of somatosensory functions have not been clearly defined.

With these reservations, stemming from the current lack of knowledge of cortical somatosensory processing and in conjunction with the limited research on the Luria-Nebraska battery to date, we offer the following principles and interpretations of impaired scores on the cutaneous section.

While impaired performances on the measures of cutaneous functions can result from lesions in various regions of the brain, primary tactile deficits are most often observed in lesions of the postcentral divisions contralateral to the side of the impairment. Frequently, lesions of the primary projection areas are accompanied by some measure of paresis in the limb contralateral to the site of the lesion. This reflects the fact that about 20% of the fibers in the primary sensory area are primary motor fibers (Luria, 1973). On occasion, disturbances of tactile functions may also be observed in lesions of the posterior parietal areas that spare the postcentral gyrus.

Luria's theoretical propositions (1966, 1973) suggest that lesions of the primary projection areas diminish the acuity of the more basic cutaneous functions, such as discrimination of sharpness (items 66 and 67) and intensity (items 68 and 69). Difficulties in localizing the source of stimulation (items 64 and 65), as well as increased two-point discrimination thresholds (items 70 and 71), are also observed. Deficits in elementary cutaneous functions are attributed to increased or unstable thresholds for the sensations or, at times, to unstable orienting responses to the cutaneous stimulation. Information contributing to more complex tactile discrimination involving the integration of tactile data, such as perceived directionality of stimulation (items 72 and 73) and tactile recognition of symbols (items 74 through 79), is analyzed in the secondary parietal areas. Lesions of the secondary divisions disrupt performance on the more complex discrimination tasks, even when more elementary cutaneous functions remain intact. Luria attributes the primary deficit in this case to an inability to simultaneously integrate bits of cutaneous information into meaningful patterns.

The first four tasks of the cutaneous section (tactile

localization, sharpness, intensity, and two-point discrimination) involve relatively elementary cutaneous skills. Impaired performance on these items reflects diminished acuity for these skills on the two body sides. The last four tasks have task requirements not present in the earlier items. Items 72 and 73 require the patient to integrate a temporal sequence of cutaneous stimulation to determine the spatial direction of stimulation. Items 74-79 require the patient to synthesize temporal stimulation to determine the spatial configuration of the stimulus sequence, then to produce a label for the configuration (geometric, numeric, or alphabetic). Thus, at least three factors influence performance on these items: integrity of elementary tactile sensation, relation of tactile stimulation to a two-dimensional coordinate system (spatial synthesis), and ability to assign a verbal label. Impaired performance on these items will result from deficits in any one of these processes, with the most severely impaired scores resulting from dysfunction in all three areas.

To determine which factor may be contributing to impairment, performance on other test sections must be examined. The contribution of deficits in elementary tactile functions can be assessed by examining performance on the first four tasks of the cutaneous section (items 64-71). Generally, the verbal requirements of items 72-79 are not demanding, but the clinician should rule out a severe naming problem by examining the patient's naming performance on the Receptive Speech and Expressive Speech scales of the battery. Also, the role of verbal processes in the performance may be assessed by readministering items 74-79, having the patient point out the tactually scribed symbol from an array of symbols presented visually. When elementary tactile functions and verbal skills are intact, a deficit in spatial-directional skills is implicated. Corroboration of a general spatial deficit may be found by reviewing the performance on stereognostic items of this section as well as on tests of visual-spatial skills in the Visual scale.

When spatial deficits are implicated, bilateral impairment may be observed with right hemisphere lesions.

When verbal deficits are evidenced, bilateral symptoms may be found with left hemisphere lesions. Bilateral impairment in tactile finger identification, particularly when accompanied by difficulties in writing, calculation, and right-left discrimination (Gerstmann syndrome), implicate the left parietal region. In relatively rare cases involving a lesion to the sematosensory transcortical fibers in the corpus callosum, a disconnection syndrome may be observed (Geschwind, 1965). In these cases the patient cannot name the symbol when it is scribed on the nondominant left hand, but the dominant right hand performance is normal. The elementary tactile abilities and general verbal and spatial skills are relatively unimpaired. The underlying defect in these cases is that, although left side cutaneous sensations are adequately analyzed in the right hemisphere, this information is not able to reach the verbal naming analyzers of the left hemisphere for a successful completion of the task.

Lesions in the left hemisphere that are outside the sensorimotor, postcentral, and posterior parietal regions usually do not produce tactile deficits per se. However, impaired performances on the items may occur, particularly with left frontal lesions. Indeed, because of generalized lowering of attentional skills and cognitive inflexibility, integrity of tactile functions is often difficult to assess in these patients. Scores may show impairment not because of defective cutaneous analyzers, but rather because of the pathological inertia and perseveration produced by the frontal disorder. Generalized cerebral disorders may produce similar response errors, and the examiner should evaluate whether such responding characterizes all of the test performance.

Other causes of poor performance on these items include peripheral injuries and neuropathies and subcortical lesions that prevent cutaneous stimulation from reaching higher cortical centers. The patient should be questioned regarding recent and remote peripheral injuries to the arms and hands, or the neck, so this information might appropriately qualify the interpretation of the test data. Generally, peripheral afferent nerve injuries produce complete loss of sensation in the corresponding anatomical distribution of the nerve. Injuries and disorders of the spinal cord may produce mixed patterns of sensory loss. Peripheral and spinal cord injuries do not produce higher cognitive deficits (e.g., spatial deficits, language disorders), but they may contribute to poor performance on the items intended to assess these higher cognitive skills to the extent that the task depends on sensations disrupted by the injury.

MUSCLE AND JOINT SENSATION

Proprioceptive stimulation is assessed by items 80 and 81 for left and for right body sides. For these items the patient may be either supine, sitting, or standing. In item 80 the patient's left arm is extended in front so it is perpendicular to the trunk of the body and bent at the elbow at an angle of 90°. The patient is then requested to place the right arm in the same position as the left. When downward drifting is observed in the stimulus arm, it will be necessary for the examiner to hold it in a fixed position for the trial. When downward drifting occurs in the response arm, it is useful to instruct the patient to inform the examiner when the arm seems to be at the same position as the stimulus arm. When downward drifting occurs, the time when the patient indicates that the positions are the same is used for the measure of accuracy. Downward drift in movement alone is not considered to reflect an incorrect response, but it should be noted for its potential clinical significance. The response is scored as incorrect if the angle difference between the two arms is greater than 10°. This roughly translates to approximately an 8 cm difference between the right and left wrists. A response is also scored as incorrect if the response arm is more than 10° in the lateral direction from the stimulus arm, even if the vertical distance difference is less than 8 cm. Responses scored as correct are assigned a value of zero, responses scored incorrect are assigned a value of 2.

Other procedures for assessing proprioceptive functions were included in the initial validation studies on the standardized battery (Golden, Hammeke, & Purisch,

1978; Hammeke, Golden, & Purisch, 1978; Purisch, Golden, & Hammeke, 1978). These procedures included an attempt to evaluate the patient's ability to perceive direction of passive movement of hands and fingers, as well as the ability to discriminate differences between two positions in which the arms were placed. The measures of directional sensation of passive movement were found to be missed so infrequently by normal and brain-injured patients that the measures did not significantly discriminate between the groups. In addition, brain-injured and schizophrenic patients were found to perform equally well on these procedures. The scoring procedures for the items assessing the ability to discriminate different arm positions with unilateral stimulation were found to be unreliable. Consequently, no differences were found between the performances of neurological, normal, and schizophrenic patients. Subsequently, the items were dropped from the battery.

Impaired performance on items 80 and 81 is attributed to disruption in deep (kinesthetic) sensations and most often reflects cortical lesions in the postcentral or posterior parietal regions of the hemisphere contralateral to the impaired side. Feedback from joints and muscles is analyzed to give the spatial position of the limbs. The difficulty in estimating the relative position of limbs is most obvious when the patient is deprived of visual cues. No disturbance in deep sensation generally is seen in lesions to the temporal or occipital regions of the brain.

When deep sensations are severely impaired, the examiner will observe a kinesthetic dyspraxia in much of the testing behavior (e.g., handling test materials, imitating the examiner's motions) that is most obvious when the patient is deprived of vision. The clinician should also examine the patient's performance on simple and dynamic oral movements (Motor scale) for evidence of oral kinesthetic apraxia.

Frontal lesions generally do not disturb deep sensation, but they may result in impaired scores on these items. To differentiate between frontal and parietal syndromes, several strategies are suggested. First of all, consistent unilateral deficits in position sense strongly suggest kinesthetic (parietal lobe) difficulties, whereas bilaterally impaired scores increase the chance that a frontal lesion is contributing to the deficit. Second, if performance on the Motor scale is significantly more impaired than performance on the Tactile scale, an anterior focus is more likely. Conversely, when tactile impairment is elevated relative to motor, a parietal focus is indicated. An examiner may want to repeat the testing procedures using finger positions, in that cortical kinesthetic dysfunction is often more pronounced in the fine motor movements of the extremities. However, the Tactile/Motor comparison does not work in all cases (for example, occipital injuries may produce the reverse pattern) and should be used cautiously, as is true of any rule suggested in this volume.

STEREOGNOSIS

Stereognosis refers to the ability to recognize an object by touch alone. This ability is evaluated in items 82–85, with measures of both verbal object identification and response latency. The patient is instructed to hold both hands out with palms up and fingers extended. A quarter is placed on the fingers of the right hand and the patient is asked to feel it and state precisely what object it is. On each trial the patient is permitted to feel the object only with the one hand.

Pure astereognosis is generally considered to spare elementary tactile sensation, so that the individual can accurately identify characteristics of the object by touch (size, weight, texture, temperature, etc.), but fails to integrate these features so as to recognize it. There is considerable controversy whether pure astereognosis exists as a clinical entity. Many researchers argue that reported cases of astereognosis have been inadequately evaluated and that difficulties in tactile naming of objects are largely due to deficits in elementary somesthesis rather than to tactile asymbolia. Others argue that astereognosis does not stem from a tactile asymbolia but is simply a modality-specific anomia resulting from the disconnection of tactile analyzing centers from cortical naming centers (Geschwind,

1965). Nonetheless, though it is rare, many well-documented cases have been reported and generally have involved injury to the posterior parietal region of the hemisphere contralateral to the impaired hand. It is highly unlikely that the clinician will observe bilateral astereognosis stemming from a unilateral hemispheric lesion, though a few cases have been reported (Hecaen & Albert, 1978).

Interpretation of poor performance on the items assessing stereognosis requires careful consideration of several potential contributing factors. First of all, the status of elementary somesthesis must be gauged from the initial items in this section. When thresholds for elementary sensations are unstable, limited tactile information is received, precluding symbolic integration of the object's characteristics. Second, the examiner should carefully observe the patient's palpation on these items to rule out disturbance in fine motor movement that hinders active palpation of the object. Lesions of the sensorimotor strip as well as peripheral injuries may impair the ability to handle the object and assess its characteristics, again precluding accurate recognition. Frontal lobe patients also show poor object palpation. In these cases fine motor skills are usually not severely impaired; rather, the ability to sustain a planned evaluation of the object's characteristics is defective, and responses are based on impulsive and premature conclusions.

Finally, the role of verbal skills, in particular naming abilities, must be considered. When areas involved in naming located in the dominant hemisphere are injured, producing an anomic aphasia, naming difficulties are not specific to the tactile modality but are usually observed in auditory and visual presentations as apparent on other portions of the battery (e.g., Visual, Receptive Speech, and Expressive Speech scales).

To evaluate the role of verbal function in impaired performance on stereognostic items, we recommend several ancillary procedures. An attempt should first be made to assess the patient's ability to describe the object characteristics (e.g., size, weight, texture, presence of sharp edges, corners). The patient may also be asked to draw a picture of the object or to point it out from an array of objects or pictures. Such procedures eliminate the need to recall the name of the object, but they still test object recognition. Finally, the patient may be asked to name the objects when presented visually. If he or she is unable to describe any characteristics of the object, or to draw its general form, elementary somesthesis or inactive palpation is the likely source of difficulty. Patients who are unable to name a palpated object but have no difficulty drawing it or picking it out from a group do not have object-recognition difficulties. When tactile naming difficulties are present only for the nondominant hand, a lesion of the corpus callosum should be considered.

It is highly improbable that the clinician might see a case that qualified as pure astereognosis. One would have to rule out significant contributions of disturbed elementary somesthesis, verbal skills, and motivational factors. Nonetheless, these items are useful inclusions in routine examination, in that they enable one to assess the extent to which elementary deficits impair more complex performance and provide lateralizing and localizing indicators.

Item Intercorrelations

Item intercorrelations between the Tactile scale and all other Luria items revealed numerous significant correlations ($r > .35$; $p < .0001$), as shown in Table 4.1 (Golden & Berg, 1981a). These intercorrelations demonstrate that the Tactile scale items are closely related to skills and abilities measured by other items of the battery. Several of the items that correlated highly with the first part of the scale (items 66 through 79) involve speech and writing skills. Anterior parietal dysfunction results in poor performance on such tasks, as do middle parietal injuries. The primary and secondary areas of the parietal lobes also are closely involved with speech and writing (Luria, 1966), though right parietal injuries generally do not appear to cause such severe dysfunction as left parietal injuries. Additionally, this section of the scale is highly correlated

with various object identification and action identification tasks, functions that are ascribed to the right parietal areas (Hecaen & Angelergues, 1962; Luria, 1973).

Other abilities that are closely related with items 66–79 are concept formation, reading skills, expressive language, memory, arithmetic symbol manipulation, acoustic analysis, and arithmetic computations. All these abilities are generally localized in the parietotemporo-occipital areas (Brain, 1941; Luria, 1966, 1973; Benson & Weir, 1972; Golden, 1978). This region of the brain is responsible for integrating information from all sensory modalities (Golden, 1978). Thus it comes as no surprise that items that measure the ability to detect and localize cutaneous sensation are correlated with other Luria items representing a wide variety of skills and abilities.

Items 80 and 81 are directly concerned with muscle and joint sensations. These are sensitive to injuries in not only the anterior but also the posterior parietal lobe (Golden, Purisch, & Hammeke, 1979). These items demonstrate a high degree of association with items involving motor skills, opening the possibility of some posterior frontal lobe involvement in the sensory-motor strip area. In addition, item 81 is correlated with object identification and writing skills, further suggesting localization in the parietotemporal area.

Of note is the fact that items 76 through 80 did not demonstrate significant correlations with other Luria test items. The lack of correlation suggests that these items are unique in the neuropsychological abilities they tap. Golden, Purisch, and Hammeke (1979) have noted that patients who have trouble with these items manifest damage in and around the angular gyrus. Thus these items may prove highly specific to dysfunction in that area.

The final four items on the Tactile scale (items 82–85) involve stereognostic perception. These items, again, are highly related to motor, visual naming, arithmetic, spatial organizational, writing, and concept formation abilities, all of which can be affected by parietotemporal injuries (e.g., Luria, 1966, 1973; Golden, 1978).

The items on the Tactile scale, in combination with the

Table 4.1: **Item Intercorrelations with Tactile Scale**

Item	r*	Item	Description
64	.35	103	Phonemic hearing—writing
64	.36	142	Repeat *house–ball–chair; ball–chair–house*
64	.36	205	Write 14, 17, 19, 109, 1023
65	.35	8	With your eyes closed, place your left hand in same position I place your right hand in
65	.37	20	Touch your right ear with your left hand
65	.36	110	Name objects from pictures
65	.44	177	Copy *B, L, ℒ, 𝒟, ℬ*
65	.42	178	Copy *pa, an, pro, pre, sti*
66	—		No correlations ≥.35 with items from other scales
67	.43	113	Point to the picture that shows: typewriting; mealtime; summer
68	.36	51	If I knock hard, you knock gently; if I knock gently, you knock hard
68	.38	110	Name objects from pictures
68	.38	113	Point to the picture that shows: typewriting; mealtime; summer
68	.35	210	Which is larger: 17 or 68; 23 or 56; 189 or 201?
69	.38	6	With your eyes closed, place your left hand in the same position I place it in (thumb against fifth finger)
69	.39	8	With your eyes closed, place your left hand in same position I place your right hand in (thumb against middle finger)
69	.35	29	Stick out your tongue as far as possible and keep it there
69	.38	59	How many beeps in all groups together?
69	.37	108	Point to eye; nose; ear
69	.41	110	Name objects from pictures
69	.38	112	What do *cat, bat, pat* mean?
69	.35	133	Repeat *a, i, m, b, sh*
69	.35	142	Repeat *house–ball–chair; ball–chair–house*
69	.39	205	Write 14, 17, 19, 109, 1023
70	.41	1	Using your right hand, touch your fingers in turn with your thumb while you count them

*r = correlation

Table 4.1: **Item Intercorrelations with Tactile Scale**   *Continued*

Item	r*	Item	Description
70	.41	2	Same as #1 with left hand
70	.39	3	Clench your right hand and then stretch your fingers as quickly as you can
70	.35	11	Right hand fingers extended in sagittal plane touching chin
70	.36	21	Clench your right hand and extend fingers of your left hand, then reverse
70	.38	22	Tap your right hand twice and your left hand once
70	.41	48	If I knock once, you knock twice; if I knock twice, you knock once
70	.36	92	Number of errors on tasks from Raven's Matrices
70	.38	108	Point to eye; nose; ear
70	.35	227	Nonverbal visual memory
71	.39	1	Using your right hand, touch your fingers in turn with your thumb, while you count them
71	.47	2	Same as #1 with left hand
71	.39	3	Clench your right hand, then stretch your fingers as quickly as you can
71	.44	4	Same as #3 with right hand
71	.37	8	With your eyes closed, place your left hand in the same position I place your right hand in (thumb against middle finger)
71	.37	20	Touch your right ear with your left hand
71	.38	21	Clench your right hand and extend the fingers of your left hand, then reverse
71	.36	22	Tap your right hand twice and your left hand once
71	.41	23	Same as #22 but reverse order of hands
71	.41	48	If I knock once, you knock twice; if I knock twice, you knock once
71	.37	92	Number of errors on tasks from Raven's Matrices
71	.43	157	Name objects from pictures
71	.37	158	Name body parts from pictures
71	.38	256	Verbal analogies
72	.41	86	Name visually presented objects
72	.39	106	Phonemic hearing—conditioned reflex

*r = correlation

Table 4.1: **Item Intercorrelations with Tactile Scale** *Continued*

Item	r*		Item Description
72	.39	108	Point to eye; nose; ear
72	.37	111	Point to knee; elbow; cheekbone
72	.40	113	Point to the picture that shows: typewriting; mealtime; summer
72	.41	136	Say *house; table; apple*
72	.41	137	Say *hairbrush; screwdriver; laborious*
72	.38	140	Say *streptomycin; Massachusetts Episcopal*
72	.37	206	Read 7–9–3; 3–5–7
72	.44	210	Which is larger: 17 or 68; 23 or 56; 189 or 201?
72	.41	255	Concept formation—opposites
72	.45	258	Discursive reasoning—elementary arithmetic problems
72	.48	260	Discursive reasoning—elementary arithmetic problems
73	.40	19	Point to your left eye with your right hand
73	.40	20	Touch your right ear with your left hand
73	.44	86	Name visually presented objects
73	.51	110	Name objects from pictures
73	.39	111	Point to knee; elbow; cheekbone
73	.47	113	Point to the picture that shows: typewriting; mealtime; summer
73	.47	133	Repeat *a, i, m, b, sh*
73	.46	136	Repeat *house; table; apple*
73	.41	148	Read these words: *hairbrush; screwdriver; laborious*
73	.42	149	Read these words: *rhinoceros; surveillance; hierarchy*
73	.40	182	Write *ba; da; back; pack*
73	.42	201	Write 7–9–3; 3–5–7
73	.40	203	Write 17 and 71; 69 and 96
73	.41	205	Write 14, 17, 19, 109, 1023
73	.42	210	Which is larger: 17 or 68; 23 or 56; 189 or 201?
74	.44	1	Using your right hand, touch your fingers in turn with your thumb while you count them
74	.42	2	Same as #1 with left hand

*r = correlation

Table 4.1: **Item Intercorrelations with Tactile Scale** *Continued*

Item	r*		Item Description
74	.38	51	If I knock hard, you knock gently; if I knock gently, you knock hard
74	.38	86	Name visually presented objects
74	.40	113	Point to the picture that shows: typewriting; mealtime; summer
74	.42	203	Write 17 and 71; 69 and 96
74	.35	205	Write 14, 17, 19, 109, 1023
74	.35	208	Read 27, 34, 158, 396, 9845
74	.35	223	Memory for seven words scored for errors
75	.36	12	Left hand fingers extended in sagittal plane touching chin
75	.45	24	Draw pattern without lifting your pencil from the paper
75	.37	59	How many beeps in all groups together?
75	.40	92	Number of errors on tasks from Raven's Matrices
75	.36	95	Draw hands on blank clockface for 12:50, 4:35, 11:10
75	.37	106	Phonemic hearing—conditioned reflex
75	.40	113	Point to the picture that shows: typewriting; mealtime; summer
75	.39	157	Name objects from pictures
75	.37	158	Name body parts from pictures
75	.39	177	Copy *B, L, ℒ, 𝒟, ℬ*
75	.39	205	Write 13, 17, 19, 109, 1023
76	—		No correlations ≥.35 with items from other scales
77	—		No correlations ≥.35 with items from other scales
78	—		No correlations ≥.35 with items from other scales
79	.35	103	Phonemic hearing—writing of sounds
80	—		No correlations ≥.35 with items from other scales
81	.36	2	Using your left hand, touch your fingers in turn with your thumb while you count them
81	.43	4	Clench your left hand and then stretch your fingers until I ask you to stop

*r = correlation

Table 4.1: **Item Intercorrelations with Tactile Scale**   *Continued*

Item	r*	Item	Description
81	.37	6	With your eyes closed, place your left hand in same position I place it in (thumb against fifth finger)
81	.39	113	Point to the picture that shows: typewriting; mealtime; summer
81	.36	203	Write 17 and 71; 69 and 96
81	.37	205	Write 14, 17, 19, 109, 1023
82	.42	1	Using your right hand, touch your fingers in turn with your thumb while you count them
82	.41	3	Clench your right hand and then stretch your fingers until I ask you to stop
82	.39	5	With your eyes closed, place your right hand in same position I place it in (thumb against fifth finger)
82	.38	33	Rapid, repeated oral movements
82	.48	86	Name visually presented objects
82	.38	87	Name objects from pictures
82	.39	90	Name overlapping objects from pictures
82	.39	92	Number of errors on tasks from Raven's Matrices
82	.37	103	Phonemic hearing—writing of sounds
82	.40	112	What do *cat, bat, pat* mean?
82	.43	113	Point to the picture that shows: typewriting; mealtime; summer
82	.43	116	Point to picture of object used to light fire
82	.43	157	Name objects from pictures
82	.44	158	Name body parts from pictures
82	.42	178	Copy *pa, an, pro, pre, sti*
82	.41	202	Write IV and VI; IX and XI
82	.41	205	Write 14, 17, 19, 109, 1023
82	.40	219	What is the missing number? 12 − ( ) = 8; 12 + ( ) = 19
82	.45	251	Concept formation—logical relationships
82	.42	255	Concept formation—opposites
83	.39	3	Clench your right hand, then stretch your fingers until I ask you to stop
83	.37	40	Copy square—score for quality
83	.39	86	Name visually presented objects

Table 4.1: **Item Intercorrelations with Tactile Scale**   *Continued*

Item	r*	Item	Description
83	.36	90	Name overlapping objects in picture
83	.36	98	Time taken to identify number of blocks in a stack including hidden blocks
83	.36	157	Name objects from pictures
83	.39	170	Complex systems of grammatical expressions
84	.41	1	Using your right hand, touch your fingers in turn with your thumb while you count them
84	.38	2	Same as #1 with left hand
84	.38	6	With your eyes closed, place your left hand in the same position I place it in (thumb against fifth finger)
84	.39	10	Do as I do. Left hand placed under chin with fingers bent
84	.40	33	Rapid, repeated oral movements
84	.43	86	Name visually presented objects
84	.39	87	Name objects from pictures
84	.40	91	Name overlapping objects in picture
84	.44	92	Number of errors on tasks from Raven's Matrices
84	.44	113	Point to the picture that shows: typewriting; mealtime; summer
84	.49	116	Point to picture of object used to light fire
84	.38	137	Repeat *hairbrush; screwdriver; laborious*
84	.57	157	Name objects from pictures
84	.43	158	Name body parts from pictures
84	.42	218	What is the missing sign? 12 ( ) 2 = 20; 10 ( ) 2 = 12; 10 ( ) 2 = 8; 10 ( ) 2 = 5
84	.42	219	What is the missing number? 12 − ( ) = 8; 12 + ( ) = 19
84	.40	256	Verbal analogies
85	.36	2	Using your left hand, touch your fingers in turn with your thumb while you count them
85	.39	4	Clench your left hand, then stretch your fingers until I ask you to stop
85	.42	6	With your eyes closed, place your left hand in the same position I place it in (thumb against fifth finger)
85	.38	40	Draw triangle—score for quality

*r = correlation

Table 4.1: **Item Intercorrelations with Tactile Scale** *Continued*

Item	r*	Item	Description
85	.36	106	Phonemic hearing—conditioned reflex
85	.44	157	Name objects from pictures
85	.35	239	Time to rearrange a series of pictures into correct sequence
85	.35	241	Time to rearrange a series of pictures into correct sequence

Table 4.2: **Tactile Factor Structure**

Item	Factor 1	Factor 2
64	65	−30
65	56	−44
66	44	−41
67	38	−46
68	61	−42
69	52	−42
70	46	−63
71	46	−69
72	67	−27
73	57	−21
74	61	−37
75	54	−42
76	49	−37
77	43	−39
78	30	−25
79	46	−41
80	35	−27
81	42	−36
82	49	−73
83	33	−70
84	47	−73
85	34	−67

*r = correlation

Table 4.3: **Items on Tactile Factor 1**

Loading	Item	Description
.65	64	Tell me where I am touching you (right hand).
.56	65	Left hand.
.61	68	(With the head of a pin on the back of the patient's wrist, depress the skin approximately 3 mm, saying "This is hard," then depress the skin approximately 1 mm, saying "This is soft.") Now, the touch you feel, is it hard or soft?
.52	69	Scoring (left hand).
.46	70	How many points do you feel? (Using a compass, begin with single point, then gradually increase separation by 5 mm on middle finger until the threshold of two-point discrimination is reached. On middle finger, spread points parallel to arms. Alternate between right and left.)
.46	71	Scoring (left hand).
.67	72	In what direction am I touching you, up or down your arm? (Alternate between right and left arms.)
.57	73	Scoring (left arm).
.61	74	I am going to trace either a cross, a triangle, or a circle on your wrist. Tell me what I am tracing.
.54	75	Scoring (left).
.49	76	(On back of wrist.) What number is this?
.46	79	Scoring (left).
.49	82	Feel this object and tell me exactly what it is.
.47	84	Scoring (left hand, errors).

Table 4.4: **Items on Tactile Factor 2**

Loading	Item	Description
.46	67	Am I touching you with the point or with the head of a pin? (Left hand scoring.)
.63	70	How many points do you feel? (Using a compass, begin with single point, then gradually increase separation by 5 mm on middle finger until the threshold of two-point discrimination is reached. Alternate between right and left.)
.69	71	Scoring (left hand).
.73	82	Feel this object and tell me exactly what it is. (Alternate between hands in this; right hand, errors.)
.70	83	Scoring (right hand, time).
.73	84	Scoring (left hand, errors).
.67	85	Scoring (left hand, time).

first 20 items on the Motor scale, are used to make up the Left-Right Hemisphere lateralization scales. A large difference in performance between left- and right-hand performance on the Tactile scale is highly indicative of lateralized brain dysfunction. An inspection of Motor scale items that correlate highly with the Tactile scale items further confirms the lateralizing aspects of the Tactile scale.

Use of item intercorrelations as an adjunct to other methods in the interpretation of Tactile scale performance deficiencies can yield a more complete picture of the extent and nature of specific brain dysfunction.

Factor Analysis

Factor analysis of the 24 items evaluating tactile functions yielded two factors. Fourteen items contributed to the first factor (See Table 4.3), the majority of which involved measures of elementary cutaneous sensation: point localization, discrimination of differential intensity, two-point discrimination, and direction of stimulation. A few items (74, 75, 76, 79, 82, 84) involved more complex tactile stimuli (recognition and naming of geometric symbols

traced on the back of the hand, or common objects placed in the hand), tasks that have been shown to be frequently related to impairment in elementary tactile sensation owing to lesions of the postcentral gyrus (Bay, 1944; Corkin, Milner, & Rasmussen, 1970). In general the items involving more complex tactile stimuli do not correlate as highly with this factor as do measures of basic cutaneous sensation. Thus the factor is thought to primarily represent elementary cutaneous sensation.

Several items (70, 71, 82, 84) in the first factor are duplicated in the second tactile factor (See Table 4.4) but load high on the second factor. The items having the highest loading on the second factor generally involve measures of stereognosis, both accuracy and response latency. These measures present a more complex tactile problem than the items of the previous factor. It is interesting that the items measuring two-point discrimination load highly on this factor. While stereognosis would intuitively depend on a synthesis of several forms of elementary sensations, perhaps it is particularly dependent on the cutaneous ability to discriminate the distance between points of stimulation.

In general, the two factors of the Tactile scale are consistent with Luria's formulation of tactile functions. The two factors correspond to elementary sensation localized to the postcentral gyrus and to a more complex, simultaneous integration of elementary sensations localized in the secondary and tertiary regions of the parietal lobes. The factors are not as clean as one would like, however, in that a few items contributing to the first factor (e.g., those measuring graphesthesia and stereognosis) would, according to Luria's formulations, fit better with the second tactile factor.

Summary

In contrast to the sequential processing of the auditory system, tactile sensations appear to be analyzed in a simultaneous fashion. Although the mechanisms of cortical processing of tactile sensation are not clearly understood, the evaluation of tactile functions nevertheless remains one of the most reliable sources of information regarding the integrity of brain structures, particularly the parietal lobes. The Tactile scale assesses elementary cutaneous and proprioceptive sensations as well as more complex tactile integrative abilities involved in stereognosis. Interpretation of performance impairment requires regard for deficits in elementary tactile functions, motor functions, verbal skills, and motivation.

5. The Visual Scale

The Visual scale of the Luria-Nebraska Neuropsychological Battery is designed to assess impairment in a broad range of visual processes, from simple recognition of familiar objects to complex visual-spatial processing. The scale consists of 14 items (86–99) and takes only a few minutes to administer and score. All items on the Visual scale employ a visual sensory stimulus, pictorial in most cases, and involve either a verbal, a manual (pointing with the finger), or a simple motor (circling the correct answer with a pencil) response. The items emphasize immediate visual and visual-spatial processing and do not rely heavily on short- or long-term memory. Some items require background knowledge of names of objects or of spatial characteristics, such as directions on a map, and the more difficult items represent new learning of visual-spatial tasks.

In general, the Visual scale is sensitive to brain damage in posterior areas, because of its utilization of visual stimulus materials and active visual tasks, and to right hemisphere lesions because it measures visual-spatial processing and spatial reasoning. It must be noted that Luria developed these measures during a period in which little was known of nondominant (right) hemisphere specialized functions, and the lateralization of cognitive functions does not play a large role in Luria's theory of brain function (Luria, 1966, 1973). Thus it is interesting that he was able to devise and select such powerful measures of right hemisphere function.

The neuropsychological assessment of visual functions has a number of inherent problems that make it difficult to develop and interpret measures of visual performance. First, and most significant, is that the visual system has no direct means for "communicating" its activity as, for example, the auditory system may communicate by using speech. In other words, the visual system is primarily involved in sensory processing rather than in motor or verbal output. This has important implications for visual assessment, because testing necessarily involves some way to evaluate the adequacy of visual processing. For example, the Bender Gestalt and the Block

Design subscale of the Wechsler Adult Intelligence Scale assess visual-spatial skills, but they also involve relatively complex motor and constructive skills in their response modalities. Thus apparent deficits on visual measures could reflect impairment in the means by which patients communicate their visual activity rather than impairment in the visual process itself. Common solutions to this problem are to simplify communication of the results of the visual activity and to assess similar visual skills using both verbal and motor response modalities. However, these approaches tend to limit the complexity of the visual task at the same time that they simplify the response requirement.

A second problem is that the visual system, though it is often viewed as a passive sensory apparatus, is actually an active processing system capable of very complex activity. Deficits in complex visual activity must be assessed with the same care as simple visual recognition, since deficits may appear only on higher-level visual tasks. For example, it is very difficult to assess the process of voluntary eye movement and patterns of visual scanning, though these are important *active* aspects of the visual process.

Finally, it is difficult to devise tasks requiring complex visual activity that are free of verbal mediation, or that cannot be solved using verbal rather than visual-spatial processing. The Category test of the Halstead-Reitan battery is an example of a test that has a strong visual-spatial component (particularly the fifth and sixth subtests) but that also assesses verbal and logical-analytical skills despite a simple motor response modality. These concerns are important both to ensure the ''purity'' of assessing visual processes alone and to detect visual deficits in the presence of unimpaired verbal ability.

Assessment of Visual Perception

The Visual scale items demonstrate Luria's approach to assessment of visual processing while avoiding these common problems. The first four items of the Visual scale (items 86–89) are visual recognition tasks of increasing difficulty.

VISUAL PERCEPTION OF OBJECTS AND PICTURES

Subjects are asked in item 86 to name four common objects: a pencil, an eraser, a rubber band, and a quarter. Next, in item 87, they are to identify somewhat less common objects from pictures. Item 88 requires that subjects again name common objects, but in this item the difficulty of the task is increased because the images initially seen are blurred. The final item in this section of the scale, item 89, has patients identify objects from high-contrast photographs. These items depend heavily upon verbal naming functions and are therefore sensitive to left temporoparietal lesions. Failures in visual recognition on these early items may reflect visual agnosia or impaired verbal naming functions that would produce difficulties with all items presented in the visual modality. Several of these early items are on the Left Sensorimotor Localization scale (McKay and Golden, 1979), which reflects sensitivity of these items to disturbances in visual scanning mechanisms involving eye movements controlled by cortical areas slightly anterior to the sensorimotor cortex.

Items 90 and 91 require rapid recognition of outlines of common objects drawn superimposed on each other. These items are sensitive to deficits in the ability to pick out relevant from irrelevant cues and to synthesize the relevant features into a recognized pattern. Successful performance on these items requires relatively intact visual-spatial perception, visual recognition, and naming skills. Thus these items assess secondary visual processes that are generally localized in right parieto-occipital areas. They also assess the ability to separate parts from the whole gestalt, a deficit common to secondary visual injuries in either hemisphere.

Consistent failure on items 86–91 should alert the test interpreter to relatively serious problems in basic visual analysis and may reflect visual agnosia in which the patient finds it difficult to recognize even familiar objects visually. Items 90 and 91 are particularly sensitive to disturbances of secondary visual processes, characterized by difficulties in visually analyzing disparate cues in a complex pattern and integrating this information into a recognized object or pattern. Visual agnosia may be reflected in grossly inaccurate guesses about the objects represented in these early Visual scale items. If the patient finds it difficult to attend to more than one visual cue at a time, he will have unusual difficulty with items 90 and 91, and this difficulty may be associated with recognition of a very small number of objects on these tasks.

Items 92 and 93 were taken by Luria (1966) from Raven's Standard Progressive Matrices. In item 92 the patient is asked to look at a series of geometric designs with a segment of each design missing. The patient's task is to visually analyze each design and select from six alternatives the one that will correctly complete it. Item 93 is the total time needed to complete the task. Recognizing the piece that completes a complex visual pattern requires intact visual-analytic and synthesizing skills. It is therefore a highly sensitive measure of right hemisphere functioning that assesses a broad range of visual-spatial skills. Failure may reflect dysfunction in various right hemisphere areas, including frontal areas, because of the necessity of shifting strategies to complete this item (Golden & Berg, 1980f).

VISUAL-SPATIAL ORIENTATION
The next three items (94–96) are specifically intended to tap visual-spatial skills. They depend upon a fund of general information including knowledge of telling time and map directions, a consideration that may be important for low-intelligence populations. For item 94, the patient is shown four numberless clockfaces, each depicting a specific time. The patient is to tell exactly (plus or minus one minute) what time each clockface depicts. Item 95 is similar to item 94, but here the patient is given three blank clockfaces and asked to draw the position of the hands for each of three specific times. A clock is correct if the hands are drawn within two minutes of the specified time. In

item 96 the subject is shown a drawing of a compass that has no notation for directions and is asked to point out north, east, and west.

These items are on the Left Parieto-Occipital localization scale (McKay & Golden, 1979), which reflects both their visual-spatial and their analytic characteristics. Damage in posterior areas and the right hemisphere may disrupt performance on these items.

INTELLECTUAL OPERATIONS IN SPACE
The final items on the Visual scale require active visual processing and visual imagery. For item 97 the subject is shown a series of four drawings, each of which depicts a stack of blocks. The subject is then asked to state the total number of blocks in each of the stacks, with a reminder to include the ones not visible. Item 98 is the total time necessary for the subject to complete this task. The final item of the Visual scale, item 99, uses complex visual squares, each of which has a small circle in one corner and a heavy, dark base line on one side. The patient has to select from four alternatives having the heavy base line at the bottom the way the rotated square would look if it were in the same orientation as the others. Items 97 and 98 require geometric analysis and imagination of objects that must be inferred from pictures of stacks of blocks. In addition to spatial skills, this item requires complex analytical skills that are disrupted by left hemisphere lesions. Item 99 is a very complex visual task that requires imagining blocks turned to new orientations in space. Items 97–99 assess complex visual-spatial abilities and active, integrated, visual processes. As such, they are very sensitive measures of right hemisphere performance. Lesions in any right hemisphere area may disrupt performance on these tasks, including right temporal lesions that disrupt nonverbal sequential analysis.

A pattern of performance involving difficulty on the later items of the Visual scale when early items are easily completed suggests intact primary and secondary visual processes but impaired visual-spatial and spatial reasoning skills. This pattern is associated with more anterior right hemisphere damage and relatively intact right posterior areas. An exception is the individual of superior intelligence who is able to compensate for basic visual deficits on easy visual tasks, but whose deficits become apparent as the difficulty of the task increases.

As has been shown, the Visual scale is characterized by increasingly complex visual-spatial tasks, though the response requirements are kept relatively simple. Thus failure on Visual scale items can usually be attributed to problems in visual analysis rather than to impaired verbal or motor performance, particularly if naming functions, assessed by early Visual scale items, are intact.

Localization of brain damage using the Visual scale is complicated by two factors. First, visual impairment is characterized by different patterns of dysfunction, as described by Luria (1966), that can be distinguished only on the basis of careful observation of the patient's manner of approach to the Visual scale items during administration of the Luria-Nebraska. The first type of impairment involves difficulties in visual analysis stemming from failure in visual feature detection, synthesis into meaningful patterns, and recognition. This dysfunction stems from injury to secondary visual areas (Luria, 1966) in the parieto-occipital lobes, particularly in the right hemisphere. If this syndrome is specific to visual processing of letters and numbers, it suggests left rather than right parieto-occipital damage (Luria, 1966). Luria describes a second form of visual problem stemming from frontal damage. This impairment is characterized by the inability to perform *active* visual processes such as organized scanning and purposeful examination of visual cues. Patients with a frontal syndrome that interferes with visual processing show characteristics of passive visual analysis such as an unshifting gaze during examination of visual stimuli and impulsive guessing during the recognition process based upon perceptually salient (but misleading) cues. Observation of performance during administration of the Luria-Nebraska provides qualitative information for distinguishing between these forms of visual impairment.

A second limitation to localization using the Visual scale is the relatively diffuse organization of the right as compared with the left hemisphere. Semmes (1968) has noted that localization of sensorimotor deficits is greater in left than right hemisphere lesions, and speculated that this reflects a more diffuse, heteromodal, and integrative organization of the right hemisphere. This was confirmed by Gur, Packer, Hungerbuhler, Reivich, Obrist, Amarnek, and Sackheim's (1980) finding, using regional cerebral blood flow techniques, that the right hemisphere has a greater relative amount of white than gray matter compared with the left hemisphere. Since white matter is involved in transfer of information across regions within the hemisphere, this implies a neuroanatomical basis for inferring more diffuse, integrative organization of the right hemisphere.

These considerations imply that deficits on the Visual scale may be difficult to localize within the right hemisphere, compared, for example, with receptive language deficits in the left hemisphere. This difficulty is confirmed by item analysis of the Visual scale. Performance on almost all the Visual scale items may be impaired by lesions in primary and secondary visual processing areas, as well as oculomotor frontal areas. In addition, the items tapping complex visual-spatial skills tend to be sensitive to almost any focal or diffuse right hemisphere lesion. Localization of focal lesions in primary visual processing areas is better accomplished by studying discrete sight losses (hemianopsia or quadrantanopsia) in different areas of the patient's visual field (see Luria, 1966) and the presence of reliable visual suppressions.

Right hemisphere parietal lesions may be associated with dramatic clinical signs of unilateral spatial neglect in which patients ignore the left side of the body or fail to attend to objects in the left visual field. This dysfunction would be apparent on the Luria-Nebraska, primarily from incomplete drawings on the Motor scale and a Writing scale characterized by failure to include the left sides of figures or letters. Focal right temporal and frontal lesions may selectively disrupt picture arrangement performance on the Intellectual scale, as well as producing degraded

Table 5.1: **Item Intercorrelations with Visual Scale**

Item	r*	Item	Description
86	.41	72	Determine whether stimulus is moving up or down right arm
86	.44	73	Same as #72—left arm
86	.43	84	Stereognosis—left hand errors
86	.46	110	Name objects from pictures
86	.51	112	What do *cat, bat, pat* mean?
86	.44	113	Point to the picture that shows: typewriting; mealtime; summer
86	.43	115	Whose watch is this (examiner's)? Whose is this (patient's)?
86	.43	124	Which is correct: Spring comes before summer, or Summer comes before spring?
86	.41	129	If Arnie hits Tom, which boy is the victim?
86	.46	133	Repeat *a, i, m, b, sh*
86	.41	142	Say *house-ball-chair; ball-chair-house*
86	.47	143	Say the sounds that go with *a, i, m, b, sh*
86	.42	152	Read *hat-sun-bell*
86	.46	158	Name body parts from pictures
86	.43	159	Name objects from description
86	.46	160	Count from 1 to 20
86	.44	178	Copy *pa, an, pro, pre, sti*
86	.48	201	Write 7-9-3; 3-5-7
86	.45	208	Read 27, 34, 158, 396, 9845
86	.42	209	Read vertically printed numbers
87	.40	33	Rapid, repeated oral movements
87	.39	84	Stereognosis—left hand errors
87	.38	127	Which of two cards is lighter; less light; darker; less dark
87	.36	222	Serial 13 subtraction from 100
87	.43	236	Description of events occurring in a picture
87	.35	257	Which word of four does not belong in the same group as the other three?
88	.40	157	Name visually presented objects
89	.35	157	Name visually presented objects
90	.39	82	Stereognosis—right hand errors
90	.47	110	Name objects from pictures
90	.51	112	What do *cat, bat, pat* mean?

*r = correlation

Table 5.1: **Item Intercorrelations with Visual Scale**   *Continued*

Item	r*	Item	Description
90	.59	113	Point to the picture that shows: typewriting; mealtime; summer
90	.37	118	Point to specified objects
90	.37	123	Draw a cross beneath a circle; a circle to the right of a cross
90	.41	129	If Arnie hits Tom, which boy is the victim?
90	.38	157	Name objects from pictures
90	.42	158	Name body parts from pictures
90	.41	159	Name objects from description
90	.38	203	Write 17 and 71; 69 and 96
90	.40	208	Read 27, 34, 158, 396, 9845
90	.42	210	Which is larger: 17 or 68; 23 or 56; 189 or 201?
90	.39	223	Serial 13 subtraction 100
90	.41	261	Time to solve elementary arithmetic problems
91	.42	110	Name objects from pictures
91	.43	112	What do *cat, bat, pat* mean?
91	.45	113	Point to the picture that shows: typewriting; mealtime; summer
91	.39	150	Read *cat-hat-bat*
91	.40	158	Name body parts from pictures
91	.42	208	Read 27, 34, 158, 396, 9845
91	.39	210	Which is larger: 17 or 68; 23 or 56; 189 or 201?
91	.39	215	How much is: 27 + 8; 44 + 57; 31 − 7; 44 − 14?
92	.41	1	Using your right hand, touch your fingers in turn with your thumb while you count them
92	.40	2	Same as #1 with left hand
92	.39	3	Clench your right hand, then stretch your fingers until I ask you to stop
92	.40	4	Same as #3 with left hand
92	.42	22	Tap your right hand twice and your left hand once
92	.41	54	Determine whether groups of tones are same or different
92	.42	59	How many beeps in all groups together?

*r = correlation

Table 5.1: **Item Intercorrelations with Visual Scale**   *Continued*

Item	r*	Item	Description
92	.44	84	Stereognosis—left hand errors
92	.46	157	Name visually presented objects
92	.41	208	Read 27, 34, 158, 396, 9845
92	.43	210	Which is larger: 17 or 68; 23 or 56; 189 or 201?
93	—		No correlations ≥.35 with items from other scales
94	.39	21	Clench right hand and extend fingers of left, then reverse
94	.36	106	Phonemic hearing—conditioned reflex
94	.37	217	In your head, subtract the number above from the one below
94	.37	218	What is the missing sign? 10 ( ) 2 = 20; 10( )2 = 12; 10( )2 = 8; 10( )2 = 5
94	.36	219	What number is missing? 12 − ( ) = 8; 12 + ( ) = 19
94	.40	220	Mental calculations: 27 + 34 + 14; 158 + 396
95	.42	62	Reproduce rhythm
95	.41	123	Draw a cross beneath a circle; a circle to the right of a cross
95	.40	203	Write 17 and 71; 69 and 96
95	.40	204	Write 27, 34, 158, 396, 9845
95	.41	208	Read 27, 34, 158, 396, 9845
95	.42	209	Read vertically printed numbers
95	.42	215	How much is: 27 + 8; 44 + 57; 31 − 7; 44 − 14?
95	.45	218	What sign is missing? 10 ( ) 2 = 20; 10( )2 = 12; 10( )2 = 8; 10( )2 = 5
95	.44	219	What number is missing? 12 − ( ) = 8; 12 + ( ) = 19
95	.42	220	Mental calculations: 27 + 34 + 14; 158 + 396
95	.43	221	Serial seven subtraction from 100
95	.42	222	Serial 13 subtraction from 100
96	—		No correlations ≥.35 with items from other scales
97	.39	59	How many beeps in all groups together?
97	.39	217	In your head, subtract the number above from the one below
97	.38	219	What number is missing? 12 − ( ) = 8; 12 + ( ) = 19
97	.38	220	Mental calculations: 27 + 34 + 14; 158 + 396
97	.37	256	Verbal analogies
97	.42	268	Discursive reasoning—complex arithmetic problems
98	—		No correlations ≥.35 with items from other scales
99	.38	1	Using your right hand, touch your fingers in turn with your thumb while you count them
99	.35	33	Rapid, repeated oral movements
99	.35	40	Draw triangle—score for quality
99	.37	51	If I knock hard, you knock gently; if I knock gently, you knock hard
99	.36	52	Tell me whether two tones are the same or different
99	.35	106	Phonemic hearing—conditioned reflex
99	.37	117	Simple sentences—conflicting instructions
99	.36	123	Draw a cross beneath a circle; draw a circle to the right of a cross
99	.41	157	Name visually presented objects
99	.40	221	Serial seven subtraction from 100
99	.45	223	Memory for seven words scored for errors
99	.38	229	Put hand in three positions as demonstrated
99	.36	241	Rearrange pictures into correct sequence—time to complete
99	.41	262	Discursive reasoning—elementary arithmetic problems
99	.40	268	Discursive reasoning—complex arithmetic problems

*r = correlation

performance on visual-spatial items on the Visual scale. Localization of brain damage using the Visual scale is made more difficult by relatively diffuse functional organization of the right hemisphere, and the localization process for visual deficits is aided by extra clinical tests and examination of certain items on the Motor, Writing, and Intellectual scales of the Luria-Nebraska.

Item Intercorrelations

Numerous significant correlations ($r > .35$; $p < .0001$) among Visual scale items and other Luria-Nebraska battery items demonstrate that each of the items on the scale is closely associated with abilities measured by other Luria-Nebraska items (Golden & Berg, 1981b).

As we noted earlier in this chapter, items 86 and 87 require naming and are thus quite sensitive to left hemisphere disorders, particularly those occurring in the temporoparietal region (Luria, 1966). It is not surprising, therefore, that these items (86 and 87) correlate most strongly with items requiring visual naming abilities and conceptualization abilities as well as reading and writing skills. All these abilities and skills can be localized to some extent in what Luria (1966) refers to as the tertiary temporo-occipital area of the left hemisphere. This region of the brain is responsible for the integration of auditory and visual information (Luria, 1966, 1973). Additionally, further evidence for parietal lobe involvement can be seen in the correlations of items requiring somatosensory information processing as well as verbal, motor, and stereognostic abilities with these Visual scale items (Luria, 1973; Roland, 1976; Golden, 1978).

Items 88–91 demand intact spatial abilities that are associated with intact right parieto-occipital functioning (Luria, 1966; Lewis, Golden, Moses, Osmon, Purisch, & Hammeke, 1979). This series of items demonstrates significant correlations with items requiring both left and right hemisphere functioning, such as sensory information processing, visual naming or recognition of objects and

numbers, and items requiring the use of arithmetical relations and operations. These correlations suggest involvement of the temporoparietal region of the left hemisphere in the region of the angular gyrus, since this area is responsible for integration of information from all sensory modalities (Golden, 1978). Disorders of this region may result in the disruption of the ability to associate names to objects (Butters & Brody, 1969). Dysfunction of the left secondary areas of the occipital lobes can lead to an inability to read or recognize numbers or letters (Ajax, 1964; Benson, Segarra, & Albert, 1974; Greenblatt, 1973; Lhermitte & Beauvois, 1973). Golden (1978) has noted that lesions of the right occipital secondary areas are likely to cause disorders of spatial relations with no loss in verbal skills.

Item 92, a strong measure of visual spatial organization and right hemisphere function, is highly correlated with simple hand movements, a frontal lobe function. This suggests that this item also requires frontal lobe involvement, particularly in terms of the mental flexibility ascribed by Luria (1973) to the frontal regions of the brain. Frontal lobe dysfunction, especially in the tertiary regions, can cause patients to lose this mental flexibility, so they find it difficult to change activities or alternate actions (Drewe, 1974; Malmo, 1974; Milner, 1963).

Items 94–96 require spatial orientation and are especially related to right hemisphere functions as long as receptive language functions remain intact, as is evidenced by the items that correlate highly with this section of the Visual scale. Arithmetic abilities are also strongly related to these items, suggesting involvement of the right parietal regions.

Although item 97 is especially sensitive to right hemisphere functions, deficits in performance may be seen in more moderate to severe left hemisphere disorders (Golden, Purisch, & Hammeke, 1979). Items requiring conceptualization, more complex arithmetic abilities, and analysis of rhythmic patterns are correlated with this item and tend to be left hemisphere functions (Luria, 1966; Lackner & Teuber, 1973; Benson & Weir, 1972).

Table 5.2: **Visual: Rotated Factor Matrix**

Item	Factor 1	Factor 2	Factor 3
86	*41*	21	08
87	*49*	31	18
88	*62*	−01	24
89	*51*	10	09
90	*48*	29	06
91	*48*	29	03
92	*44*	32	08
93	21	07	34
94	16	*64*	08
95	33	*55*	20
96	12	*41*	02
97	17	*55*	32
98	07	16	*74*
99	*45*	28	26

Item 99 is highly sensitive to right hemisphere dysfunction (Golden, Purisch, & Hammeke, 1979). Not surprisingly, therefore, visual-spatial abilities, tone analysis, memory, and arithmetic skill are all highly correlated with this item. Losses in the secondary area of the right temporal lobe may disturb both visual and auditory pattern analysis involved in all of these items (Kimura, 1963; Meier & French, 1965b). The right temporal area is especially important for rhythmic patterns that cannot be translated into a verbal code (Kimura, 1963; Luria, 1973; Milner, 1971; Warrington & James, 1967).

The Visual scale is highly useful in determining the localization of brain injury in the right hemisphere. However, the item intercorrelations demonstrate that left hemisphere dysfunction may also interfere with performance on these items. Poor performance on Visual scale items therefore must be carefully scrutinized in the interpretive process lest one be misled.

Factor Analysis

Factor analysis of the Visual scale showed clear factors emerging for that scale, as is seen in Table 5.2 (Golden, Purisch, Sweet, Graber, Osmon, and Hammeke, 1980).

Eight of the visual items loaded on the first visual factor. In a strikingly close correspondence to Luria's theory, most of these items (Table 5.3) have been specifically identified by Luria (1966) as measures of the visual perceptual process. Consequently, Golden, Purisch, Sweet, Graber, Osmon and Hammeke (1980) have labeled this factor visual perception. Each of the items that occur on this factor presents visual stimuli that must be identified in various ways. As one progresses through the items, however, they become increasingly more difficult, requiring a greater degree of active analysis and discrimination of relevant cues.

Visual factor 2 (Table 5.4) comprises four items, each of which appear to measure spatial orientation. The factor analysis again supports one of Luria's contentions—that visual-spatial ability is a separately measurable function distinct from visual perception. Most of the items were specifically intended by Luria to measure visual-spatial ability. Thus, the factor has been labeled visual-spatial perception.

The last factor, visual factor 3, shows significant loading on only one item: item 98, the overall time involved in responding to the visual-spatial task on item 97 (Table 5.5). This factor appears to the speed of the visual-spatial perceptual process that consists of several components—examining and analyzing the visual stimulus, identifying relevant cues, relating significant features, and integrating these features into recognizable patterns. Such a detailed process takes time, and the more complex visual-spatial stimuli require even more time. Since item 98 appears to represent a specific factor, it appears that impairment of visual-spatial perception can be measured not only in terms of accuracy but also in terms of the speed of the process. This factor has been called visual-spatial perceptual speed (Golden, Purisch, Sweet, Graber, Osmon, & Hammeke, 1980).

Table 5.3: **Items on Visual Factor 1**

Loading	Item	Description
.41	86	(Examiner presents objects one at a time.) What do you call this object?
.49	87	(Examiner presents pictures one at a time.) What is this picture supposed to be?
.62	88	(Examiner presents pictures one at a time.) What is this picture supposed to be?
.51	89	(Examiner presents pictures one at a time.) What is this picture supposed to be?
.48	90	What objects can you make out in this picture?
.48	91	What objects can you make out in this picture?
.44	92	The upper part of this card has a design with a piece missing. All of the smaller pieces below it have the right shape to fit the part missing in the design above. Put your finger on the piece with the design that will complete the pattern of the larger design.
.45	99	At the left of this paper there is a square with a circle in one corner. Notice the heavy dark line on one side of the square. This is the base line. Now look at these squares and notice that each square has a circle in one corner and the bottom of each square is a heavy line, the base line. By using the base line as a reference point, you can tell which square is just like the sample. Now I want you to circle the letter under the square that is just like the sample.

Table 5.4: **Items on Visual Factor 2**

Loading	Item	Description
.64	94	Tell me exactly what time these clocks tell.
.55	95	Draw the hands of a clock if the time is 12:50, 4:35, 11:10. Make sure you draw the minute hand longer than the hour hand.
.41	96	If this compass were on a map, which way would be north? east? west?
.55	97	This drawing shows a stack of blocks. When I show you the card, tell me how many blocks make up that stack. Be sure to include both the blocks you see and those you don't see.

Table 5.5: **Items on Visual Factor 3**

Loading	Item	Description
.74	98	Scoring (time for # 97).

Summary

The Visual scale is designed to evaluate a wide range of visual functions and is thus highly sensitive to right hemisphere dysfunction as well dysfunction in the posterior portions of the brain. A number of problems are inherent in the neuropsychological evaluation of visual functions; but, if carefully analyzed, the Visual scale can offer a tremendous amount of information concerning specific brain dysfunction.

6. Receptive Speech

The Receptive Speech scale consists of 33 items designed to detect impairment of receptive speech from basic to complex manifestations. The term receptive speech refers to perception of speech sounds, understanding of the meaning of words and phrases, and ultimately understanding of consecutive speech.

The most basic level of receptive speech involves phonemic hearing, of which speech sound discrimination is a fundamental factor. This process requires an intact auditory system. It is known that even a relatively slight decrease in auditory skills in childhood may hamper sound discrmination, thus interfering with speech development. Adequate auditory activity is therefore a prerequisite for differentiating speech sounds. Hence it is important to determine the intactness of hearing before assessing receptive speech.

Phonemic Hearing

To investigate phonemic hearing one must investigate several of the cerebral processes that underlie receptive speech as a whole. These processes include acoustic analysis articulation, pitch discrimination, and stability of acoustic traces (Luria, 1966). Items used for this include the writing and repetition of phonemes (100–105), discrimination of speech sounds (106), and discrimination of pitch changes (107).

Typically, the integrity of phonemic hearing is appraised by relatively simple methods. On the LNNB the patient is asked to repeat simple, isolated sounds (*b, p, m*) (100) or to repeat and distinguish pairs of sounds (item 102), including different disjunctive phonemes (*m–p, p–s*), and similar-sounding phonemes (*b–p, d–t, k–g, r–l*)(102). To increase the difficulty the individual is given a series of three sounds or simple syllables in item 104, incorporating either disjunctive phonemes (*a–o–a, u–a–i, bi–ba–bo, bi–bo–ba*) or correlating phonemes (*m–s–d, b–p–b, d–t–d*)(104). For each of the items listed above (100, 102, 104), the patient is also required to write the letters that each of the sounds represents (items 101, 103, 105). The first series of items measures the ability to discriminate simple speech sounds, whereas the second series additionally examines the retention of phonemic traces.

Testing discrimination of speech sounds by asking the patient to repeat sounds encompasses both phonetic auditory discrimination and the pronunciation of the corresponding sounds. These tasks yield uniform results only when the pronunciation is not hindered by expressive speech problems (Luria, 1966). Thus the discrimination of speech sounds must also be tested by other means to avoid improper conclusions owing to impaired motor aspects of speech. This is a particularly important when the intactness of the motor aspect of speech is in doubt.

A number of techniques can be used to evaluate speech sound discrimination without using motor speech. In one instance (item 106) the patient's capacity is studied using the conditioned reflex principle. The patient is instructed to raise the right hand during the pronunciation of one sound (ba) and the left hand when a similar sound is pronounced (pa). A more sensitive variant of this test (item 107) is somewhat more complex. Different sounds (b and p) are pronounced at the same pitch while identical sounds (b and b) are pronounced at different pitches, and the patient is asked to determine whether the letters pronounced are the same or different. This variant is used to determine which component—phonemic or tonal— allows the discrimination of speech sounds.

Deficiencies in phonemic hearing are a basic symptom of a lesion of the posterior temporal lobe of the left (dominant) hemisphere (Luria, 1966). Such problems can be identified using items 100-107. Extensive lesions may lead to difficulties with very different phonemes (Luria, 1966). In less severe cases the patient may still be able to differentiate some phonemes but not closely related ones. Individuals with motor or kinesthetic deficits (chaps. 2 and 4) may also show problems with these items. These patients will have trouble repeating sounds that are very different acoustically but are pronounced in similar ways.

They may show problems in attempting to switch between phonemes or may perseverate on a single sound. This becomes especially serious when several sounds must be repeated sequentially. This is especially seen in patients with a dysfunction of the frontotemporal regions of the left hemisphere (Luria, 1966). Right temporal lobe lesions will frequently impair the ability to reproduce rhythms, but the ability to discriminate speech sounds remains.

Word Comprehension

The second stage in the analysis of the receptive speech is the evaluation of word comprehension. To understand words, one must have relatively accurate phonemic hearing, and one must understand relationships between words, objects, actions, and other classes represented by words. Words can be misinterpreted as a result of defective phonemic hearing or as a result of temporo-occipital lesions that disturb the relationships of words to their meaning (Luria, 1966).

In investigating word comprehension (items 108-112), the examiner presents individual words that must be defined either verbally or by pointing at objects or pictures of objects. Item 108 asks that the patient "find" items that are not directly visible (eye, nose, ear). A more sensitive variant of this task appears in item 109, where word comprehension is studied by frequent repetition of the same words (point to eye-nose-ear-eye-nose). Repeating a word may cause it to lose its meaning for the patient (Luria, 1966). In item 110 the patient is asked to point out a named object from among seven pictures. Since the ease with which the patient interprets the word and points to the appropriate picture largely depends on the number of alternatives available, the number of pictures from which selection is made has a direct effect on performance. A patient with a mild disturbance of word comprehension may be able to select the correct answer from three alternatives but not from a greater number. For item 111 the patient is asked to point to body parts using somewhat more complicated and less familiar words (knee, elbow, cheekbone). The final item in this section of the scale (item 112) requires the patient to define words that differ by one phoneme (e.g. *cat, bat, pat*).

When performing these items, individuals with lesions of the left temporal lobe demonstrate obvious problems. Either they fail to understand the words clearly or they rapidly lose the meanings after a few repetitions of the word series. The loss of word meaning increases with the number of words presented at any one time. This symptom is characteristic of a lesion of the middle portions of the left temporal region, associated with the syndrome of acoustic-mnestic aphasia (Luria, 1966). Although these patients may understand individual words, they begin to have problems as soon as groups of words are presented.

Patients with the kinesthetic form of motor aphasia generally do not have difficulty with word meanings but they may have trouble if they try to pronounce words aloud to clarify the meaning. Individuals with frontal motor aphasia will understand individual words providing that articulatory difficulties do not arise and that pathological inertia does not interfere with transfer from one verbal form to another (Luria, 1966).

Patients with frontal and frontotemporal lesions typically can understand individual words but have problems with words presented in succession. They may continue to give the same word meaning even when the words are different (perseveration of word meaning).

Simple Sentence Comprehension

To understand sentences one must understand individual words, but this is not all. In addition to understanding the basic structure of sentences, one also must be able to remember series of words forming sentences and to inhibit premature conclusions from only one part of the sentence. If the latter ability is missing, comprehension of a sentence is replaced by a guess at its meaning.

To investigate the understanding of simple sentences one begins by giving the patient a series of simple phrases and asking him to find, after each presentation, a picture illustrating the event described by the phrase (item 113). Next one presents instructions whose meaning is not limited to the objects mentioned in them (items 114–116). Executing such instructions requires analysis of the corresponding speech structures (e.g., "Whose watch is this [examiner's]? Show me what is used to light the fire [3 pictures illustrating a stove, firewood, and matches are shown]. Patients who have a tendency to follow the instructions without analysis may understand them as isolated words. In one task, for example, they may point to the object (watch), but not indicate that the watch belongs to the examiner, and in the other task they may point to the fire rather than the object that lights it.

Additionally, this section of the Receptive Speech scale contains sentences with successively conflicting instructions (item 117: "If it is night now, point to the gray card; if it is day now, point to the black card"; and, "If it is day now, point to the black card; if it is night now, point to the gray card"). Inability to overcome the well-established direct association (night-black; day-gray) and to carry out the instruction may also lead to fragmentary perception of meaning.

Comprehending a sentence with no complex grammatical structures usually presents little difficulty to individuals with brain lesions, since the simple sentence represents the most common and firmly established unit of conversational speech. Even when the brain-damaged individual is unable to comprehend the meaning of individual words, familiar sentences may still be understood.

Sentence comprehension may, however, be limited. An increase in complexity can increase the difficulty of understanding a sentence. Patients with lesions of the temporal lobes may show problems after a small increase in complexity. Individual words are lost, the sentence is fragmented, and the patient may comprehend only words presented out of context.

A second factor is related to the need to inhibit guesses at meaning. The chance of guessing rather than truly understanding is especially great if the meaning is different from what the patient is familiar with. Familiar fragments may evoke associations not in agreement with the meaning of the sentence. Responses of this kind may be seen in patients with generalized cerebral dysfunction and in patients with specific frontal or frontotemporal lesions.

Logical Grammatical Structures

At a certain stage of speech development, grammatical forms begin to appear that reflect not only isolated objects, actions, or qualities, but also the complex relations between them (Luria, 1966). In a developed language, such relations are denoted by familiar methods such as the system of inflections, the order of the words in the sentence, and the various auxiliary words (prepositions, conjunctions, etc.) that act as special devices for transmitting relationships (Luria, 1966). In some instances these devices conflict with the simpler direct connotation of objects and actions. For instance, in the expression ''father's brother'' (item 122) we are concerned not with either a father or a brother, but with a third person, an uncle. In the sentences ''The boy hit the ball'' and ''The ball hit the boy,'' the same objects and actions are directly mentioned, but the arrangement of the words gives radically different meanings. In the construction ''a cross beneath a circle,'' it is not just two objects that are mentioned but also the spatial relation between them.

It is possible that a system of connections expressed by certain grammatical devices may conflict with the order of actions directly presumed from the order of words in the sentence (Luria, 1966). This can be easily seen in the command ''Point to the key with the pencil.'' When performing this task, the individual must not follow the order of the words given in the sentence, but rather must start by attending to the object mentioned last.

Understanding logical-grammatical structures is a highly complex process. To grasp the meaning of a grammatical construction it is essential to understand the meaning of the words as well as the structures combining these words. This requires integration of the elements of the sentence in a simultaneous rather than a consecutive procedure.

When investigating the comprehension of logical grammatical structures, one should avoid long phrases with complex structure, since such phrases require memorization of their elements, and this contaminates the results. For analysis of the degree to which a patient can still understand logical-grammatical relationships, it is most useful to employ the simplest sentences that can still express a given relationship.

In the Luria-Nebraska, the investigation of logical-grammatical structures starts with items devised to assess the understanding of simple inflective constructions (items 118, 119, 120). Three items are placed in front of the patient (a pencil, a key, and a comb), and instructions are given in three variations using the same operative words in different logical-grammatical relations. In item 118 the patient is asked to point to two named objects: ''Point at the pencil; point at the key.'' The patient is next given instructions incorporating the same words, but placed in special relation to each other by instrumental prepositions (item 119)—''Point with the key toward the pencil; point with the pencil toward the key.'' This includes not only the meaning of words but also the relations expressed by the prepositions. In the final item (120), the instructions are further complicated by requiring analysis of the word order and inversion of the action—''Point to the pencil with the key; now, point to the comb with the pencil.'' Before this can be done correctly, the patient must inhibit the initial impulse to carry out the action in the order in which the objects are named.

Patients with different types of cerebral dysfunction will experience various degrees of difficulty in carrying out these tasks. A patient with a lesion of the left temporal lobe and manifestations of acoustic aphasia is frequently unable to perform even the first of these items (Luria, 1966). Since such patients easily lose the meaning of the words presented, they cannot repeat them. Obviously, loss of the meaning of words is also a handicap in understanding more complex sentences.

Patients with lesions of the parieto-occipital region of the left hemisphere may interpret the phrase "with the pencil toward the key" agrammatically as the construction "pencil-key." They point separately to the two objects named, paying no attention to the relation established by the inflective structure of the phrase. A defect of this type, however, develops only from relatively severe lesions of this region (Luria, 1966), and those with less severe lesions will perform this task reasonably well.

Patients with lesions of the frontal regions of the brain can carry out the first two items but frequently have trouble with the third item (120). The tendency to follow the order of words in the sentence causes them both to ignore and to be unaware of the need for inversion. The patient performs the instruction according to the order in which the objects are named. This performance may be so well maintained and so persistent that the patient continues to follow the order of the words even after an explanation is given. However, these tests are relatively complex in character, and their performance involves a number of processes, which makes analysis of results difficult. Therefore to detect deficits, complicating factors are reduced to a minimum.

In contrast, difficulties characteristically encountered by patients with an inability to comprehend grammar—agrammatism—require other types of items that involve specialized operations of simultaneous synthesis. Such items utilize the attributive genitive case, prepositional constructions, and certain comparative constructions as in items 121–131 (Luria, 1966). In item 121 the patient is given a picture of a woman and a girl and asked to point to the "daughter's mother." Item 122 requires the patient to ascertain whether "father's brother" and "brother's father" are the same person. Patients with a disturbance in simultaneous synthesis are usually unable to grasp these phrases as single conceptual entities. In response to item 121, they may point to each picture individually. Item 122

confuses them, and they conclude that the two expressions have the same meaning. Attempts to obtain a precise definition of the phrases are often unsuccessful because of the difficulties these patients experience as soon as they try to reach beyond the nominative function of the words (Luria, 1966).

Items 123 and 124 investigate the comprehension of prepositional constructions by using spatial relations. In this section of the scale, the patient first is asked to draw a "cross beneath a circle" and "a circle to the right of a cross." Next, in a variant of this item, the patient is asked to determine which is correct: "Spring comes before summer" or "Summer comes before spring."

Luria (1966) notes that, as a rule, patients with manifestations of semantic aphasia experience great difficulty with these items because the analysis of such spatial relations is especially complex for them. Luria goes on to say that they usually exhibit well-defined symptoms of receptive agrammatism, grasping the meaning of individual words but understanding the instruction "Draw a cross beneath a circle" to mean "Draw a cross and a circle beneath it."

Patients with lesions of the temporal regions of the cortex and the concomitant loss of the meaning of words may understand the necessary logical grammatical relations but forget the shapes when performing the task. These patients may substitute alternate shapes.

Individuals with lesions of the frontal lobes may be able to understand the necessary logical-grammatical relationship but be unable to solve the problem. For example, after successfully completing a number of problems of the type "Draw a cross beneath a circle," such individuals are not able to "Draw a circle to the right of a cross" but perseverate by reproducing the established pattern (Luria, 1966). Patients with a marked frontal lobe syndrome cannot grasp the essence of the problem; they may draw both figures at the same place or repeat the same figure over and over.

Items 123–128 investigate patients' comprehension of comparative constructions and are carried out like other items in this section of the scale. In item 125 the patient is asked to determine "which boy is shorter, if John is taller than Peter." This task requires not only comprehension, but also mental inversion. In a variant, item 126 asks the patient to state which of the two constructions—"A fly is bigger than an elephant" or "An elephant is bigger than a fly"—is correct. Item 127 requires the determination of which of two cards is "lighter," "less light," "darker," and "less dark." In item 128 the patient is told that "Mary is lighter than Jane but darker than Sue," and then asked which girl is lightest. Even if grammatical disorders are only latent, such a task will generally be beyond the capabilities of such patients. Having understood the significance of the relationship "Mary is lighter than Jane," the patient is unable to reach the necessary conclusion. Luria (1966) claims that in such cases not even an arrangement of cards with pictures of three girls with different hair colors or of cards with girls' names written on them improves performance, and that combining this complex construction into a single system remains impossible.

A similar form of task used to examine the understanding of inverted grammatical constructions is seen in items 129, 130, and 131. In some of these structures, the order of the words does not correspond to the order of the actions.

Such sentences (e.g., item 129—"If Arnie hit Tom, which boy was the victim?" item 130—"If I had breakfast after I sawed wood, what did I do first?") cannot be understood correctly from their direct syntax. Like several of the items in this section, they may be interpreted only when the other requirements for this process (i.e., ability to understand word meaning, ability to engage in goal-directed activity) are present.

Item 132, the final item on the scale, is designed to analyze the comprehension of complex grammatical structure, including subordinate constructions, distant phrases, and so on. All of these logical-grammatical constructions have in common the factor of verbal expression of spatial relations. Patients with lesions of the parieto-occipital re-

gions understand the individual components of such expressions but cannot understand the overall expression.

The use of these items is important in detecting mild manifestations of receptive agrammatism, true forms of which occur with lesions of the left inferior temporal and parieto-occipital areas (Luria, 1966). This disorder leads to the syndrome of semantic aphasia. The mechanism responsible for these disturbances is not yet known, but they appear to be based on defects of special forms of simultaneous (spatial) synthesis represented in language and performed within the parietal-occipital cerebral regions.

Item Intercorrelations

A comparison of the Receptive Speech scale items with all other Luria-Nebraska items yields a number of significant correlations ($r > .35$; $p < .0001$), as illustrated in Table 6.1. (Golden & Berg, 1981c).

While all items on this scale have the common requirement of understanding speech, there are also a number of other specific and general factors that differentiate each item from others on the scale. The intercorrelations demonstrated that each of the Receptive Speech scale items is closely related to skills tapped by other Luria test items.

Items 100–107 involve the comprehension of simple phonemes. It is important to note which individuals can either say or write the phonemes, but not both. The ability to repeat phonemes but not write them suggests impairment in the area of the angular gyrus, while the ability to write but not say phonemes suggests an expressive rather than a receptive speech disorder (Golden, Purisch, & Hammeke, 1979). The item intercorrelations with these first seven items confirm involvement of the angular gyrus and the right hemisphere areas implicated by poor performance on item 107. Also, the intercorrelations strongly suggest a much broader left temporoparietooccipital involvement with these receptive speech processes that extends well beyond the area of the angular gyrus.

Table 6.1: **Item Intercorrelations with Receptive Speech Scale**

Item	r*	Item	Description
100	.41	134	Repeat *sp, th, pl, str. awk*
100	.35	137	Repeat *hairbrush; screwdriver; laborious*
100	.37	223	Memory for seven words scored for error
101	—		No correlations ≥ .35 with items from other scales
102	.41	134	Repeat *sp, th, pl, str, awk*
102	.36	157	Name objects from pictures
102	.35	218	What sign is missing? 10 ( ) 2 = 20; 10 ( ) 2 = 12; 10 ( ) 2 = 8; 10 ( ) 2 = 5
102	.41	223	Memory for seven words scored for error
103	.35	64	Cutaneous sensation—right side
103	.37	82	Stereognosis—right hand errors
103	.36	84	Stereognosis—left hand errors
103	.38	134	Repeat *sp, th, pl, str, awk*
103	.36	178	Copy *pa, an, pro, pre, sti*
103	.35	179	Write words from memory—visual presentation
103	.40	197	Read sentences
103	.38	227	Draw geometric shapes from memory
103	.39	256	Verbal analogies
104	.37	133	Repeat *a, i, m, b, sh*
104	.41	134	Repeat *sp, th, pl, str, awk*
104	.36	179	Write words from memory—visual presentation
104	.40	218	What sign is missing? 10 ( ) 2 = 20; 10 ( ) 2 = 12; 10 ( ) 2 = 8; 10 ( ) 2 = 5
104	.40	230	Visual memory for words
104	.37	256	Verbal analogies
105	.38	134	Repeat *sp, th, pl, str, awk*
105	.35	144	Read *sp, th, pl, str, awk*
105	.37	148	Read *hairbrush; screwdriver; laborious*
105	.47	183	Write *wren; knife*
105	.44	197	Read sentences
105	.37	204	Write 27, 34, 158, 396, 9845
105	.36	218	What sign is missing? 10 ( ) 2 = 20; 10 ( ) 2 = 12; 10 ( ) 2 = 8; 10 ( ) 2 = 5
105	.46	223	Memory for seven words scored for error

*r = correlation

Table 6.1: **Item Intercorrelations with Receptive Speech Scale**

Continued

Item	r*	Item	Description
105	.40	227	Draw geometric shapes from memory
105	.36	257	Verbal analogies
106	.39	2	Using your left hand, touch your fingers in turn with your thumb while you count them
106	.38	8	With your eyes closed, place your left hand in the same position as I place your right hand in (thumb against middle finger)
106	.41	12	Left hand fingers extended in sagittal plane touching chin
106	.40	23	Tap your left hand twice and your right hand once as quickly as you can
106	.38	48	If I knock once, you knock twice; if I knock twice, you knock once
106	.38	51	If I knock hard, you knock gently; if I knock gently, you knock hard
106	.39	59	How many beeps in all groups together?
106	.38	70	Two-point tactile discrimination—right hand
106	.39	72	Determine whether stimulus is moving up or down right arm
106	.42	84	Stereognosis—left hand errors
106	.39	86	Name visually presented objects
106	.43	133	Repeat *a, i, m, b, sh*
106	.39	170	Complete sentences (visual stimulus, verbal response)
106	.40	205	Write 14, 17, 19, 109, 1023
106	.37	223	Memory for seven words scored for error
106	.38	257	Verbal analogies
107	.41	257	Verbal analogies
108	.41	34	Show me how to chew
108	.40	72	Determine whether stimulus is moving up or down right arm
108	.36	73	Same as #72 with left arm
108	.43	136	Repeat *house; table; apple*
108	.55	201	Write 7-9-3; 3-5-7
108	.43	205	Write 14, 17, 19, 109, 1023
108	.51	206	Read 7-9-3; 3-5-7
108	.46	210	Which is larger: 17 or 68; 23 or 56; 189 or 201?

*r = correlation

Table 6.1: **Item Intercorrelations with Receptive Speech Scale**

Continued

Item	r*	Item	Description
108	.47	258	Discursive reasoning—elementary arithmetic problems
109	.37	33	Rapid, repeated oral movements
109	.35	54	Determine whether two groups of tones are same or different
109	.36	205	Write 14, 17, 19, 109, 1023
109	.35	223	Memory for seven words scored for error
110	.41	69	Cutaneous sensation—left side
110	.51	73	Determine whether stimulus is moving up or down left arm
110	.38	75	Identify shapes drawn on left wrist
110	.47	86	Name visually presented objects
110	.47	90	Name overlapping objects in picture
110	.42	91	Name overlapping objects in picture
110	.46	133	Repeat *a, i, m, b, sh*
110	.49	181	Write *f, t, h, l*
110	.53	203	Write 17 and 71; 69 and 96
110	.45	204	Write 27, 34, 158, 396, 9845
110	.42	208	Read 27, 34, 158, 396, 9845
110	.46	210	Which is larger: 17 or 68; 23 or 56; 189 or 201?
110	.49	258	Discursive reasoning—elementary arithmetic problems
111	—		No correlations ≥.35 with items from other scales
112	.51	86	Name visually presented objects
112	.51	90	Name overlapping objects in picture
112	.43	91	Name overlapping objects in picture
112	.43	137	Repeat *hairbrush; screwdriver; laborious*
112	.43	146	Read *cat; dog; man*
112	.49	150	Read *cat-hat-bat*
112	.49	158	Name body parts from pictures
112	.45	160	Count from 1 to 20
112	.49	163	Say the days of the week backward starting with Sunday
112	.45	201	Write 7-9-3; 3-5-7
112	.46	205	Write 14, 17, 19, 109, 1023

Table 6.1: **Item Intercorrelations with Receptive Speech Scale**

Continued

Item	r*	Item	Description
112	.45	206	Read 7-9-3; 3-5-7
112	.44	208	Read 27, 34, 158, 396, 9845
112	.58	210	Which is larger: 17 or 68; 23 or 56; 189 or 201?
112	.42	251	Concept formation—logical relationships
112	.45	258	Discursive reasoning—elementary arithmetic problems
113	.49	67	Cutaneous sensation—left side
113	.46	73	Determine whether stimulus is moving up or down left arm
113	.45	84	Stereognosis—left hand errors
113	.58	90	Name overlapping objects in picture
113	.45	91	Name overlapping objects in pictures
113	.45	142	Repeat *house-ball-chair; ball-chair-house*
113	.47	158	Name body parts from pictures
113	.48	159	Name objects from description
113	.45	177	Copy *B, L, ℒ, 𝒟, ℬ*
113	.45	178	Copy *pa, an, pro, pre, sti*
113	.46	181	Write *f, t, h, l*
113	.47	201	Write 7-9-3; 3-5-7
113	.48	203	Write 17 and 71; 69 and 96
113	.49	205	Write 14, 17, 19, 109, 1023
113	.53	206	Read 7-9-3; 3-5-7
113	.55	207	Read IV, VI, IX, XI; 17, 71, 69, 96
113	.48	209	Read vertically printed numbers
113	.46	258	Discursive reasoning—elementary arithmetic problems
114	—		No correlations ≥.35 with items from other scales
115	.41	19	Point to left eye with right hand
115	.38	20	Touch right ear with left hand
115	.48	34	Show me how to chew
115	.36	72	Determine whether stimulus is moving up or down right arm
115	.35	73	Same as #72 using left arm
115	.43	86	Name visually presented objects

*r = correlation

Table 6.1: **Item Intercorrelations with Receptive Speech Scale**

Continued

Item	r*	Item	Description
115	.42	158	Name body parts from pictures
115	.41	159	Name objects from description
115	.46	206	Read 7-9-3; 3-5-7
115	.44	210	Which is larger: 17 or 68; 23 or 56; 189 or 201?
116	.43	82	Stereognosis—right hand errors
116	.40	84	Stereognosis—left hand errors
116	.36	86	Name visually presented objects
116	.37	90	Name overlapping objects in picture
117	.36	99	Intellectual operations in space
117	.36	220	Mental computation: 27 + 34 + 14; 158 + 396
117	.37	223	Memory for seven words scored for error
117	.41	233	Memory for sentences
117	.39	234	Memory for paragraphs
117	.41	251	Concept formation—logical relationships
117	.36	256	Verbal analogies
117	.37	261	Time taken to solve elementary arithmetic problems
118	.38	34	Show me how to chew
118	.36	86	Name visually presented objects
118	.35	203	Write 17 and 71; 69 and 96
119	.38	86	Name visually presented objects
119	.39	159	Name objects from description
119	.36	201	Write 7-9-3; 3-5-7
119	.39	204	Write 27, 34, 158, 396, 9845
119	.98	205	Write 14, 17, 19, 199, 1023
119	.39	210	Which is larger: 17 or 68; 23 or 56; 189 or 201?
119	.38	258	Discursive reasoning—elementary arithmetic problems
120	.35	86	Name visually presented objects
120	.37	203	Write 17 and 71; 69 and 96
120	.38	204	Write 17, 34, 158, 396, 9845
120	.36	205	Write 14, 17, 19, 109, 1023
120	.36	210	Which is larger: 17 or 68; 23 or 56; 189 or 201?

Table 6.1: **Item Intercorrelations with Receptive Speech Scale**

Continued

Item	r*	Item	Description
121	.36	72	Determine whether stimulus is moving up or down right arm
121	.38	73	Same as #72 using left arm
121	.35	138	Repeat *rhinoceros; surveillance; hierarchy*
121	.41	146	Read *cat; dog; man*
121	.36	154	Repeat sentences
121	.46	203	Write 17 and 71; 69 and 96
121	.38	205	Write 14, 17, 19, 109, 1023
121	.35	214	How much is: 7 − 4; 8 − 5?
121	.38	255	Concept formation—opposites
122	—		No correlations ≥.35 with items from other scales
123	.37	23	Tap your left hand twice and your right hand once as quickly as you can
123	.38	87	Name objects from pictures
123	.38	90	Name overlapping objects in picture
123	.41	95	Draw hands on blank clockfaces for: 12:50, 4:35, 11:10
123	.38	148	Name body parts from pictures
123	.38	159	Name objects from description
123	.39	163	Say the days of the week backward starting with Sunday
123	.41	205	Write 14, 17, 19, 109, 1023
123	.43	210	Which is larger: 17 or 68; 23 or 56; 189 or 201?
123	.40	223	Memory for seven words scored for errors
123	.47	230	Write words from memory after visual presentation
123	.41	248	Concept formation—definitions
124	.39	19	Point to your left eye with your right hand
124	.42	20	Touch your right ear with your left hand
124	.43	86	Name visually presented objects
124	.43	147	Read *house; table; apple*
124	.38	159	Name objects from description
124	.38	163	Say the days of the week backward starting with Sunday
124	.48	205	Write 14, 17, 19, 109, 1023

r = correlation

Table 6.1: **Item Intercorrelations with Receptive Speech Scale**

Item	r*	Item	Description
124	.45	208	Read 27, 34, 158, 396, 9845
124	.57	210	Which is larger: 17 or 68; 23 or 56; 189 or 201?
124	.40	258	Discursive reasoning—elementary arithmetic problems
125	.37	176	Phonetic analysis—e.g., what is the second letter in *cat*? first letter in *match*?
125	.45	203	Write 17 and 71; 69 and 96
125	.46	204	Write 27, 34, 158, 396, 9845
125	.36	219	What number is missing? 12 − ( ) = 8; 12 + ( ) = 19
126	.36	191	Which of the letters *B, J,* or *S* stands for *John*?
126	.43	210	Which is larger: 17 or 68; 23 or 56; 189 or 201?
127	—		No correlations ≥.35 with items from other scales
128	—		No correlations ≥.35 with items from other scales
129	.42	25	Show me how to pour and stir tea
129	.42	58	How many beeps do you hear?
129	.41	59	How many beeps in all groups together?
129	.41	86	Name visually presented objects
129	.41	90	Name overlapping objects in picture
129	.42	142	Repeat *house–ball–chair; ball–chair–house*
129	.45	159	Name objects from description
129	.44	204	Write 27, 34, 158, 396, 9845
129	.41	205	Write 14, 17, 19, 109, 1023
129	.41	209	Read vertically printed numbers
129	.45	210	Which is larger: 17 or 68; 23 or 56; 189 or 201?
129	.42	214	How much is: 7 − 4; 8 − 5?
129	.42	219	What number is missing? 12 − ( ) = 8; 12 + ( ) = 19
129	.42	261	Time to solve elementary arithmetic problems
130	.35	95	Draw hands on blank clockface for: 12:50, 4:35, 11:10

*r = correlation

Table 6.1: **Item Intercorrelations with Receptive Speech Scale**   *Continued*

Item	r*	Item	Description
130	.35	95	Draw hands on blank clockface for: 12:50, 4:35, 11:10
130	.36	204	Write 27, 34, 158, 396, 9845
130	.35	208	Read 27, 34, 158, 396, 9845
130	.35	219	What number is missing? 12 − ( ) = 8; 12 + ( ) = 19
130	.35	220	Mental computation: 27 + 34 + 14; 158 + 396
130	.39	256	Verbal analogies
130	.38	257	Verbal analogies
131	—		No correlations ≥.35 with items from other scales
132	.35	254	Concept formation—opposites

*r = correlation

Items 100–107 demonstrate high correlations with items requiring both audioverbal and visual memory. Specific disturbances of audioverbal memory are a typical feature of lesions of the left temporal areas, while visual memory disorders are frequently found in temporo-occipital injuries (Luria, 1973; Meyer, 1959; Milner, 1958). Items requiring intact sensorimotor area functioning in both hemispheres are also highly related to this section of the scale, suggesting anterior parietal lobe involvement in phonemic analysis of speech. Other indicators of left temporoparietooccipital involvement that are correlated with items 100–107 include reading skills, writing skills, concept formation abilities, and arithmetic symbol comprehension and manipulation (Benson & Wier, 1972; Golden, 1978; Luria, 1966, 1973; Zurif & Ramier, 1972).

Item 106 demonstrates involvement with frontal lobe functioning as well as with the temporoparietooccipital area, particularly during the output phase of the task. In addition to requiring obvious sensorimotor and kinesthetic functions, intentionality of movement appears to be a requirement for the task, as does the ability to carry out verbal instructions as motor acts. Both of these have been associated with left frontal lobe dysfunction (Golden, 1978; Luria, Pribram, & Homskaya, 1964).

Items 108-116 involve understanding simple words and sentences. These items are meant to determine whether the patient is correctly hearing and interpreting what is said, a left temporal lobe function (Kimura, 1961; Lansdell, 1970; Neff & Goldberg, 1960). Injury to the primary left temporal area can result in "word deafness," in which the patient cannot understand speech (Gazzaniga, Glass, Sarno, & Posner, 1973), but there is no accompanying deficit in writing, reading, or other cognitive processes (Jerger, Lovering, and Wertz, 1972). This is an important distinction, since a number of Luria items that significantly correlate with this segment of the Receptive Speech scale do involve reading, writing, concept-formation, and arithmetic skills. Poor performance on these items, then, would point to a more posterior cerebral injury. Additionally, a number of item intercorrelations suggest right hemisphere involvement, particularly of the parietal area, in the performance of these items. Poor performance on these specific items (110, 113, 115, 116) may indicate right parietal dysfunction, since lesions of the posterior divisions of the right hemisphere may disturb the visual recognition of objects (Luria, 1973).

Beginning with item 117 and continuing through the end of this scale, the individual is required to respond to increasingly difficult instructions. All these items can be affected by injury to the left hemisphere, but several can also be affected by right hemisphere dysfunction. Items 118, 119, 120, and 123, for example, require some spatial orientation on the part of the patient. If the patient appears to understand the sentence or instruction but is unable to correctly carry out the spatial tasks, the possibility of right hemisphere dysfunction cannot be overlooked. This is further demonstrated by the items correlating highly with items 118, 119, 120, and 123 that require visual naming, comparisons of numbers, and other tasks demanding spatial organization, all of which are typically localized in the right hemisphere (Golden, 1978; Luria, 1966, 1973). Parietotemporooccipital functions of the left hemisphere

such as writing, reading, concept formation, and discursive reasoning also are related to the functions tapped by items 118, 119, 120, and 123. The item intercorrelations further show, as noted by Luria (1973), involvement of the secondary areas of the left temporal lobe (Meyer & Yates, 1955; Golden, 1978).

Items in the last section of this scale (items 121, 122, 125, 126-132) are especially sensitive to damage in the parieto-occipital areas of the left hemisphere, though they may be affected by a simple lack of understanding in the patient resulting from injuries to the left temporal lobe or the angular gyrus (Golden, Purisch, & Hammeke, 1979). Several of the items in this series demonstrate a significant correlation with right temporoparietooccipital functions including visual naming, spatial organization, and musical skills of pitch and rhythm discrimination and reproduction (Hecaen & Angelergues, 1962; Luria, 1973; Milner, 1958). These items also correlate highly with tasks requiring writing, arithmetic skills, reading, and verbalized concept formation, which tend to be left hemisphere functions. That items requiring intact motor functions and items involving ability to solve problems presented verbally demonstrated significant correlations with some of the items in this section of the scale suggests some frontal lobe involvement. Luria (1973) has noted that patients with frontal lesions show disturbances in tests involving the solution of verbal problems, particularly complex ones.

Factor Analysis

Factor analysis of the Receptive Speech scale of the Luria-Nebraska Neuropsychological Battery derived two factors, as can be seen in Table 6.2 (Golden, Purisch, Sweet, Graber, Osmon, & Hammeke, 1980). In this discussion of receptive speech, Luria considered two primary aspects that needed to be assessed. The first aspect was the ability to perceive speech sounds accurately and meaningfully. The first factor (Table 6.3) derived from the Recep-

Table 6.2: **Receptive Speech: Rotated Factor Matrix**

Item	Factor 1	Factor 2
100	*41*	10
101	*38*	03
102	*77*	04
103	*88*	10
104	*75*	05
105	*72*	09
106	*42*	25
107	*35*	20
108	09	03
109	24	23
110	17	14
111	07	07
112	22	*44*
113	09	21
114	05	03
115	−02	12
116	14	*39*
117	16	25
118	05	05
119	03	18
120	05	−03
121	14	00
122	07	00
123	08	*65*
124	−01	14
125	15	30
126	13	21
127	00	21
128	09	04
129	09	*58*
130	15	17
131	08	09
132	04	27

Table 6.3: **Items on Receptive Factor 1**

Loading	Item	Description
.41	100	Repeat exactly the sound you hear.
.38	101	Now write down the letter of the alphabet that each sound represents.
.77	102	Repeat the two sounds you hear: *m–p, p–s, b–p, d–t, k–g, r–l*
.88	103	Write down the letter each sound represents.
.75	104	Now there will be three sounds; repeat them.
.72	105	Write down all the letters each sound represents.
.42	106	If you hear *ba,* please raise your right hand; if you hear *pa,* please raise your left hand.
.35	107	Now you will hear two letter sounds. Tell me whether the letters you hear are the same or different: *b–p* (pronounced at same pitch); *b–b* (pronounced at different pitches).

tive Speech scale does indeed support Luria's contention that speech sound perception is a primary neuropsychological ability. Eight items load significantly on this factor. All are intended to assess speech sound perception. For each item, single phonemes or a series of phonemes are spoken and are to be identified in various ways. In this way, deficits in any one manner of responding are not able to prevent assessment of this factor.

The second aspect of receptive speech identified by Luria is verbal comprehension. Luria distinguished three aspects of this ability: comprehension of words, of simple sentences, and of complex sentences. The second receptive speech factor (Table 6.4) that emerged consists of only four items out of several designed to evaluate verbal comprehension. That so few of these intended items loaded on this factor sheds doubt on the validity of verbal comprehension as an identifiable unitary underlying variable. Even if Luria's further breakdown into word, simple sentence, and complex sentence comprehension is considered, these items were still not all intended to assess the same subtype of verbal comprehension. However, two of these items that show the highest loading on this factor, items 123 and 129, were both intended by Luria to assess comprehension of complex verbal structures. In both, the general ability to consider simultaneously and relate all the verbal elements of the sentence underlies accurate comprehension. This would indicate that a specifically identifiable ability underlying speech comprehension is simultaneous processing. Thus, factor 2 is called verbal comprehension–simultaneous processing.

Table 6.4: **Items on Receptive Factor 2**

Loading	Item	Description
.44	112	What does (*word*) mean? (*cat; bat; pat*)
.39	116	(Place cards left to right.) Show me what is used to light a fire.
.65	123	Draw a cross beneath a circle; now draw a circle to the right of a cross.
.58	129	If Arnie hit Tom, which of the boys was the victim?

Unfortunately, this leaves few clues to the relationship of the remaining 21 items of the scale. Although all require verbal comprehension, they also individually require a wide variety of subskills for verbal comprehension, such as inverted grammatical structure, syntactic analysis, spatial analysis, logical relations, temporal sequencing, prepositional interpretation, and so on. Golden, Purisch, Sweet, Graber, Osmon, & Hammeke, (1980) note that it appears that each of the remaining items formed their own single-item factors rather than coming together under a more general verbal comprehension factor. These findings suggest that each of these abilities is more independent than Luria suggested and that they are mediated by functional systems that are demonstrably different from one another. However, before we reach such conclusions, further research is necessary to determine if the current factor structure is replicable.

Summary

Overall, the Receptive Speech scale is extremely sensitive to the presence of brain dysfunction. The scale appears to be much more easily elevated by damage to the left hemisphere. The item intercorrelations suggest that the scale may also be elevated by damage to the right hemisphere. There is some evidence that anterior dysfunction in the right hemisphere can cause specific elevations on the Receptive Speech scale (e.g., Lewis, Golden, Moses, Osmon, Purisch, & Hammeke, 1979), and the intercorrelations and factor analysis support this notion to some degree. It may be that this elevation is due to the possible involvement of the right frontal areas in the understanding of basic English phonemes, perhaps through the analysis of pitch, rhythm, and complex spatial syntax. This, however, requires further investigation.

7. Expressive Speech

This scale consists of 42 items (133–174) intended to assess impairment of expressive speech from basic to complex manifestations. The most elementary level of verbalization assessed is reflective speech. Items at this level (133–156) require oral repetition or reading of visually presented models. Spontaneous verbalization is not required. The primary abilities needed are accurate auditory perception, retention, articulation, and smooth transition from one articulation to the next. Items at this level require the repetition of simple and complex phonemes and words, series of words and phrases, and sentences. Most items are also presented visually so they may be read.

Representing a higher level of verbal expression is the naming of objects, assessed by items 157–159. Nominative speech is more complex and less automatic than reflective speech and may show impairment in the absence of reflective speech deficits. Nominative speech requires that appropriate verbal labels be provided without a direct acoustic or symbolic model. In addition to accurate perceptual and articulatory abilities, one must be able to recall an object's name and to select this name from other possible alternatives that are mentally generated. Items at this level require the patient to identify familiar and unfamiliar pictures and to name objects from verbal descriptions.

Narrative speech represents the highest level of verbal expression and is assessed by the remaining items (160–174). Narration requires active generation of new verbal associations expressed by a system of syntax. Conversely, reflective and nominative speech are reactive forms of expression not requiring new verbal associations. Narration may be elicited as a response to an external stimulus or extemporaneously. The active generation of narrative speech requires that a plan or intention be translated into a verbal form through internal speech with its predicative structure (Luria, 1966). No such plan or intention is required for either reflective or nominative speech. Items at this level require the forward and backward narration of common serial expressions, the description of pictorial and verbal presentations, extemporaneous expression, and expression based upon the analysis and synthesis of complex grammatical systems.

Reflective Speech

In investigating reflective speech one can assess the integrity of several basic neuropsychological processes underlying expressive speech as a whole—namely, acoustic analysis, articulation, smooth motor expression, and stability of acoustic traces (Luria, 1966). Tasks include the repetition of speech sounds (133, 134), words (135-142), and sentences (154, 155, 156). Several of these items are also presented for reading (143-153).

Impairment of any of the aforementioned neuropsychological processes will result in characteristic disturbances at the various levels of repetitive speech. However, the integrity of all of these processes is not necessary at all levels. Rather, hierarchical organization exists in which an increasing number of neuropsychological abilities are required as items become more demanding (Luria, 1966). For example, stability of acoustic traces (the memory component) is more crucial for repetition of sentences than of words.

The most basic items of this section requiring the repetition of speech sounds demand functional integrity of acoustic analysis and articulation. Impairment of these processes will also be reflected in more complex forms such as words and sentences. However, in disturbances of latent articulation or acoustic analysis, not reflected in speech sound production, difficulty in word repetition will appear only as conditions become complex (Luria, 1966). Therefore words to be repeated proceed from simple and familiar words to acoustically complex and unfamiliar words.

Other abilities are required for accurate repetition as the demands become greater. Each word represents a complex of sounds, so that the patient must switch smoothly from one to the next. In addition, it is necessary to inhibit the verbalization of conflicting associations elicited by any word. A memory factor is introduced when the number of words is increased, as in sentences and series of phrases.

Items to be read rather than repeated alter the stimulus from auditory to visual. This controls for the confounding effects of auditory acuity in repetition tasks, and it eliminates the memory component needed for repetition of sentences. Impaired performance on these items may result from a lesion that also causes a repetitive speech deficit. On the other hand, impaired visual perceptual processes may result in reading deficits. A discussion of these latter factors will be reserved for the section on reading disorders.

Articulation of Speech Sounds

Examining the items will make the preceding discussion clearer. To begin, items 133 and 134, entailing repetition of speech sounds, require functional integrity of the articulatory and acoustic analytic processes. Accurate articulation requires that motor impulses be precisely addressed to the vocal musculature. An intact afferent feedback system providing information on the placement of the musculature is vital to this process. Lesions of the inferior portion of the sensorimotor and postcentral area disrupt the somesthetic and kinesthetic impulses that constitute this afferent system. In this condition, known as afferent motor dysphasia, articulemes (sounds produced by articulatory movements) are confused. In milder instances only similar articulemes are substituted, for example, the labials *m* and *b*. Severe impairment is reflected by a complete breakdown of articulation (Luria, 1973).

A breakdown of acoustic analysis or phonemic discrimination also impairs repetition of speech sounds. This impairment results from a lesion of the secondary areas of the auditory cortex in the posterior superior temporal gyrus (Wernicke's area). In these cases of sensory dysphasia, spoken sounds become confused, and an incorrect repetition follows. Milder cases involve only the substitution of similar-sounding phonemes, for example, *b* being repeated as *p* (item 133). The more complex speech sounds of item 134 make greater demands on phonemic discrimination and may elicit a latent disorder not reflected in item 133. In addition, the greater complexity of item 134 may result in errors due to pathological inertia, to be discussed below.

Item 135 presents pairs of open and closed monosyllabic words. Impairment of articulation or of acoustic analysis of individual sounds will likewise be reflected in these more complex stimuli and manifested in the substitution of articulemes or phonemes. Patients with phonemic discrimination difficulties often repeat another word with similar phonetic composition, a literal paraphasia—for example, *three* is substituted for *tree*. In other cases phonemic discrimination may be so impaired that the word becomes uninterpretable and there are obvious signs of confusion.

In addition to increasing the complexity of the acoustic stimuli, item 135 also assesses the integrity of a third neuropsychological process, the ability to transfer smoothly from one articuleme to the next. For this to occur, the afferent impulse responsible for a previous articuleme must be inhibited before the new one is initiated. The inability to inhibit the previous impulse, that is, pathological inertia, results from a lesion of the inferior premotor area (Broca's area). In this disorder, the patient could repeat a sound were it not for the perseveration of the previous sound. Errors of this type are exemplified by the repetition of *see-see* for *see-seen,* and *tree-tree* or *tree-treek* for *tree-trick.*

It is possible that pathological inertia will, albeit rarely, be manifested on item 134. This item presents habitual speech sound combinations that have assumed the character of verbal automatisms and thus presumably each require single impulses. If these verbal automatisms disintegrate, a separate impulse will be needed for each constituent sound, which will be subject to pathological inertia. This condition would indicate severe disturbances in the neurodynamics that make fluent expressive speech possible.

Reflected (Repetitive) Speech: Single Words and Series of Words

Latent disorders of acoustic analysis, articulation, or motor transition may become evident on this next series of items. Items 136, 137, 138, and 140 require single-word repetition (with the exception of *Massachusetts Episcopal* of item 140). These words proceed from relatively familiar and acoustically simple to less familiar and acoustically complex. Of course, difficulties apparent on "easier" items will intensify as items become more demanding. For instance, a breakdown of phonemic discrimination when attempting to repeat *house* (136) will result in a literal paraphasia or obvious signs of confusion, such as, "I don't understand! What did you say?" Interestingly, expressions of confusion may be pronounced with ease though repetition of the stimulus item is impaired (Luria, 1966).

Deficits in latent articulation and motor transition will similarly be exposed as words become less familiar or acoustically more demanding. An exception to this occurs when a particular word has, through exposure, become an automatism for a particular individual. In these cases the impairment might even be evident on the simplest repetition item (and of course manifested as items become more demanding) but not show up on a relatively more complex stimulus.

Items 139, 141, and 142 each present a series of three words. This lengthening of the stimulus demands the integrity of a fourth neuropsychological process, acoustic-verbal memory, in addition to the processes already discussed. Item 139 presents the acoustically similar words *cat-hat-bat.* Items 141 and 142 each present two different sequences of the same three words.

Acoustic-verbal memory is distrubed by lesions of the middle and inferior segments of the temporal lobe. Often no more than one or two words can be retained at any one time, as the patient helplessly recognizes. Forgetting the words in the series results not only in omissions but often in perseverations and contaminations of previous words in the series. For example, item 140 may reveal impairment by the reply *bell–sun–bell* or contamination by the reply *hat–sell–sun*.

Retaining the proper order of the word series also becomes difficult with a disturbance of acoustic-verbal memory. This phenomenon is evident when all three words are correctly recalled but are repeated in different order. However, a correct repetition of the sequence may become an inert stereotype, repeated in the same order even when the task requires a change of order. This type of neurodynamic inertia is revealed by perseveration of the rearranged order of the second series.

Acoustic-verbal memory is further taxed by the sentences in items 154–156. Whereas items 154 and 155 present single sentences increasing in length and complexity, item 156 places the highest demands on acoustic-verbal memory with a series of three sentences given together. Latent disorders not evident with word series are revealed by these items. Words are forgotten, and only fragments are repeated. Often the general meaning is gleaned although the words are forgotten, resulting in sentence substitution such as "It is hot out" for "The weather is fine today" (154) or verbal paraphasias for individual words. Contamination of sentences frequently occurs and is especially evident on item 156—for example, "The house is shining, the moon is sweeping. . . ."

The following discussion focuses upon the reading of several of the items presented for repetition in items 143–153. As we stated earlier, reflective speech also entails reading several of the items. It is expected that qualitatively similar difficulties in acoustic analysis, motor transition, and articulation experienced during repetition will remain evident. If errors of these kinds are absent in reading while found in repetition, this casts doubt upon the diagnosis of the underlying disorder gleaned from repetition. In essence, the reading items serve as a useful validity check of the repetition errors caused by these types of impairment.

On the other hand, reading presents different conditions than does repetition and thus requires different neuropsychological abilities. Auditory stimuli are replaced by visual ones, which eliminates the influence of auditory acuity and acoustic-verbal memory. Reading disturbances may also be evident owing to impairment in visual or spatial impairments. These are not primary expressive speech deficits, and discussion of them will be reserved for the section on disorders of reading.

Nominative Speech

Nominative speech requires that one select the correct word without a direct verbal model. Word finding is the basis of higher levels of spontaneous speech and must be investigated in its isolated form to discover any primary deficits. The ability to name objects depends upon the integrity of several processes, including analysis of the acoustic properties of the word brought to mind, stability of the acoustic trace, and selection of the appropriate word based on its defining characteristics and clear visual images.

Items 157 and 158 present pictures of objects (157) or parts of the body (158) for identification. Correct performance on both items requires integrity of the same neuropsychological processes mentioned above. However, identifying body parts may prove more difficult, since they are pictured apart from the rest of the body, removing contextual cues.

Impairment of acoustic analysis by lesions of the superior region of the temporal lobe hampers attempts to express the correct word. While an acoustic trace may be elicited, the patient is unable to identify the correct sounds. Attempts to say the word result in literal paraphasias using phonemically similar sounds (Luria,

1966). For instance, for *stapler* (157), *shapler, spatler, saptler, satpler,* and so on.

Instability of acoustic traces owing to lesions of middle and inferior divisions of the left temporal lobe leads to word amnesia. These patients visually recognize the object, but their attempts to retrieve the appropriate verbal label are often futile. Verbal paraphasias are common in which the object can often be described functionally or conceptually or named by words in a similar category (Luria, 1966). For instance, attempts to identify *elbow* (158) may result in a response such as, "a joint . . . to bend your arm . . . shoulder . . . no," and so forth.

Word amnesia may not be revealed in the retrieval of names of objects presented singly. A testing of the limits procedure in which several pictures are presented simultaneously often uncovers a latent impairment of this type; often perseveration on the first-named object will occur. An item that presents several pictures simultaneously, such as item 110 of the Receptive Speech scale, may be used for this purpose.

Lesions of the frontotemporal region, additionally affecting Broca's area, add the difficulty of pathological inertia. In these cases perseveration of previously given names may occur. Confounding this state is instability of acoustic traces, in which the patient may not become sufficiently aware of the perseveration and does not self-correct.

Another type of word amnesia is found with lesions of the parieto-occipital region of the cortex. Patients in this group, like those with middle temporal lesions, may recognize the object but cannot find the appropriate label. Verbal paraphasias are common. The difference between these two groups is revealed when the patient is prompted with the initial sounds of the word. Patients suffering from parieto-occipital lesions typically can identify the object with this procedure whereas middle temporal lesioned patients cannot.

The underlying neuropsychological impairment involved in the word amnesia with lesions of the parieto-occipital region is not clearly understood. The most likely explanation appears to be that this cortical region is a tertiary association area in which information from the optic, verbal-auditory, and tactile-kinesthetic analyzers is integrated. The appropriate verbal label for an object must be selected from the network of possible visual, spatial, and acoustic choices, and semantically, visually, acoustically, or spatially similar alternatives must be inhibited. Perhaps prompting with initial sounds allows the exact selection of the word from the general category of objects with similar defining characteristics (Luria, 1973).

A final condition for successful identification is the ability to form a clear visual image of the object to be named. Lesions of the temporo-occipital region result in optic dysphasia, producing a blurred image that cannot be verbally identified. The pictured objects or body parts of items 157 and 158 may thus not be identifiable. An attempt to establish a clearer visual image may help to overcome this difficulty. Items presenting progressively clearer visual images appear on the Visual scale (item 88).

Item 159 requires the same neuropsychological abilities discussed above, but it differs from the preceding two items in that identification must be accomplished from functional description rather than from a visual model. Without the need for direct visual perception, emphasis is on forming an internally rather than an externally generated mental image and is closer to the processes represented by word finding or spontaneous speech. As above, integrity of the temporo-occipital area is vital to forming the visual image even when a visual model is lacking. Breakdown of this integrity differs from visual impairment resulting from a lesion of the secondary optic association area. The primary effect of a lesion in this latter area is optic agnosia and thus is classified as a perceptual rather than a speech-related disorder (Luria, 1973).

Narrative Speech

Neuropsychological processes contributing to narrative speech are assessed by items 160–174. Narration is the higher form of verbal expression and depends on many of the more basic abilities already discussed for appropriate execution. Phonemic discrimination is needed to decipher verbal acoustic traces, and stable acoustic traces are needed to ensure word recall, understanding, and sequencing. Afferent feedback is necessary for proper articulation, and of course smooth transition ensures fluency.

Yet, despite the integrity of these basic processes, narration may still be impaired, since it requires even higher and more complex abilities. Unlike reflective and nominative speech, narration operates without visual or acoustic models. Rather, internal ideas and associations must be translated into an external expression. Furthermore, this expression requires an appreciation of proper grammatical structure (Luria, 1966).

Two crucial aspects of coherent narrative speech are fluency and spontaneity. Basic fluency is assessed by items 160–163, in which the patient recites forward and backward the numbers 1 through 20 and the days of the week. These are rather automatic and habitual series, not requiring grammatical structure and thus cannot be considered narration in the true sense. Dysfluency on any of these sequences may result from a disturbance of any of the processes previously discussed and perhaps already discovered at an earlier level of this section. For example, an instability of acoustic traces may result in the patient's forgetting the place in the sequence, leading to omissions or to repetitions of previous numbers or days. Reversing the sequence is not habitual and places greater emphasis upon stable acoustic traces, resulting in further difficulties of this type. For example, "Sunday, Saturday, Thursday, . . . Wednesday . . . Wednesday . . ." and so on.

Dysfluency with these habitual series certainly indicates fluency problems in the more demanding narrative speech process measured by items 164–167, which require description of a picture (164), paraphrasing of a short story (166), and a short extemporaneous speech (168). In addition to fluency, spontaneity of expression is measured by the time it takes to transform thoughts into verbal expression (165, 167, 169).

Narrative fluency is disrupted by a lesion of Broca's area even when not severe enough to create efferent motor dysphasia. The manifestations of this type of disorder resemble the telegraphic speech of the young child. Nominative speech is preserved, but there is difficulty verbalizing the ancillary predicative connecting words. Luria (1966) theorizes that this results from a disturbance in the "predicative function of speech" owing to lesions of the anterior speech regions of the cortex. In essence, internal speech (thinking), which is greatly contracted compared with verbal expression, cannot be expanded upon by using predicative speech structures. The resulting expression sounds disjointed and dysfluent, consisting of individual nominative words. For example, in describing the picture in item 164, a patient with an injury to this area might say, "Man . . . here . . . and water . . . man there . . . helping."

Spontaneity of speech may also be impaired, as reflected in longer reaction times. No deficit is present in the formation of thoughts; rather, the slowness reflects difficulty and effort in expressing these thoughts.

Lesions anterior to Broca's area, in the prefrontal region of the cortex, result in a qualitatively distinct narrative disturbance. In this disorder, internal speech can be expanded and expressed in a fluent and grammatically correct manner. The difficulty is an inability to formulate original internal speech associations. In this disturbance, called dynamic dysphasia, narration requiring original thought is impossible (Luria, 1966.)

The patient with dynamic dysphasia can repeat questions in an echolalic manner and even answer questions that contain the wording for the reply (e.g., "Is it a nice day today?" "Yes, it is a nice day today"). Automatic or stereotyped phrases, similarly not requiring the generation of new associations, can be spoken fluently. Thus items 160 and 162, involving well-ingrained series, are easily recited. The reversal of these series, however (161, 163), requires the active formation of new associations and thus creates severe problems.

A patient with dynamic dysphasia cannot successfully generate extemporaneous reflections upon the stimuli presented in items 164, 166, and 188, and verbal productivity will be low. Latent forms of this disorder will be reflected in longer reaction times (165, 167, 169) owing to the difficulty in generating associations to the stimuli.

The ability to form verbal associations among the words in a phrase or sentence consistent with acceptable grammatical requirements is the essence of meaningful narrative speech. Thus far the items of this section have considered solely the fluency and spontaneity of narration. Items 170–174 assess appreciation of grammatical structure—the ability to select and arrange words to fit into sentences in a way that is meaningful and grammatically appropriate.

Item 170 provides three sentences, each with a word omitted. The sentences get progressively more difficult as the word to be supplied becomes less obvious, requiring greater analysis of the entire sentence. Specifically, the first sentence presents a choice of three words; the second sentence requires insertion of an obvious word into a simple sentence without choices provided; and the third sentence requires a word that can be supplied only after careful analysis and synthesis of the elements of the sentence. Item 171 assesses the time required to analyze the sentences in the formulation of the missing words.

Item 172 presents the three words *automobile, wood,* and *garage* and asks for a sentence including them. This task requires the patient to establish an original idea for thematically relating the words and then to provide connecting links between the words. In other words, the basic structural or substantive links of the sentence are provided and the predicative connectors must be supplied.

Finally, in the last items all the words of a sentence are supplied in disarranged sequence and the patient must arrange them meaningfully. This task requires a thorough appreciation of grammatical structure so that the words can be grouped appropriately. Item 173 measures the adequacy of the final production, and item 174 measures the automacy of the process by the time needed to complete the task.

Each of the items 170–174 requires an appreciation of the grammatical structure of a sentence. This is impaired by lesions of the anterior divisions of the cortex, including Broca's area, and of the postfrontal areas anterior to the premotor cortex. Disturbance on these items combined with good performance on earlier items not requiring an appreciation of grammatical structure or the generation of associative links between words is often a good indication of a lesion in this region.

Of course lesions of other parts of the cortex can affect performance on these items as well; the effects are evident in reflective or nominative disabilities, probably uncovered on earlier items. For example, a patient with a parieto-occipital injury might be able to appreciate the meaning and grammatical structure of the sentences of item 170 but would be unable to retrieve the required word owing to dysnomia, the nature of which already has been discussed. Similarly, injuries to Wernicke's area or the postcentral cortex will each result in characteristic disturbances probably manifested on earlier items, such as literal or verbal paraphasias, slurring, and word contaminations.

There are important qualitative differences in the narrative speech of patients with injuries of the posterior versus the anterior divisions of the cortex. The former often have trouble retrieving words, especially nominatives, leading to omissions or verbal paraphasias. Predicative links are provided easily. Just the opposite is seen with lesions to the anterior cortex which results in telegraphic speech. These patients have trouble providing predicative links but supply nominative words with relative ease.

Anterior and posterior injuries also are distinguished by the degree to which the appropriate intonation and rhythm of narration are preserved. In general, patients with anterior lesions speak in a rather unexpressive monotone; patients with posterior lesions have a normal sense of intonation and rhythm. Even when words are omitted or paraphasias substituted, they still have the lively inflection characteristic of normal speech.

Table 7.1: **Item Intercorrelations with Expressive Speech Scale**

Item	r*	Item	Description
133	.35	69	Cutaneous sensation—left side
133	.42	72	Determine whether stimulus is moving up or down right arm
133	.47	73	Same as #72 with left arm
133	.46	86	Name visually presented objects
133	.38	90	Name overlapping objects in picture
133	.43	106	Phonemic hearing—conditioned reflex
133	.46	110	Name objects from pictures
133	.43	112	What do *cat, bat, pat* mean?
133	.43	113	Point to the picture that shows: typewriting; mealtime; summer
133	.43	210	Which is larger: 17 or 68; 23 or 56; 189 or 201?
134	.38	84	Stereognosis—left hand errors
134	.41	100	Repeat single phonemes
134	.41	102	Repeat phoneme pairs
134	.39	103	Write phoneme triplets
134	.42	104	Repeat phoneme triplets
134	.38	105	Write phoneme triplets
134	.38	112	What do *cat, bat, pat* mean?
134	.38	234	Memory for sentences
135	.38	73	Determine whether stimulus is moving up or down left arm
135	.38	112	What do *cat, bat, pat* mean?
135	.36	204	Write 27, 34, 158, 396, 9845
135	.43	205	Write 14, 17, 19, 109, 1023
135	.37	210	Which is larger: 17 or 68; 23 or 56; 189 or 201?
135	.35	214	How much is 7 − 4; 8 − 5?
136	.40	72	Determine whether stimulus is moving up or down right arm
136	.46	73	Same as #72 with left arm
136	.36	86	Name visually presented objects
136	.43	108	Point to: eye; nose; ear
136	.35	110	Identify objects from pictures by pointing
136	.39	201	Write 7-9-3; 3-5-7

r = correlation

Table 7.1: **Item Intercorrelations with Expressive Speech Scale** *Continued*

Item	r*	Item	Description
136	.39	210	Which is larger: ≥ 17 or 68; 23 or 56; 189 or 201?
136	.44	211	Which is larger: 189 or 201; 1967 or 3002?
136	.44	258	Discursive reasoning—elementary arithmetic problems
136	.44	260	Discursive reasoning—elementary arithmetic problems
137	.41	25	Show me how to pour and stir tea
137	.35	69	Cutaneous sensation—left side
137	.35	70	Two-point tactile stimulation—right hand
137	.40	72	Determine whether stimulus is moving up or down right arm
137	.37	110	Identify objects from pictures by pointing
137	.43	112	What do *cat, bat, pat* mean?
137	.37	123	Draw a cross beneath a circle; draw a circle to the right of a cross
137	.37	178	Copy *pa, an, pro, pre, sti*
137	.35	198	Read sentences
137	.40	205	Write 14, 17, 19, 109, 1023
137	.39	233	Memory for sentences
138	.36	1	Using right hand, touch fingers in turn with thumb while you count them
138	.38	92	Number of errors on tasks from Raven's Matrices
138	.35	121	Show, by pointing, who is the daughter's mother
138	.38	195	Read *insubordination; indistinguishable*
138	.35	198	Read sentences
138	.37	233	Memory for sentences
138	.39	253	Concept formation—logical relationship
138	.42	255	Concept formation—opposites
138	.38	256	Verbal analogies
139	—		No correlations ≥ .35 with items from other scales
140	.37	51	If I knock hard, you knock gently; if I knock gently, you knock hard

r = correlation

Table 7.1: **Item Intercorrelations with Expressive Speech Scale**

Continued

Item	r*	Item	Description
140	.39	72	Determine whether stimulus is moving up or down right arm
140	.36	200	Time taken to read paragraph
140	.40	210	Which is larger: 17 or 68; 23 or 56; 189 or 201?
140	.36	219	What number is missing? 12 − ( ) = 8; 12 + ( ) = 8; 12 + ( ) = 19
140	.42	230	Visual memory for words
141	—		No correlations ⩾.35 with items from other scales
142	.40	72	Determine whether stimulus is moving up or down right arm
142	.38	73	Same as #72 with left arm
142	.39	110	Identify objects from picture by pointing
142	.41	112	What do *cat, bat, pat* mean?
142	.45	113	Point to the picture that shows: typewriting; mealtime; summer
142	.39	119	Point with the key toward the pencil; point with the pencil toward the key
142	.39	129	If Arnie hit Tom, which boy was the victim?
142	.45	203	Write 17 and 71; 69 and 96
142	.44	205	Write 14, 17, 19, 109, 1023
142	.52	210	Which is larger: 17 or 68; 23 or 56; 189 or 201?
143	.36	90	Name overlapping objects in picture
143	.35	204	Write 27, 34, 158, 396, 9845
144	.46	176	Phonetic analysis—e.g., what is the second letter in *cat*? the first letter in *match*?
144	.41	183	Write *wren; knife*
144	.44	185	Write words and phrases
144	.37	189	What word is made by these letters: *s–t–o–n–e; k–n–i–g–h–t*?
144	.44	200	Time taken to read paragraph
144	.44	202	Write IV and VI; IX and XI
144	.42	218	What sign is missing? 10 ( ) 2 = 20; 10 ( ) 2 = 12; 10 ( ) 2 = 8; 10 ( ) 2 = 5
144	.44	227	Draw geometric shapes from memory
144	.40	235	Logical memorizing—recall by visual aid

*r = correlation

Table 7.1: **Item Intercorrelations with Expressive Speech Scale**

Continued

Item	r*	Item	Description
144	.40	254	Concept formation—logical relationships
144	.46	256	Verbal analogies
145	.43	178	Copy *pa, an, pro, pre, sti*
145	.40	182	Write *ba; da; back; pack*
145	.43	193	Read *juice; bread; bonfire; cloakroom; fertilizer*
145	.42	198	Read sentences
145	.49	204	Write 27, 34, 158, 396, 9845
145	.43	205	Write 14, 17, 19, 109, 1023
145	.41	209	Read vertically printed material
145	.46	210	Which is larger: 17 or 68; 23 or 56; 189 or 201?
145	.40	219	What number is missing? 12 − ( ) = 8; 12 + ( ) = 19
146	.43	112	What do *cat, bat, pat* mean?
146	.41	121	Show, by pointing, who is the daughter's mother
146	.44	190	Tell me what you see: *K, S, W, R, T*
146	.42	193	Read *juice; bread; bonfire; cloakroom; fertilizer*
146	.42	198	Read sentences
146	.44	203	Write 17 and 71; 69 and 96
146	.41	204	Write 27, 34, 158, 396, 9845
146	.43	205	Write 14, 17, 19, 109, 1023
146	.48	206	Read 7-9-3; 3-5-7
146	.43	208	Read 27, 34, 158, 396, 9845
146	.42	210	Which is larger: 17 or 68; 23 or 56; 189 or 201?
146	.44	211	Which is larger: 189 or 201; 1967 or 3002?
146	.42	214	How much is 7 − 4; 8 − 5?
147	.42	73	Determine whether stimulus is moving up or down left arm
147	.49	112	What do *cat, bat, pat* mean?
147	.42	113	Point to the picture that shows: typewriting; mealtime; summer
147	.43	124	Which is correct: Spring comes before summer, or Summer comes before spring?

*r = correlation

Table 7.1: Item Intercorrelations with Expressive Speech Scale

Continued

Item	r*	Item	Description
147	.40	193	Read *juice; bread; bonfire; cloakroom; fertilizer*
147	.45	198	Read sentences
147	.42	201	Write 7-9-3; 3-5-7
147	.43	203	Write 17 and 71; 69 and 96
147	.45	204	Write 27, 34, 158, 396, 9845
147	.45	205	Write 14, 17, 19, 109, 1023
147	.51	206	Read 7-9-3; 3-5-7
147	.43	208	Read 27, 34, 158, 396, 9845
147	.53	210	Which is larger: 17 or 68; 23 or 56; 189 or 201?
147	.44	214	How much is 7 − 4; 8 − 5?
147	.43	258	Discursive reasoning—elementary arithmetic problems
148	.39	62	Reproduce rhythm
148	.41	176	Phonetic analysis; e.g., what is the second letter in *cat*? first letter in *match*?
148	.39	183	Write *wren; knife*
148	.46	189	What word is made by the letters: *s-t-o-n-e; k-n-i-g-h-t*
148	.43	193	Read *juice; bread; bonfire; cloakroom; fertilizer*
148	.43	195	Read *insubordination; indistinguishable*
148	.39	199	Read paragraph—score for errors
148	.39	204	Write 27, 34, 158, 396, 9845
148	.40	254	Concept formation—logical relationships
149	.37	176	Phonetic analysis; e.g., what is the second letter in *cat*? first letter in *match*?
149	.43	187	Number of words written in 60 seconds on a specified topic
149	.38	193	Read *juice; bread; bonfire; cloakroom; fertilizer*
149	.44	195	Read *insubordination; indistinguishable*
149	.37	199	Read paragraph—score for errors
149	.39	200	Time needed to read paragraph
149	.37	202	Write IV and VI; IX and XI
149	.38	235	Logical memorizing—recall by visual aid
149	.38	256	Verbal analogies
150	.40	59	How many beeps in all groups together?
150	.38	69	Cutaneous sensation—left side
150	.38	91	Name overlapping objects in picture
150	.45	112	What do *cat, bat, pat* mean?
150	.40	113	Point to the picture that shows: typewriting; mealtime; summer
150	.42	177	Copy *B, L, ℒ, 𝒟, ℬ*
150	.44	178	Copy *pa, an, pro, pre, sti*
150	.41	198	Read sentences
150	.40	204	Write 27, 34, 158, 396, 9845
150	.42	205	Write 14, 17, 19, 109, 1023
150	.42	206	Read 7-9-3; 3-5-7
150	.45	208	Read 27, 34, 158, 396, 9845
150	.41	210	Which is larger: 17 or 68; 23 or 56; 189 or 201?
151	.43	176	Phonetic analysis; e.g., what is the second letter in *cat*? first letter in *match*?
151	.39	185	Write words and phrases
151	.41	189	What word is made by these letters: *s-t-o-n-e; k-n-i-g-h-t*?
151	.54	195	Read *insubordination; indistinguishable*
151	.45	200	Time taken to read paragraph
151	.42	219	What number is missing? 12 − ( ) = 8; 12 + ( ) = 19
151	.41	247	Understanding of thematic texts
151	.39	254	Concept formation—logical relationships
152	.42	86	Name visually presented objects
152	.40	113	Point to the picture that shows: typewriting; mealtime; summer
152	.39	178	Copy *pa, an, pro, pre, sti*
152	.49	206	Read 7-9-3; 3-5-7
152	.40	210	Which is larger: 17 or 68; 23 or 56; 189 or 201?
153	.38	86	Name visually presented objects
153	.37	185	Write words and phrases
153	.41	198	Read sentences

*r = correlation

Table 7.1: **Item Intercorrelations with Expressive Speech Scale**

Continued

Item	r*	Item	Description
153	.42	204	Write 27, 34, 158, 396, 9845
153	.39	205	Write 14, 17, 19, 109, 1023
153	.39	206	Read 7-9-3; 3-5-7
153	.48	210	Which is larger: 17 or 68; 23 or 56; 189 or 201?
153	.38	214	How much is: 7 − 4; 8 − 5?
153	.38	219	What number is missing? 12 − ( ) = 8; 12 + ( ) = 19
154	.36	72	Determine whether stimulus is moving up or down right arm
154	.36	121	Show, by pointing, who is the daughter's mother
154	.39	203	Write 17 and 71; 69 and 96
154	.40	204	Write 27, 34, 158, 396, 9845
154	.45	205	Write 14, 17, 19, 109, 1023
154	.42	210	Which is larger: 17 or 68; 23 or 56; 189 or 201?
155	.36	106	Phonemic hearing—conditioned reflex
155	.35	195	Read *insubordination; indistinguishable*
155	.45	223	Memory for seven words scored for error
155	.39	230	Write words from memory after visual presentation
155	.39	232	Retention and retrieval of words—homogeneous interference
155	.45	233	Memory for sentences
155	.37	235	Logical memorizing—recall by visual aid
156	.37	59	How many beeps in all groups together?
156	.35	90	Name overlapping objects in picture
156	.39	123	Draw a cross beneath a circle; draw a circle to the right of a cross
156	.36	189	What word is made by these letters: *s-t-o-n-e; k-n-i-g-h-t*?
156	.36	195	Read *insubordination; indistinguishable*
156	.37	205	Write 14, 17, 19, 109, 1023
156	.36	210	Which is larger: 17 or 68; 23 or 56; 189 or 201?
156	.35	221	Serial seven subtraction from 100
156	.36	222	Serial 13 subtraction from 100

*r = correlation

Table 7.1: **Item Intercorrelations with Expressive Speech Scale**

Continued

Item	r*	Item	Description
156	.43	223	Memory for seven words scored for errors
156	.40	230	Write words from memory after visual presentation
156	.47	233	Memory for sentences
156	.37	256	Verbal analogies
157	.41	1	Using your right hand, touch your fingers in turn with your thumb while you count them
157	.43	2	Same as #1 with left hand
157	.38	3	Clench your right hand and then stretch your fingers as quickly as you can
157	.40	21	Clench your right hand and extend fingers of left hand, then reverse
157	.39	22	Tap your right hand twice and your left hand once
157	.44	33	Rapid, repeated oral movements
157	.43	71	Two-point tactile discrimination—left hand
157	.51	84	Stereognosis—left hand errors
157	.44	85	Stereognosis—left hand time
157	.48	87	Name objects from pictures
157	.40	88	Name objects from pictures
157	.41	99	Intellectual operations in space
157	.41	187	Number of words written in 60 seconds on a specified topic
157	.49	218	What sign is missing? 10 ( ) 2 = 20; 10 ( ) 2 = 12; 10 ( ) 2 = 8; 10 ( ) 2 = 5
157	.42	227	Draw geometric shapes from memory
157	.42	235	Logical memorizing—recall by visual aid
157	.44	241	Time needed to rearrange picture into a meaningful sequence
158	.36	71	Two-point tactile discrimination—left hand
158	.37	75	Identify shapes drawn on back of left wrist
158	.44	82	Stereognosis—right hand errors
158	.44	83	Stereognosis—right hand time
158	.43	84	Stereognosis—left hand errors
158	.46	86	Name visually presented objects
158	.42	90	Name overlapping objects in picture
158	.40	91	Name overlapping objects in picture

*r = correlation

Table 7.1: **Item Intercorrelations with Expressive Speech Scale**

Continued

Item	r*	Item	Description
158	.49	112	What do *cat, bat, pat* mean?
158	.47	113	Point to the picture that shows: typewriting; mealtime; summer
158	.42	115	Whose watch is this (examiner's)? Whose is this (patient's)?
158	.43	206	Read 7-9-3; 3-5-7
159	.41	90	Name overlapping objects in picture
159	.48	113	Point to the picture that shows: typewriting; mealtime; summer
159	.41	115	Whose watch is this (examiner's)? Whose is this (patient's)?
159	.35	119	Point with the key toward the pencil; point with the pencil toward the key
159	.45	129	If Arnie hit Tom, which boy was the victim?
159	.36	191	Which of these letters, *B, J,* or *S,* stands for *John*?
159	.35	193	Read *juice; bread; bonfire; cloakroom; fertilizer*
159	.37	197	Read sentences
159	.40	201	Write 7-9-3; 3-5-7
159	.44	203	Write 17 and 71; 69 and 96
159	.41	204	Write 27, 34, 158, 396, 9845
159	.46	205	Write 14, 17, 19, 109, 1023
159	.40	206	Read 7-9-3; 3-5-7
159	.41	207	Read IV, VI, IX, XI; 17, 71, 69, 96
159	.41	208	Read 27, 34, 158, 396, 9845
159	.51	210	Which is larger: 17 or 68; 23 or 56; 189 or 201?
159	.41	213	How much is: 3 + 4; 6 + 7?
159	.42	219	What number is missing? 12 − ( ) = 8; 12 + ( ) = 19
159	.43	251	Concept formation—logical relationships
159	.43	252	Concept formation—logical relationships
159	.43	255	Concept formation—opposites
159	.42	258	Discursive reasoning—elementary arithmetic problems
159	.46	261	Time needed to solve elementary arithmetic problems

*r = correlation

Table 7.1: **Item Intercorrelations with Expressive Speech Scale**

Continued

Item	r*	Item	Description
160	.46	86	Name visually presented objects
160	.45	112	What do *cat, bat, pat* mean?
160	.41	204	Write 27, 34, 158, 396, 9845
160	.40	205	Write 14, 17, 19, 109, 1023
160	.41	210	Which is larger: 17 or 68; 23 or 56; 189 or 201?
161	.38	203	Write 17 and 71; 69 and 96
161	.37	204	Write 27, 34, 158, 396, 9845
161	.38	205	Write 14, 17, 19, 109, 1023
161	.37	208	Read 27, 34, 158, 396, 9845
161	.40	209	Read vertically printed numbers
161	.39	210	Which is larger: 17 or 68; 23 or 56; 189 or 201?
162	.35	72	Determine whether stimulus is moving up or down right arm
162	.40	73	Same as #72 with left arm
162	.41	112	What do *cat, bat, pat* mean?
162	.36	124	Which is correct: Spring comes before summer, or Summer comes before spring?
162	.43	180	Write your first and last name
162	.41	201	Write 7-9-3; 3-5-7
162	.41	204	Write 27, 34, 158, 396, 9845
162	.43	205	Write 14, 17, 19, 109, 1023
162	.41	206	Read 7-9-3; 3-5-7
162	.45	208	Read 27, 34, 158, 396, 9845
162	.45	210	Which is larger: 17 or 68; 23 or 56; 189 or 201?
162	.47	258	Discursive reasoning—elementary arithmetic problems
163	.38	59	How many beeps in all groups together?
163	.38	95	Draw hands on blank clockface for 12:50, 4:35, 11:10
163	.39	123	Draw a cross beneath a circle; draw a circle to the right of a cross
163	.39	129	If Arnie hit Tom, which boy was the victim?
163	.36	190	Tell me what you see here: *K, S, W, R, T*
163	.45	204	Write 27, 34, 158, 396, 9845

*r = correlation

Table 7.1: **Item Intercorrelations with Expressive Speech Scale**

Continued

Item	r*	Item	Description
163	.43	205	Write 14, 17, 19, 109, 1023
163	.40	207	Read IV, VI, IX, XI; 17, 71, 69, 96
163	.45	208	Read 27, 34, 158, 396, 9845
163	.45	212	How much is: 3×3; 5×4; 7×8?
163	.45	214	How much is: $7 - 4$; $8 - 5$?
163	.44	219	What number is missing? $12 - (\ \ ) = 8$; $12 + (\ \ ) = 19$
164	—		No correlations $\geqslant$.35 with items from other scales
165	—		No correlations $\geqslant$.35 with items from other scales
166	—		No correlations $\geqslant$.35 with items from other scales
167	—		No correlations $\geqslant$.35 with items from other scales
168	—		No correlations $\geqslant$.35 with items from other scales
169	—		No correlations $\geqslant$.35 with items from other scales
170	.39	83	Stereognosis—right hand time
170	.37	210	Which is larger: 17 or 68; 23 or 56; 189 or 201?
170	.35	259	Time taken to solve elementary arithmetic problems
171	.35	200	Time taken to read paragraph
171	.35	223	Memory for seven words scored for errors
172	—		No correlations $\geqslant$.35 with items from other scales
173	.36	218	What sign is missing? $10 (\ \ ) 2 = 20$; $10 (\ \ ) 2 = 12$; $10 (\ \ ) 2 = 8$; $10 (\ \ ) 2 = 5$
173	.35	223	Memory for seven words scored for errors
173	.40	235	Logical memorizing—recall by visual aid
173	.41	256	Verbal analogies
174	.36	218	What sign is missing? $10 (\ \ ) 2 = 20$; $10 (\ \ ) 2 = 12$; $10 (\ \ ) 2 = 8$; $10 (\ \ ) 2 = 5$
174	.36	223	Memory for seven words scored for errors
174	.38	235	Logical memorizing—recall by visual aid
174	.35	254	Concept formation—logical relationships
174	.39	256	Verbal analogies

*r = correlation

Item Intercorrelations

A number of significant correlations ($r > .35$; $p < .0001$) are noted when correlating items from the Expressive Speech scale with all other Luria-Nebraska items, as can be seen in Table 7.1.

Expressive speech functions are typically considered to be localized in the frontal, temporal, and parietal regions of the left hemisphere, as we noted at length earlier in this chapter. Items 133, 134, and 135 require the functional integrity of articulatory and acoustic analytic processes. Accurate articulation requires intact afferent feedback systems as well as intact efferent motor systems. Lesions of the inferior portion of the sensorimotor and postcentral areas can disrupt the somesthetic and kinesthetic components of this system (Luria, 1966). Not surprisingly, therefore, a number of items that correlate highly with items 133 and 134 demand intact somatosensory and kinesthetic feedback routes for good performance. In addition, these items are closely associated with Luria items that require the repetition of phonemes. The secondary area of the left temporal lobe (Brodmann's areas 21 and 22) is responsible for the analysis and integration of speech and the decoding of language phonemes (Luria, 1966, 1973; Zurif & Ramier, 1972). Other items that correlate with this section of the Expressive Speech scale include those tapping such functions as audioverbal memory, writing, arithmetic comparisons, and simple computation, all of which have been reported to be left temporoparietooccipital functions (Benson & Wier, 1972; Golden, 1978; Golden, Purisch, & Hammeke, 1979; Luria, 1973).

Items 136–142 require word repetition. As the words to be repeated increase in difficulty, articulatory deficits are more likely to be apparent, suggesting a lesion of the primary area of the left frontal lobe (Golden, 1978). If speech sounds are slurred, the possibility of kinesthetic damage must not be overlooked since it would suggest parietal lobe dysfunction (Golden, Purisch, & Hammeke,

1979). Indeed, several of the items correlating significantly with this portion of the scale indicate that the possibility of parietal lobe involvement in either the left or the right hemisphere must be entertained where poor performance is noted on items 136-142. These items demonstrated a close relationship with Luria items requiring intact cutaneous sensation, kinesthetic feedback, and spatial organization, as well as with such abilities as reading, writing, concept-formation, naming, arithmetic reasoning and memory. Thus, poor performance of these items may indicate generalized left hemisphere dysfunction.

For items 143-153, the patient is asked to repeat the same material as in items 133-142 but after reading rather than hearing it. Reading disturbances will obviously hinder performance on these items (143-153), and, as would be expected, Luria items requiring intact reading skills correlate highly with this section. Additionally, writing and naming skills appear to be closely related to these items. Disorders of the left temporoparietooccipital areas, especially in the region of the angular gyrus, may lead to a loss of reading skills. Injuries to this area may also disrupt writing skills and cause loss of the ability to associate names and objects (Butters & Brody, 1969). Items tapping memory, a temporal lobe function (Golden, 1978), also correlate with this section of the Expressive Speech scale.

Other abilities that demonstrate a significant relationship with items in this scale include arithmetic reasoning and tasks demanding the ability to attend as well as to follow instructions. These abilities are typically considered to fall in the domain of the frontal lobe. A patient with frontal lobe dysfunction may be unable to put verbal instructions into action, particularly when the instructions are symbolic or complex (Luria, Pribram, & Homskaya, 1964). The item intercorrelations further suggest that either the left or the right frontal region may be involved in the dysfunction.

Items 154-156 require intact audioverbal memory, which is disturbed by lesions of the middle and inferior regions of the temporal lobe (Luria, 1966). Lesions in the general area of the temporoparietooccipital region typically can interfere with verbal memory (Warrington, Logue, & Pratt, 1971). Further evidence of the importance of memory to correct performance is seen in other items requiring intact memory function, which correlate significantly with this section of the scale. Writing, reading, rhythmic pattern analysis, naming, and spatial organizational abilities additionally appear to be related to performance of these items, further underscoring the role played by the temporoparietooccipital area of the brain.

Correct performance of items 157 and 158 relies upon processes of the temporal lobe (Luria, 1973). These items correlated highly with several items requiring visual naming. They also show a distinct relationship with frontal and parietal lobe functions, including spatial organization, cutaneous sensation, kinesthetic feedback, simple motor movements, and oral praxis (Luria, 1973; Golden, 1978).

Visual naming, reading skills, basic arithmetic skills, and concept-formation all correlate significantly with item 159 and support a temporo-occipital localization. Additionally, tasks involving discursive reasoning appear to bear some relationship to this item, suggesting involvement of the frontal lobe. Luria (1966) notes that discursive reasoning requires a preliminary formation of new systems of association, a frontal lobe function.

Difficulties on items 160-163, demanding varying forms of automatic speech, are typically associated with frontal lobe damage, usually in the left hemisphere (Luria, 1966). This may be particularly true for items 161 and 163, which require reversal of the two series. Reversals of associations such as these demand the active formation of new associations. Thus frontal lobe injury may result in great difficulties with those tasks. However, significant correlations with items requiring writing and reading of numbers as well as with items requiring visual naming suggests left temporoparietooccipital involvement.

No one item of the series 164-169 demonstrated significant correlations with other Luria-Nebraska items not part of the Expressive Speech scale. This suggests that these items may be relatively pure indexes of expressive speech function. In these items the patient is asked to generate extemporaneous reflections upon the stimulus material. Narrative expressive speech begins with an intention or plan, which must be recoded into a verbal form and molded into a speech expression. Lesions of the left tertiary areas of the frontal lobe may result in a complete loss of voluntary speech (Luria, 1958; Zangwill, 1966).

The final section of the scale (items 170–174) involves complex systems of grammatical expression. Each item demands an appreciation of the grammatical structure of a sentence. This ability is impaired by lesions of the anterior divisions of the cortex, including Broca's area, and the frontal areas anterior to the premotor cortex. The item intercorrelations with this section indicate that injuries in other parts of the cortex may also affect performance on these items. The correlations with other Luria-Nebraska items requiring intact cutaneous sensation, memory, reading skills, arithmetic abilities, and concept-formation clearly suggest that damage to the temporoparieto-occipital area will hamper performance on items 170–174.

The intercorrelations suggest that expressive speech is highly complex and multidetermined and cannot easily be localized to one region of the brain. Several items from the Receptive Speech scale correlate highly with the Expressive Speech scale; this suggests that there is significant overlap between expressive and receptive speech functions.

Factor Analysis

Factor analysis of the Expressive Speech scale of the Luria-Nebraska Neuropsychological Battery yields five distinct factors, as seen in Table 7.2.

The first factor (Table 7.3) consists of six items. Each requires the reading of familiar, rather simply pronounced words. Reading difficulties are relatively rare on these items owing to their familiarity and automatic recognition. Basic articulatory difficulties are revealed by errors on these items, and these are typically the effect of dysarthria

Table 7.2: **Expressive Speech: Rotated Factor Matrix**

Item	Factor 1	Factor 2	Factor 3	Factor 4	Factor 5
133	21	02	52	06	01
134	08	03	54	31	11
135	14	12	45	14	14
136	30	00	42	−06	05
137	13	04	74	14	10
138	13	−02	48	38	−01
139	16	00	44	06	06
140	15	04	56	26	06
141	04	00	54	09	03
142	21	11	54	08	−01
143	23	16	07	31	−03
144	23	12	20	50	03
145	46	03	14	17	03
146	72	01	10	16	03
147	72	−01	19	14	04
148	37	10	22	49	04
149	12	09	15	55	14
150	59	04	13	07	06
151	16	16	20	52	04
152	62	−04	14	24	−03
153	62	−01	12	15	00
154	17	07	37	12	01
155	14	09	27	51	05
156	14	08	31	34	05
157	16	15	23	28	17
158	19	02	07	18	17
159	39	11	24	18	01
160	31	05	23	00	08
161	33	17	15	−02	14
162	27	08	12	−02	04
163	46	08	16	04	15
164	02	11	19	08	−04
165	06	−05	08	−02	73
166	06	10	07	18	−09
167	19	03	04	14	75
168	13	10	04	21	−09
169	−08	−01	11	05	71
170	20	12	10	18	04
171	04	23	13	23	06
172	10	05	14	28	−03
173	02	94	06	17	00
174	02	86	10	18	−05

Table 7.3: **Items on Expressive Factor 1**

Loading	Item	Description
		Read these words:
.46	145	See-seen; tree-trick
.72	146	Cat; dog; man
.72	147	House; table; apple
.59	150	Cat-hat-bat
.62	152	Hat-sun-bell
.62	153	House-ball-chair

Table 7.4: **Items on Expressive Factor 2**

Loading	Item	Description
		Repeat after me:
.52	133	a, i, m, b, sh.
.54	134	sp, th, pl, str, awk.
.45	135	See-seen; tree-trick.
.42	136	House; table; apple.
.74	137	Hairbrush; screwdriver; laborious.
.48	138	Rhinoceros; surveillance; hierarchy.
.44	139	Cat-hat-bat.
.56	140	Streptomycin; Massachusetts Episcopal.
.54	141	Hat-sun-bell; hat-bell-sun.
.54	142	House-ball-chair; ball-chair-house.

Table 7.5: **Items on Expressive Factor 3**

Loading	Item	Description
		Read these words:
.50	144	sp, th, pl, str, awk.
.49	148	Hairbrush; screwdriver; laborious.
.55	149	Rhinoceros; surveillance; hierarchy.
.52	151	Streptomycin; Massachusetts Episcopal.

Table 7.6: **Items on Expressive Factor 4**

Loading	Item	Description
.73	165	Tell me what's happening in this picture. Scoring: number of words in 5 seconds.
.75	167	I am going to read this short story out loud. Follow along carefully, because when I'm through I'm going to take the card away and then you'll have to tell the story back to me in your own words. Scoring: number of words in 5 seconds.
.71	169	Please make a short speech about the conflict between the generations. Scoring: number of words in 5 seconds.

Table 7.7: **Items on Expressive Factor 5**

Loading	Item	Description
.94	173	The words on this card can make a sentence if they are arranged correctly. I want you to arrange them so they do make a sentence. Scoring: errors.
.86	174	Scoring: time.

or a form of expressive dysphasia. As such, this factor is called automatic articulation—reading.

The second factor shows significant loading on ten items (Table 7.4). Each requires verbal repetition or echoing of words spoken by the examiner, and, like those contributing to factor 1, they may be seen to assess articulation. However, unlike factor 1, not all the words are acoustically simple. Rather, many are multisyllabic, unfamiliar, or acoustically complex. Reading these more difficult words presents a more arduous task of acoustic processing. Repeating them, on the other hand, requires only a basic degree of processing, since mere echoing is possible. Errors, as with factor 1, most likely represent problems in basic articulation, the effect of dysarthria or a form of expressive dysphasia. This factor thus has been called automatic articulation—echoing. With the first two factors measuring basic articulation through different response modalities—reading and repetition—the examiner can assess articulation even when profound dyslexia or visual impairment prevents reading or when hearing loss prevents echoing.

Expressive factor 3 consists of four items, as can be seen in Table 7.5. These items present complex or unfamiliar sounds or words to be read. This requires greater active acoustic processing than does the echolalic repetition of some of the same words also included under factor 2. Similarly, much greater active processing is required when reading these unfamiliar or complex items of factor 3 than when reading the familiar and similar sounds and words included under factor 1.

Golden, Purisch, Sweet, Graber, Osmon, and Hammeke, (1980) note that the differences represented by the first two factors and the third factor are often seen clinically in brain-damaged individuals. They often retain the ability to clearly pronounce words and phrases that are familiar and habitually spoken, but words and phrases that are less often spoken, and therefore not habitual, present great problems in articulation. Producing these nonhabitual expressions requires a much more deliberate and conscious effort of acoustic analysis and synthesis. It is this active process underlying articulation that appears to be measured by factor 3, which has been called active articulation (Golden, Purisch, Sweet, Graber, Osmon, & Hammeke, 1980) to distinguish it from the more passive and reactive form of articulation represented by the first two factors.

Three items make up the fourth factor of the Expressive Speech scale (Table 7.6). In each of these items, a stimulus is used to elicit a verbal response. The intention is to measure verbal fluency, on the assumption that a more fluent response is also more wordy. However, this may not always be true, as when a response is given disjointedly but is spoken quickly with many words. As a result, this factor has been labeled verbal productivity rather than verbal fluency.

The fifth expressive speech factor identified shows significant loadings on two items (Table 7.7). These items measure ability to organize a scrambled series of words into a meaningful sentence and the time needed to accomplish this. This is a difficult task that assesses verbal ability at a very high level. To perform this task the patient must combine and organize verbal material in a way that is meaningful and grammatically acceptable. In general, a high degree of what Golden, Purisch, Sweet, Graber, Osmon, and Hammeke (1980) refer to as "language sense" is needed, not only to organize the words appropriately, but also to do so semiautomatically rather than by conscious trial and error. This factor has therefore been called verbal organization, reflecting the underlying ability to organize and combine speech into meaningful and grammatically correct expressions.

Summary

The specific effects of localized lesions on reflective, nominative, and narrative speech have been described. Of course brain injuries that have resulted in generalized behavioral deficits will affect speech processes as well. For example, injuries to the prefrontal divisions produce a characteristic lack of spontaneity in behavior as a whole, including a decrease in speech initiative. This needs to be distinguished from the lack of initiative found in dynamic dysphasia, in which speech processes are selectively impaired. Diffuse injuries, especially those affecting subcortical structures involved in the regulation of cortical tone, result in a generalized disturbance of neurodynamics. The patient easily becomes fatigued, memory traces become less stable, and the general level of performance tends to diminish as testing proceeds.

8. Reading and Writing Scales

The construction of the Reading and Writing scales of the Luria-Nebraska Neuropsychological Battery provides for evaluation of these scales as complex mental functions. These scales assess reading and writing as the conjoined, synchronous, and integrated work of multiple areas of the brain. Successful performance depends on the integrity and contributions of a variety of areas of the cortex. This format allows the practitioner to assess which aspects of these complex cortical functions are impaired in particular patients and provides information useful for localizing when used in conjunction with other data from the battery.

Performance on the Writing scale of the Luria is sensitive to dysfunctions that have historically been labeled dysgraphias and spelling dyspraxias. Deficits in motor, tactile, and spatial functions as well as in expressive and receptive language skills will be reflected in performance on this scale (Golden & Berg, 1980a). Reading deficits have traditionally been associated with occipital lobe lesions. Performance on the Reading scale however, may be disrupted by disturbances of multiple cortical areas. Reading, as a complex language skill, will be sensitive to damage impinging on that system. Deficits in attention and intent, as mediated by the frontal lobe, may disturb reading skills in a distinctive manner.

Special Considerations in the Evaluation of the Writing Process

Written speech is a special type of language skill that is developed as a result of training. The neuropsychological nature of writing tasks changes with the sophistication and facility of the writer as well as with the nature of the task. Children learning to write utilize different neuropsychological processes to reach a goal than do adults. Adults write most words as total units, without considering the acoustic makeup of the word or the motor makeup of the individual letters. For the child just learning to write, the process is taught and completed as a complex cycle of unconnected acts that are sequentially linked but are not smooth or automatized.

Four major systems are involved in writing:

1. the acoustic system
2. the sensorimotor system
3. the visual-spatial system
4. the intentional/attentional system.

Roughly, these systems depend on integrity of the temporal area, the sensorimotor area (pre- and postcentral), the tertiary area of the parietal, occipital, and temporal zones, and the frontal area. At a peripheral level, adequate auditory acuity and muscle control are required.

The process of writing, both from dictation and spontaneously, begins with acoustic analysis of the word. The word must be broken up into its constituent phonemes (individual sound units). Acoustic analysis must be accurate enough to perceive relatively fine differences between sounds, and the writer must attend to essential phonemic elements while neglecting unessential and phonetically irrelevant aspects. Acoustic analysis includes recognition of the order of phonemes within the overall matrix of the word or phrase. Phonemic hearing, as required for accurate acoustic analysis, is mediated by the posterior third of the first temporal gyrus (Luria, 1966, 1973).

Research indicates that quick and accurate articulatory movement plays an important role in analyzing the sound composition of words (Luria, 1966). When children are just learning to write they say words aloud to assist in phonemic decoding. It has been demonstrated (Luria, 1966) that when articulation is not permitted young children make many more mistakes in writing. Individuals with lesions of the postcentral region of the sensorimotor cortex (e.g., those with kinesthetic [afferent] aphasia) lose the specificity and clarity of articulatory movements, a deficit that can be expected to interfere with learning to write or with writing unfamiliar words.

Writing from dictation requires, in addition to adequate phonemic discrimination, the ability to acoustically perceive and preserve the correct sound sequence within words. One must inhibit the influence of components of the sound system that are not in a critical position. This capacity is disturbed by any diminution in the process of active inhibition, such as occurs with lesions of the frontal lobe (Luria, 1966).

The sensorimotor system is active in the writing process as the perceived phonemes are translated to graphemes (the written symbols for sounds). For children just learning to write the graphemes of their language, each stroke of each letter requires a special impulse and intent. Letters are not initially constructed as smooth, integrated wholes, but are drawn as series of single elements. The control needed to form each element correctly requires postcentral integrity.

Gradually writing is transformed into a smooth kinetic melody in which the progressive activation and inhibition of muscle groups replaces the conscious drawing of individual components. The writer is no longer conscious of the construction of single elements but operates in terms of words and sentences. The development of these fluid kinetic patterns of behavior requires integrity of the premotor zone of the cortex.

Though the letters of our language are so familiar to accomplished readers and writers that we rarely think about their spatial qualities, initially the child must learn the peculiar and specific optic-spatial requirements of each letter. Spatial orientation differences between letters must be discriminated and responded to appropriately. Deficits in the parieto-occipital area of the cortex will interfere with the ability to accurately analyze visual-spatial information (Luria, 1966, 1973). Deficits in visual-spatial organization will lead to disturbances in copying, such as mirror-image writing and directional confusion.

Writing from dictation requires an additional step not necessary in copying. The child learning to write must consciously ascertain the grapheme associated with the phoneme he has discriminated, which requires integrity of the acoustic-optic system as mediated by the left angular gyrus.

Clearly, learning to write requires the integration of

numerous skills and the integrity of multiple units of the cortex. The child performs these tasks step-by-step. Observing young children as they copy letters reveals the laboriousness of this task. When the multiple steps of acoustic analysis and association of the grapheme with phoneme are added, its enormous complexity becomes apparent.

Cortically intact adults copy and write from dictation with ease and with little conscious awareness of the steps involved. With practice, given the integrity of all the units required for adequate performance, writing becomes automatized and fluid. Competent writers rarely experience the need for phonetic analysis; they write phrases and words as smooth kinetic units.

Luria (1966, 1973) notes that the character of cortical relationships is not consistent throughout the development of a function. The effect of a lesion of a particular area of the cortex upon a given cognitive function differs depending on how developed the skill was before the insult. Disturbances of relatively elementary sensory and integrative processes in childhood will have a devastating effect upon the development of higher cognitive functions, since these serve as the foundation for more complex skills. Luria (1966) states that after the development of higher functional systems, disturbances of elementary sensory and integrative processes will have a more limited effect, and may be compensated for by other previously elaborated systems.

In assessing impairments in writing, it is important to keep in mind the developmental ontogenetic change in the process. When brain damage secondary to trauma, aging, tumors, vascular changes, and such occurs after writing has been established as a smooth, automatized function, writing of established words and phrases may remain unimpaired. In spite of the integrity of this higher-level cortical function, careful examination of the patient's attempts to write words that are not overlearned and that require utilization of the basic sensory and integrative processes used by younger writers may reveal impairments. Writing must be assessed as both an analytic and an automatized

process. These data are necessary for understanding the psychological processes employed in writing and provide an analysis of an individual patient's impairment which is useful for localization and rehabilitation.

In assessing the process of writing English one must take into account the peculiarities of the language. Luria notes that writing different languages entails different patterns of cortical organization (1966). Although there is a phonetic system that is useful in the analysis of written English, a good deal of our spelling is based upon conventions that must be learned by rote. In assessing the writing of meaningful English the examiner must be sensitive to whether the patient is encountering difficulties with the analytic and synthetic aspects of writing or with the idiosyncratic features of our language.

The writing section of the Luria-Nebraska Neuropsychological Battery may be divided into three sections: phonetic analysis (items 175–176), simple copying writing (items 177–180), and copying writing—complex forms (items 180–187).

INVESTIGATION OF PHONETIC ANALYSIS

The first two items of the Writing scale (items 175 and 176) emphasize phonetic analysis. Item 175 requires that the patient state how many letters make up certain words. Four words are presented, varying from a simple monosyllabic word such as *cat* to more complex words such as *hedge,* where the task of discriminating individual sounds is made more difficult by the presence of elided consonants and multiple vowels.

A disruption of phonemic hearing, as in sensory aphasia, may lead to difficulty in stating the number of sounds in a word (Luria, 1966). Lesions of the posterior third of the first temporal gyrus are associated with sensory aphasia. Deficits are particularly notable when individual sounds must be picked out of complex units, as this task requires.

We have noted that children use kinesthetic feedback from articulation to assist in acoustic analysis. Adults with impairments in phonemic discrimination may also resort to articulating the words in this way. Though accurate performance assisted by articulation is not scored as an error, the examiner should note this behavior if it persists throughout testing. Such data will be useful in attaining a thorough understanding of the patient's assets and liabilities.

Item 176 requires the patient to identify individual sounds and accurately assess their relative positions within a word. Initially a phonetically simple word such as *match* is presented. The patient is asked to identify its first letter. Then words with sound blends are presented. These tasks require adequate phonemic analysis. Discerning the position of a sound within a word requires that the patient not only separate the sound from the matrix of the whole word but also correctly attend to and discriminate the temporal relation of sounds. Identifying the sound within the word is crucial to spelling unfamiliar words.

The complexity of this task renders it sensitive to a wide variety of disorders. The ability to analyze words phonetically has been shown to be related to the skills of reading and copying printed text, spelling simple words, performing arithmetic calculations, writing numbers from dictation, determining logical relations, and performing subtraction of serial sevens (Golden and Berg, 1980a). Effective discrimination of phonemes and assessment of the order of sounds within a word may be disrupted by lesions of the posterior third of the first temporal gyrus. Such patients have difficulty both in identifying isolated phonemes from the sound complex and in stating the order of sounds within a word. Such an impairment is often accompanied by difficulties in synthesizing a whole word from the series of sounds (as required by item 188 in the Reading scale), and in discriminating similar-sounding phonemes (as required in the Receptive Language scale).

A defect in phonetic analysis also may be associated with a lesion of the postcentral area of the cortex. Such patients exhibit kinesthetic (afferent) motor aphasia. Though they can analyze the number of sounds within a word more easily than can patients with sensory aphasia, they have difficulty determining the positions of sounds within a word. Failures in discrimination of speech sounds are secondary to the defective articulatory analysis of sound. Such patients cannot easily and precisely organize buccal-oral movement. Errors in the discrimination of speech sounds in such patients typically involve phonemes with similar articulatory patterns, such as *l, n, b,* and *m.* Difficulties with kinesthetic control of oral movement will also be evidenced on the Motor scale.

Dysfunctions in phonetic analysis may also result from a lesion of the premotor area of the left hemisphere (Luria, 1966). Such patients cannot perform motor acts as smooth kinetic units and often cannot inhibit perseveration of movement. Patients with efferent (kinetic) motor aphasia secondary to such lesions find it particularly difficult to ascertain the order of sounds within a word. They often identify the most strongly accented sound in the word as being the first phoneme. This disturbance in ascertaining the order of sounds is evident even in relatively mild or latent forms of efferent motor aphasia.

Patients with lesions of the prefrontal zones of the cortex demonstrate impairment in stability of intention and weakness in inhibition of initial stimuli. This deficit interferes with their ability to complete adequate phonetic analysis. They make gross mistakes in perceiving the temporal organization of sounds within a word (Luria, 1966). The deficits seen with such disorders are often associated with impetuous attempts to guess the correct answer.

It should be noted that the items used to assess phonetic analysis on the Writing section of the Luria-Nebraska Neuropsychological Battery require that the patient identify the letter—that is, the specific optic-spatial symbol—associated with a sound. Patients who have adequate phonemic analytic skills as demonstrated on the Receptive Language section of the Luria but are unable to identify the particular grapheme associated with the discriminated phoneme will be unsuccessful at these tasks. Such difficulties are rare, but when present they occur in patients with lesions of the left angular gyrus. Such patients may also be impaired on nonautomatized mathematical tasks (Benson & Wier, 1972; Luria, 1966, 1973).

Patients with writing deficits secondary to difficulties with phonemic analysis will not necessarily have impairment of the motoric component of writing. Those with only a defect of phonemic analysis can copy words and phrases and can readily write from dictation overlearned words and symbols that have become established as optic ideograms.

SIMPLE WRITING AND COPYING

The items in this section emphasize the motor components of writing. An individual's performance on these tasks can be more adequately interpreted in conjunction with performance on the Motor scale.

Item 177 acquires that patients copy, in their own handwriting, letters presented both in standard printing and in script. The chief purpose of this task is to ascertain whether they can easily recognize the letters by attending to key features of the stimului and can perform the motor act of writing. This task emphasizes the visual-motor aspect of writing. The examiner must attend to the quality of the motor reproduction. Smooth, facile reproduction is qualitatively far different from labored drawing of the letters.

Patients with classic optic agnosia secondary to disturbances of the secondary area of the visual cortex may fail to synthesize the intricate details of the script letters into a whole and may not recognize them. They may draw the letters piecemeal. Patients with optic agnosia will also demonstrate deficits on the Visual and Reading scales.

Motor disturbances may distort the process of copying letters. Patients with efferent motor apraxia (a disturbance of the premotor area) may draw the letters as unconnected parts because they fail to produce smooth kinetic patterns of movement. Such a disturbance should also be evident on the manual items of the Motor scale.

Visual-spatial disturbances such as mirror writing should be noted. Such distortions may be part of a more general picture of spatial apractic agnosia secondary to lesions of the parieto-occipital area of the cortex.

Item 178 requires the patient to copy simple syllables such as *an* and *pre*. This task allows the examiner to evaluate the same skills assessed in the copying of single letters. In addition the patient's writing a series of letters allows the examiner to assess the ability to switch from element to element within the syllable. Patients with lesions in the premotor zone have difficulty changing smoothly from one letter to another, since the kinetic organization of motor movement is compromised by such lesions. Each movement takes active planning, and time limits may not be met.

If the lesion extends deeper into the brain so that it involves connections between the premotor region and the basal motor ganglia in addition to the premotor area itself, the previously described changes in ability to complete complex motor movements are accompanied by perseveration (Luria, 1966), so the patient cannot discontinue a single movement once it has begun. Such patients may repeat the same letter over and over, unable to switch to the next grapheme, or they may add unnecessary strokes to a single grapheme. Patients with this difficulty will have trouble inhibiting movement on other items on the battery, such as some of the copying and rhythm tasks.

Item 180, in which patients are asked to write their own first and last names, further emphasizes the integrity of automatized writing. Most patients, even those with very little education, write their names as inert motor stereotypes. The examiner will quickly be alerted to disturbances in the motor component of writing if this is performed laboriously. Failure to execute this task as a smooth, overlearned motor pattern is associated with premotor deficits.

Item 179 requires that the patient write three words after viewing them for five seconds. This task assesses the stability of memory traces (Luria, 1966). Lesions of the frontal and frontotemporal areas of the cortex may lead to instability of memory traces, making patients unsuccessful on this task. Perseveration on a single word in the series, or substitution of words from earlier in the subtest, may occur owing to pathological failure to inhibit irrelevant memories. Inability to evaluate one's own success on other sections of the Luria-Nebraska battery, such as the Memory or Motor scales, may corroborate the hypothesis that frontal lobe deficits are disrupting performance on this task.

COPYING AND WRITING: COMPLEX FORMS

The next section of the Writing scale requires the patient to write letters, sounds, words, and phrases from dictation. Spontaneous writing is required as well. On these tasks the acoustic-analytic and synthetic aspects of the writing process are combined with the motor components, requiring more sophisticated forms of writing.

In item 181 the patient is asked to write individual letters of the alphabet from dictation, recoding the sounds heard into the appropriate graphemes. Disturbances may occur either in the auditory analysis of the sound or in the act of putting the configuration on paper. Patients who have had difficulty with acoustic analysis on the initial section on this scale may demonstrate the same disturbance on this task. The examiner should be alert to unusually long latency periods between stimuli and responses. Rearticulation, either aloud or subvocally, may be used by patients with temporal lobe lesions. Such lesions will make it difficult for them to perceive differences between sounds, though they may be able to perform adequately using the kinesthetic feedback provided by articulation.

Long latency periods may also indicate difficulty in ascertaining which graphemes are associated with the phonemic pattern discriminated. Patients with lesions of the tertiary area of the parieto-occipital zone have defects in the integration of visual and auditory stimuli. This will also be evident in their performance on the Reading scale and on other tests requiring the integration of sensory data such as stereognosis.

The patient's ability to write simple open syllables and words, such as *ba* and *pack,* is evaluated through item 182. Items 183 and 184 require that increasingly more complex and less familiar words be written from dictation.

Correct performance in writing nonsense syllables depends heavily upon adequate acoustic analysis. Patients

rarely have a visual memory of these syllables, and they cannot rely upon firmly established motor stereotypes. Performance on tasks requiring writing simple overlearned words may reveal acoustic-articulatory deficits, but it is more likely to illuminate difficulties in the optic-spatial, motor components of writing.

Writing the more complicated, unfamiliar words required by item 184 utilizes the entire complex, multifaceted process of writing. Errors should be analyzed to determine if they are part of a pattern of errors both within the scale and on the battery as a whole.

Because these complex words tend to be unfamiliar and cannot be written as automatized stereotypes, the patient must apply acoustical analysis to identify the specific phonemes that make them up, and the order in which the phonemes are used. Patients with lesions in the left temporal lobe may have trouble with this. Their pattern of performance within the scale will be distinctive in that they may not manifest any difficulty on those tasks emphasizing the visual-motor components of writing or on items that can be completed as inert motor stereotypes. Such patients will have difficulty on tests of receptive language and on spelling items emphasizing acoustic analysis.

Patients with afferent aphasia, a deficit of the kinesthetic basis of speech secondary to damage to the postcentral area of the cortex, may also have trouble with acoustic analysis. They fail to distinguish differences adequately because articulatory substitutions go uncorrected, secondary to distortion in the kinesthetic feedback. Such patients are likely to confuse letters that are articulated in a similar manner, such as *n, l,* and *b,* rather than letters with similar sounds such as *b* and *p.* The latter type of confusion is more typical of the errors associated with sensory (temporal lobe) aphasia.

Patients with lesions of the premotor area may also have difficulty writing unfamiliar and more complicated words. Though the capacity for acoustic analysis remains intact, these patients cannot maintain smooth kinetic patterns of movement, which disrupts the ability to switch from articuleme to articuleme. They characteristically have trouble determining the position of phonemes within a word, and transposition of graphemes when writing is common. Disorders of the premotor zone disrupt the motor component of writing in a similar manner. There is marked inertia of the motor analyzer, and the required letters may be replaced by perseverative repetition of unnecessary movements as the patient attempts to write them.

Lesions of the tertiary parietal area will be reflected in the writing of the complex words, since they cannot ordinarily be written as motor stereotypes. Errors resulting from such lesions reflect difficulty in multimodal integration. The patient may know exactly what sound is to be written but be unable to identify the appropriate grapheme. Patients with lesions in this area have difficulty writing complex words because of visual spatial deficits. As previously noted, they may be expected to demonstrate a pattern of deficits on the battery that reflects difficulty in simultaneously integrating stimuli from different sensory modalities.

Item 185 requires writing series of words and short phrases. This item emphasizes the role of the frontal area in writing. Though all the skills required by the earlier items are necessary in writing phrases and series of words, such items tend to elicit manifestations of disturbances in intentionality and self-evaluation. Weakness in the regulation of behavior by speech is evidenced as patients with frontal lobe disorders begin to perseverate upon a single portion of the stimulus. Such patients easily become fatigued, and micrographia may result.

The spontaneous writing required by item 186 represents the most sophisticated form of the writing process. To complete this item successfully the patient must complete the entire sequence of turning thoughts into internal speech, which is then recoded as written signs. For success on this item the entire functional system for writing must be intact, including the capacity to exert selective control over what is written, a function of the frontal area of the cortex.

Special Considerations in the Evaluation of Reading

Like writing, reading is a complex language skill that is systematically taught rather than learned spontaneously. Reading, in its most sophisticated form, is the opposite process from writing. The fluent reader translates visual-spatial symbols into internal language that then can be expressed verbally.

Reading, like spelling, may be done at a variety of levels. The child who struggles to "sound out" *cat* from *c-a-t* will, and accurately so, be said to be reading. Neuropsychologically, however, this is a different process from that used by an adult who readily responds to the configuration *cat* as a sight word, with no need to resort to phonetic analysis. Competent readers respond to many words as ideograms. That is, they rapidly perceive the written symbol as familiar and associate it with a spoken word without resorting to vocalization.

Individuals with intact reading skills vary their approach to reflect the demands of the material. At times they will need to "sound out" unfamiliar words. This process, as has been mentioned, is neuropsychologically different from sight-reading. Both are reading, though, and investigation of the two processes will help us to understand individual patterns of neuropsychological strengths and deficits. Sensitive interpretation of the Reading scale requires the examiner to attend to both the patient's performance on the Reading scale as a whole and the pattern of intrascale scatter. In addition the examiner must attend to the relationship between performance on the Reading scale and performance on the rest of the battery as a whole.

INVESTIGATION OF READING

The Reading scale may be broken down into four major sections: phonetic synthesis (items 188–189); analysis and perception of letters (items 190–191); reading—syllables and words (items 192–196); reading—phrases and whole texts (items 197–200).

Adequate reading skills require integrity of the peripheral visual system. The examiner should be alert to the possibility that a patient may have a visual acuity defect and need glasses or to the presence of a peripheral visual handicap.

PHONETIC SYNTHESIS

Item 188 requires that the patient state what sound is made by a series of letters presented one by one. For example, "What sound is made by the letters g–r–o?" To succeed on this task the patient must associate a sound with each letter, then synthesize those sounds into a whole. This is what children do when, in teaching them to read, we tell them to "sound out" a word.

Synthesizing sounds into a single syllable requires integrity of the premotor region of the cortex. Lesions in this area produce kinetic (efferent) motor aphasia, a disturbance in the smooth chain of articulatory movements in which the constant inhibition and modification of the mechanism is disrupted. In addition, the dynamic structure of language as a whole may be disturbed (Luria, 1966). The determinative values of patterns of speech no longer operate, and the fluency of articulation and grammar decreases. Patients with kinetic motor aphasia differ from those with kinesthetic motor aphasia in that they can still pronounce individual sounds. Impairment in the synthesis of individual sounds into a whole, which may be partly attributable to pathological inertia of the motor analysis system, is the hallmark of kinetic aphasia.

Lesions of the left frontal and frontotemporal divisions of the cortex also may be evidenced by difficulty with phonetic synthesis. Patients with frontal syndromes have unstable phonetic traces and find perception of the temporal organization of phonemes difficult. Their performance is often marked by impulsive guesses at the correct response. Impulsiveness and failure to evaluate one's own behavior are other manifestations of frontal syndrome.

Lesions of the tertiary area of the temporoparieto-occipital area will also affect phonetic synthesis in the absence of any deficits in articulation or phonemic discrimination. Such patients have considerable trouble as-

certaining the proper position of sounds within a word and synthesizing sounds presented individually because of a deficit in the basic process of simultaneous perception of stimuli (Luria, 1966). These lesions will be accompanied by other deficits indicative of instability of the sound images of words, such as anomia and difficulty in understanding complex speech constructions.

Patients with lesions of the secondary area of the temporal lobe also have trouble synthesizing discrete sounds into a unified whole. Their underlying deficit is based upon the disintegration of the sound structure of speech associated with acoustic agnosia (Luria, 1966). They can be expected to demonstrate other signs of a disorder of phonemic hearing (for example, deficits on the Receptive Language scale) and the associated disturbances in the conceptual basis of speech.

Item 189 asks that patient to identify the word made by a series of letters presented individually. For example, "What word is made by the letters k–n–i–g–h–t?"

This task, like the previous one, requires synthesis of sound units into a whole, and the same cortical units are used. The words utilized demand increased sophistication and facility with the idiosyncratic sound system of the English language, and education begins to play a role in performance. Intact, educated adults may respond correctly to item 189 without resorting to phonetic analysis and synthesis. They respond to the sequence of letters as a learned ideogram. Patients with deficits in acoustic analysis that interfere with performance on item 188 may successfully complete item 189 in an automatized fashion.

READING: ANALYSIS AND PERCEPTION OF LETTERS

Item 190 requires that the patient recognize and identify a series of printed capital letters. This primarily assesses the visual aspect of reading.

Patients with lesions of the secondary area of the visual cortex suffer from literal alexia and may not be able to read letters. Literal alexia is a variant of optic agnosia, and as such it represents a failure in the ability to recognize key stimulus features and synthesize them into a whole. Letters lose their meaning, or identification of letters becomes unstable. Patients with such a disorder may confuse letters that are similar in outline, such as *K* and *X*.

Patients with disturbance in spatial perception associated with lesions of the parieto-occipital zones of the left hemisphere do not necessarily have symptoms of visual agnosia, but they do experience a profound disturbance of spatial organization. They may have trouble recognizing letters when orientation in space is a key discriminating factor, and they may also have difficulty on other tasks emphasizing spatial orientation. This may be evidenced in mirror writing problems in reading clocks without numbers (item 94), and difficulty in orienting themselves with compass coordinates (item 96).

Although recognizing letters is considered primarily a test of visual functioning, a dysfunction of the acoustic system may also interfere with performance. Lesions of the secondary area of the temporal lobe, primarily the posterior third of the first temporal gyrus, may lead to a deficit in true reading. Such a deficit results from a breakdown in the analysis and synthesis of the phonetic aspect of speech. Although familiar words may be read easily, syllables, unfamiliar words, and individual letters may be difficult for such patients to recognize (Luria, 1966).

On item 191 the patient is asked to state which letter, *B, J,* or *S,* stands for *John.* Most adults write or read *John* in a smooth, automatized fashion with little need for acoustic analysis or conscious use of phonemic discrimination. They need only name the letter, and they may be able to do this despite difficulty in identifying individual letters owing to a disturbance in visual perception.

READING: SYLLABLES AND WORDS

On item 192 the examinee is asked to read five nonsense syllables, such as *po* and *spro,* that contain sound blends and both long and short vowel sounds. This item taps the visual, acoustic, and oral expressive aspects of reading.

The visual aspect of reading may, of course, be disrupted by optic agnosia. Luria (1966) reports that patients with acute trauma to the secondary area of the occipital zone have initially demonstrated such severe disturbances that they were unable to distinguish between line drawings and written words. Patients with visual disorders that disturb their ability to complete the synthesis necessary for visual recognition will demonstrate disorders on the Visual scale of the Luria-Nebraska.

A less obvious disturbance that occurs secondary to lesions of the anterior zone of the occipital cortex is a narrowing of the visual field. This constriction occurs not in terms of units of space but rather in the number of objects simultaneously perceived. The examiner should be alert to behavior that indicates difficulty in perceiving words as wholes. The condition of *simultaneous agnosia* makes recognition of complex visual structures impossible, though the patient may still easily recognize simple shapes and objects. Such patients may resort to reading letter-by-letter to identify a word. In these instances there is difficulty with familiar as well as unfamiliar words.

Reading syllables requires attention to spatial features, which is disturbed by lesions of the tertiary area of the cortex. Patients with lesions of the left hemisphere may have trouble reading nonsense syllables. Inversions of sounds within a word may indicate such a failure, and these patients will also show other signs of spatial disorientation.

Acoustic disorders associated with lesions of the left temporal area may significantly impair the process of reading unfamiliar words, such as the nonsense syllables in item 192. Though such patients may easily read well-established optic ideograms, they cannot complete the phonetic analysis and synthesis necessary for true reading of these complex syllables. Patients with sensory aphasia may also be expected to show deficits on the Writing and Receptive Speech scales of the Luria battery.

The oral expressive aspect of reading may be disturbed in conjunction with either kinesthetic or kinetic motor aphasia. The disturbance in reading associated with kinesthetic (afferent) motor aphasia parallels the defects manifested on the Writing and Expressive Speech scales. Impairment in the accuracy of articulation leads to a disturbance in the clarity of oral reading. Such patients have more trouble reading aloud than reading to themselves. They may have difficulty reading even single letters aloud.

Patients with kinetic motor aphasia associated with lesions of the premotor area of the cortex cannot shift smoothly from one articulation to the next. They have no trouble pronouncing individual letters, but they cannot synthesize sounds into syllables. They may spell out words letter-by-letter. This disorder differs from simultaneous agnosia in that the mechanism of the defect lies not in optic constriction but in the breakdown of smooth kinetic motor movement. Problems in the functional system of reading, associated with kinetic motor aphasia, are seen concurrently with deficits in oral motor movement on the Motor scale and the Expressive Speech scale.

On item 193 the patient is to read five words in order of increasing difficulty. A one-syllable word (e.g., *juice*) initiates the series, but later on less familiar words are presented (e.g., *fertilizer*). Some patients may recognize these words as optic ideograms, but others will truly use the analytic-synthetic process of reading.

On item 194 the patient is asked to read items that in general have been established as inert optic stereotypes requiring no true reading (for example, *U.N., U.S.A.*). Items 195 and 196 present a series of complex, most often unfamiliar words (such as *astrocytoma* and *insubordination*) that, it is anticipated, will require the entire process of acoustic and visual analysis and synthesis and oral expressive coordination that constitute true reading.

Discrepant performance on reading tasks that require active analysis and synthesis as opposed to those that can be completed as a stereotyped response to specific stimuli is of great diagnostic significance (Luria, 1966). In true reading the patient pronounces the word with facility and attempts to correct any mistakes in oral production. The skills used to decode the visual stimulus are generalizable to unfamiliar words. Such reading requires that the analytic and integrative skills of vision and hearing be intact.

Patients with oral motor deficits may have to show in ways other than speech (as in pointing to pictures) that they have read the words presented. Direct recognition of optic ideograms, on the other hand, is not true reading. Though this skill is ultimately necessary for fluent reading, the ability to instantly recognize, pronounce, and understand a written word does not prove that the patient can use the underlying skills that form the functional system of true reading. Patients with auditory or visual deficits may read overlearned words but be unable to read unfamiliar words requiring an active psychological response.

READING: PHRASES AND WHOLE TEXTS

Although the neuropsychological processes of visual and auditory analysis necessary for reading have been investigated, the comprehension aspect has not been attended to thus far. A special feature requiring consideration is that reading is a two-way process. As the reader grasps the meaning of groups of letters, he begins to anticipate the remainder of the phrase or sentence—to develop an expectation of what will follow. This expectation, based upon the meaning of what has been read, influences the reading process. Luria (1966) notes that a sign saying "Smoking Probited" in an area of fire hazards will often be read as "Smoking Prohibited."

Expectation about the remainder of the text operates in reading individual words as well as phrases. Apperception of the initial letter group may encourage an individual to guess at the rest of the word. This tendency will be exacerbated when there is weakening of the inhibitory processes with fatigue or secondary to any pathological condition of the cortex. Deficits in the capacity for true reading may precipitate guesses.

Item 197, which requires reading of two meaningful phrases (e.g., "The man went out for a walk"), can be used to evaluate whether true reading occurs or whether the patient attempts to read by guesswork. Defects in the underlying neuropsychological processes of reading may show up in the tendency to guess at what a sentence says once initial cues have been recognized. Such deficits will be evident on the simpler items of the Reading scale and on other items that require the same neuropsychological processes. For example, patients with sensory aphasia may guess at these phrases because they lack true reading skill. Such patients can be expected to manifest deficits on the phonetic analysis sections of both the Reading and the Writing scales and on the Receptive Speech scale.

Patients with frontal syndromes are notable for their random and impulsive responses, which will be evident when they attempt to read phrases. They may respond to initial cues without checking whether other available information corroborates their hypothesis. Inertia of mental processes and the tendency to make rapid judgments distort the reading process. Frontally damaged patients may be distinguished from the group described above by their pattern of reading errors based on impetuousness rather than on a defect in underlying reading skills, as evidenced earlier in the scale and on the Visual and Receptive Speech scales of the Luria-Nebraska.

Item 198 further investigates the capacity for true reading. The patient is presented with two phrases that contain incongruities (e.g., ''The boy went to bed because she was ill''). Someone who begins to make random guesses, whether because of a defect in the basic neuropsychological processes of reading or because of disinhibition secondary to frontal lobe damage, will be unable to read these phrases accurately.

In item 199 the patient is asked to read a short paragraph at about fifth-grade level of difficulty. The reading is timed, and item 200 compares the patient's speed to group norms.

Luria (1966) notes that an individual's performance on paragraph reading may be qualitatively assessed for indications of optic ataxia, which is associated with simultaneous agnosia (associated with lesions of the left parietooccipital zone). Such patients will have trouble moving smoothly from one line to the next and will tend to read odd words at random. This defect may not be observable in reading single words or short phrases.

Paragraph reading may also be disrupted by a defect in the auditory, visual, or oral expressive components of reading. Item 198 will be particularly useful in highlighting frontal lobe disturbances. Patients with such damage characteristically begin by making attempts at true reading, but they may suddenly change to guessing at the words and begin inserting irrelevant associations, with consequent disintegration of the reading process.

Item Intercorrelations

A series of intercorrelations between the Writing scale items and all other Luria-Nebraska items reveals numerous significant correlations ($r \geq .35$; $p < .0001$), as shown in Table 8.1 (Golden & Berg, 1980a).

The 13 items that compose the Writing scale have in common the requirement of writing skills, but a number of other specific factors differentiate each item from the others on the scale. The intercorrelations demonstrate that each of the Writing scale items is closely related to skills measured by other items of the battery that are not part of the same scale. Such information allows for a more specific interpretation of the specific dysfunction represented by the inability to perform a given test item.

Items 175 and 176 deal specifically with phonetic analysis of individual words. The ability to analyze words phonetically also appears to be related to the ability to read and copy printed text, spell simple words, perform arithmetic calculations, write numbers from dictation, determine logical relationships, and do serial sevens subtraction. Such disorders tend to be localized to the temporoparietooccipital area, especially in and around the angular gyrus of the left hemisphere (Luria, 1973). Kinsbourne and Warrington (1964) have observed that lesions in this area produce deficits in spatial abilities. For instance, an inability to spell may be result from placing letters in the wrong order (*cat* spelled *cta*). While deficits

Table 8.1: **Item Intercorrelations with Writing Scale**

Item	r*	Item	Description
175	.43	195	Read *insubordination; indistinguishable*
175	.42	204	Write 27, 34, 158, 396, 9845
175	.41	212	How much is: 3×3; 5×4; 7×8?
175	.41	221	Serial seven subtraction from 100
176	.47	144	Repeat *sp, th, pl, str, awk*
176	.43	151	Read *streptomycin; Massachusetts Episcopal*
176	.43	189	What word is made by these letters: *s-t-o-n-e; k-n-i-g-h-t*?
176	.45	193	Read *juice; bread; bonfire; cloakroom; fertilizer*
176	.46	195	Read *insubordination; indistinguishable*
176	.42	199	Read paragraph
176	.49	200	Time taken to read paragraph
176	.41	202	Write IV and VI; IX and XI
176	.47	204	Write 27, 34, 158, 396, 9845
176	.40	207	Read IV, VI, IX, XI; 17, 71, 69, 96
176	.42	212	How much is: 3×3; 5×4; 7×8?
176	.42	213	How much is: $3 + 4$; $6 + 7$?
176	.42	215	How much is: $27 + 8$; $44 + 57$; $31 - 7$; $44 - 14$?
176	.41	251	Concept formation—logical relationships
177	.40	6	With your eyes closed, place your left hand in the same position I place it in (thumb against fifth finger)
177	.41	51	If I knock hard, you knock gently; if I knock gently, you knock hard
177	.44	65	Cutaneous sensation—left side
177	.42	73	Determine whether stimulus is moving up or down left arm
177	.43	74	Identify shape drawn on right wrist
177	.43	95	Draw hands on blank clockface at: 12:50, 4:35; 11:10
177	.43	106	Phonemic hearing—conditioned reflex
177	.51	110	Point to picture of shoe, candle, stove
177	.40	112	What do *cat, bat, pat* mean?
177	.45	113	Point to the picture that shows: typewriting; mealtime; summer
177	.46	190	Tell me what you see here: *K, S, W, R, T*

*r = correlation

Table 8.1: **Item Intercorrelations with Writing Scale**   *Continued*

Item	r*	Item	Description
177	.42	194	Read these letters *U.N., U.S.A., U.S.S.R*
177	.51	201	Write 7-9-3; 3-5-7
177	.48	203	Write 17 and 71; 69 and 96
177	.47	204	Write 27, 34, 158, 396, 9845
177	.46	205	Read 7-9-3; 3-5-7
177	.53	208	Read 27, 34, 158, 396, 9845
177	.40	219	What is the missing number? $12 - (\ ) = 8$; $12 + (\ ) = 19$
178	.44	8	With your eyes closed, place your left hand in the same position I place my right hand in (thumb against middle finger)
178	.41	51	If I knock hard, you knock gently; if I knock gently, you knock hard
178	.41	59	How many beeps in all groups together?
178	.42	65	Cutaneous sensation—left side
178	.43	84	Stereognosis—left hand errors
178	.44	86	Name visually presented objects
178	.71	95	Draw hands on blank clockface for: 12:50; 4:35; 11:10
178	.43	145	Read *see-seen; tree-trick*
178	.44	150	Read *cat-hat-bat*
178	.42	190	Tell me what you see here: *K, S, W, R, T*
178	.46	205	Write 14, 17, 19, 109, 1023
178	.47	210	Which is larger: 17 or 68; 23 or 56; 189 or 201?
178	.45	215	How much is: $27 + 8$; $44 + 57$; $31 - 7$; $44 - 14$?
178	.43	219	What number is missing? $12 - (\ ) = 8$; $12 + (\ ) = 19$
179	.41	223	Memory for words
180	.43	162	Say the days of the week
181	.50	110	Identify objects from pictures by pointing
181	.46	113	Point to picture that shows: typewriting; mealtime; summer
181	.48	201	Write 7-9-3; 3-5-7
181	.45	203	Write 17 and 71; 69 and 96
181	.46	205	Write 14, 17, 19, 109, 1023
181	.41	206	Read 7-9-3; 3-5-7
181	.41	208	Read 27, 34, 158, 396, 9845

*r = correlation

Table 8.1: **Item Intercorrelations with Writing Scale** *Continued*

Item	r*	Item	Description
181	.41	210	Which is larger: 17 or 68; 23 or 56; 189 or 201?
182	.53	204	Write 27, 34, 158, 396, 9845
182	.43	208	Read 27, 34, 158, 396, 9845
182	.40	210	Which is larger: 17 or 68; 23 or 56; 189 or 201?
183	.42	104	Repeat phoneme triplets
183	.47	105	Write phoneme triplets
183	.41	144	Read *sp, th, pl, str, awk*
183	.42	188	What sound is made by these letters: *g–r–o; p–l–y?*
183	.44	189	What word is made by these letters: *s–t–o–n–e; k–n–i–g–h–t?*
183	.45	197	Read sentences
183	.41	203	Write 17 and 71; 69 and 96
183	.40	218	What sign is missing? 10 ( ) 2 = 20; 10 ( ) 2 = 12; 10 ( ) 2 = 8; 10 ( ) 2 = 5
184	.48	196	Read *astrocytoma; hemopoiesis*
185	.44	144	Read *sp, th, pl, str, awk*
185	.40	193	Read *juice; bread; bonfire; cloakroom; fertilizer*
185	.44	195	Read *insubordination; indistinguishable*
185	.44	199	Read paragraph
185	.55	200	Time taken to read paragraph
185	.44	204	Write 27, 34, 158, 396, 9845
185	.44	205	Read 7–9–3; 3–5–7
185	.44	207	Read IV, VI, IX, XI; 17, 71, 69, 96
185	.41	208	Read 27, 34, 158, 396, 9845
185	.44	215	How much is: 27 + 8; 44 + 57; 31 − 7; 44 − 14?
185	.41	218	What sign is missing? 2 ( ) 10 = 20; 10 ( ) 2 = 12; 10 ( ) 2 = 8; 10 ( ) 2 = 5
185	.40	227	Draw geometric shapes from memory
185	.43	251	Concept formation—logical relationships
186	.40	200	Read paragraph
187	.42	1	Using your right hand, touch your fingers in turn with your thumb while you count them

r = correlation

in this area do not interfere with the ability to do well-practiced arithmetic problems requiring only memory and not arithmetic ability (Benson & Wier, 1972; Luria, 1966), the ability to perform simple problems that do require arithmetic skills (e.g., items 212, 213, 215) may be impaired.

Items 177 and 178, in addition to assessing writing and copying skills, also appear to be influenced by deficient spatial abilities, somesthetic and motor feedback on a gross level, visual naming, and arithmetic skills. Again, these deficiencies may be localized in the left temporoparietooccipital areas in the region of the angular gyrus. Since this area is responsible for integrating information from all sensory modalities, disorders of this brain region may lead not only to a loss of reading and writing skills, but also to deficits in naming (Butters & Brody, 1969) and in the ability to understand and manipulate arithmetic symbols (Benson & Wier, 1972; Luria, 1973).

Items 179 and 180 demand simple writing and copying skills as well as short-term memory. These items are significantly correlated with items on other scales requiring automatic verbal and written responses and memory. Again, the temporoparietooccipital area is highly implicated in performance of these items. Difficulties with these two items may suggest a lesion interfering with verbal memory (Warrington, Logue, & Pratt, 1971). Luria (1966, 1973) has suggested that this is due to a disturbance in categorizing verbal material, a process essential to efficient recall. Additionally, a patient's inability to read or write his or her own name often indicates of a generalized dementia or, in some cases, a disorder of automatic writing that may occur with injuries to both hemispheres.

Items 181–186 require the patient to write from dictation material of increasing complexity. As the complexity increases, so apparently does the need for attention and concentration as well as intact auditory comprehension, as is indicated by the increasing number of significant correlations with other Luria items. Patients with tertiary frontal disorders may have difficulty attending to and concentrating on a given task.

This series of items (181–186) also correlates with the ability to repeat phonemes and write phonemes from dictation. The ability to repeat phonemes but not write them suggests impairment in the area of the angular gyrus, while the ability to write but not repeat phonemes suggests a disorder of expressive speech (Golden, Purisch, & Hammeke, 1979).

Items 183–185 are closely related to some of the more difficult Arithmetic scale items requiring number and symbol manipulation as well as more complex arithmetic calculations. Spatial deficits resulting from left parieto-occipital dysfunction and low educational level are likely to become apparent here.

The final items in this scale (186, 187) require the patient to write spontaneously about a specified topic. These items are highly correlated with tasks assessing fine motor movement, reading skills, and speed of reading. If the patient is in general able to write but has difficulty forming letters and changing from one letter to another, there could be a problem in kinesthetic feedback. If the person is simply unable to write owing to paralysis, this of course suggests a lesion in the motor strip of the posterior frontal lobe. Poor performance on these items may reflect disorders of the tertiary parietal areas responsible for, among other things, the analysis of grammatical structure.

The Reading scale yields a pattern of significant intercorrelations ($r \geq .35$; $p < .0001$) similar to that of the Writing Scale, as is seen in Table 8.2 (Golden & Berg, in press). Items 188 and 189 require the generation of sounds from letters the examiner says aloud. This task generally measures the ability to integrate letters as well as the auditory analysis functions of the temporal and parietal areas of the left hemisphere (Golden, Purisch, & Hammeke, 1979). The ability to synthesize words phonetically also appears to be significantly related to the ability to read and copy printed text and numbers, perform comparatively simple arithmetic calculations, write numbers from dictation, determine logical relations, and make numerical comparisons. Typically, deficits in these abilities tend to localize to the left temporoparietooccipital area. Also, as

Table 8.2: **Reading Scale Item Intercorrelations**

Item	r*	Item	Description
188	.38	148	Read *hairbrush; screwdriver; laborious*
188	.36	149	Read *rhinoceros; surveillance; hierarchy*
188	.39	176	Phonetic analysis; e.g., what is the second letter in *cat*; first letter in *match*?
188	.42	183	Write *wren; knife*
188	.39	204	Write 27, 34, 158, 396, 9845
188	.45	213	How much is: 3 + 4; 6 + 7?
188	.39	218	What sign is missing? 10 ( ) 2 = 20; 10( )2 = 12; 10( )2 = 8; 10( )2 = 5
188	.36	256	Verbal analogies
189	.38	117	Simple sentences—conflicting instructions
189	.39	140	Repeat *streptomycin; Massachusetts Episcopal*
189	.46	148	Read *hairbrush; screwdriver; laborious*
189	.41	151	Read *hat–sun–bell*
189	.47	159	Name objects from description
189	.44	175	How many letters are there in: *cat; trap, banana; hedge*
189	.43	176	Phonetic analysis; e.g., what is second letter in *cat;* first letter in *match*?
189	.44	183	Write *wren; knife*
189	.44	204	Write 27, 34, 158, 396, 9845
189	.39	205	Write 14, 17, 19, 109, 1023
189	.38	207	Read IV, VI, IX, XI; 17, 71, 69, 96
189	.38	210	Which is larger: 17 or 68; 23 or 56; 189 or 201?
189	.38	212	How much is: 3 × 3; 5 × 4; 7 × 8?
189	.38	213	How much is: 3 + 4; 6 + 7?
189	.39	214	How much is: 7 − 4; 8 − 5?
189	.44	219	What number is missing? 12 − ( ) = 8; 12 + ( ) = 19
189	.40	230	Write words from memory after visual presentation
189	.38	254	Concept formation—logical relationships
190	.44	146	Read *cat; dog; man*
190	.38	150	Read *cat–hat–bat*
190	.46	177	Copy B, L, ℒ, 𝒟, ℬ
190	.42	178	Copy *pa, an, pro, pre, sti*

*r = correlation

Table 8.2: **Reading Scale Item Intercorrelations**   *Continued*

Item	r*	Item	Description
190	.42	181	Write *f, t, h, l*
190	.42	201	Write 7-9-3; 3-5-7
190	.44	203	Write 17 and 71; 69 and 96
190	.40	204	Write 27, 34, 158, 396, 9845
190	.41	206	Read 7-9-3; 3-5-7
190	.55	208	Read 27, 34, 158, 396, 9845
190	.39	210	Which is larger: 17 or 68; 23 or 56; 189 or 201?
190	.37	219	What number is missing? 12 − ( ) = 8; 12 + ( ) = 19
190	.40	258	Discursive reasoning—elementary arithmetic problems
191	.36	72	Determine whether stimulus is moving up or down right arm
191	.36	74	Identify shapes drawn on right wrist
191	.36	159	Name objects from description
191	.36	177	Copy *B, L, ℒ, 𝒟, ℬ*
192	.36	105	Write phoneme triplets
192	.38	148	Read *hairbrush; screwdriver; laborious*
192	.36	179	Write words from memory after visual presentation
192	.43	183	Write *wren; knife*
193	.37	124	Which is correct: Spring comes before summer, or Summer comes before spring?
193	.42	145	Read *see-seen; tree-trick*
193	.42	146	Read *cat; dog; man*
193	.41	147	Read *house; table; apple*
193	.42	148	Read *hairbrush; screwdriver; laborious*
193	.38	149	Read *rhinoceros; surveillance; hierarchy*
193	.38	150	Read *cat-hat-bat*
193	.39	153	Read *house-ball-chair*
193	.40	182	Write *ba; da; back; pack*
193	.47	204	Write 27, 34, 158, 396, 9845
193	.40	205	Write 14, 17, 19, 109, 1023
193	.47	208	Read 27, 34, 158, 396, 9845
193	.42	213	How much is: 3 + 4; 6 + 7?
194	.42	177	Copy *B, L, ℒ, 𝒟, ℬ*
194	.38	178	Copy *pa, an, pro, pre, sti*
194	.41	203	Write IV and VI; IX and XI
194	.36	205	Write 14, 17, 19, 109, 1023
194	.36	207	Read IV, VI, IX, XI; 17, 71, 69, 96
194	.37	208	Read 27, 34, 158, 396, 9845
194	.35	211	Which is larger: 189 or 201; 1967 or 3002?
195	.39	129	If Arnie hit Tom, which boy was the victim?
195	.39	144	Read *sp, th, pl, str, awk*
195	.43	148	Read *hairbrush; screwdriver; laborious*
195	.44	139	Read *cat-hat-bat*
195	.54	151	Read *streptomycin; Massachusetts Episcopal*
195	.43	175	How many letters are there in: *cat; trap; banana; hedge?*
195	.46	176	Phonetic analysis; e.g., what is the second letter in *cat;* first letter in *match?*
195	.39	179	Write words from memory after visual presentation
195	.44	185	Write words and phrases to dictation
195	.40	207	Read IV, VI, IX, XI; 17, 71, 69, 96
195	.41	221	Serial seven subtraction from 100
195	.39	222	Serial 13 subtraction from 100
195	.40	223	Memory for seven words scored for error
195	.43	247	Understanding of thematic texts
195	.38	251	Concept formation—logical relationships
195	.38	253	Concept formation—logical relationships
195	.39	254	Concept formation—logical relationships
196	.35	244	Understanding of thematic texts
197	.40	103	Phonemic hearing—writing
197	.36	104	Repeat phoneme triplets
197	.44	105	Write phoneme triplets
197	.38	147	Read *house; table; apple*
197	.38	150	Read *cat-hat-bat*
198	.36	112	What do *cat, bat, pat* mean?
198	.37	144	Read *sp, th, pl, str, awk*
198	.42	145	Read *see-seen; tree-trick*
198	.42	146	Read *cat; dog; man*

*r = correlation

Table 8.2: **Reading Scale Item Intercorrelations**   *Continued*

Item	r*	Item	Description
198	.44	147	Read *house; table; apple*
198	.38	148	Read *hairbrush; screwdriver; laborious*
198	.41	150	Read *cat–hat–bat*
198	.41	153	Read *house–ball–chair*
198	.38	178	Copy *pa, an, pro, pre, sti*
198	.41	204	Write 27, 34, 158, 396, 9845
199	.37	144	Read *sp, th, pl, str, awk*
199	.39	148	Read *hairbrush; screwdriver; laborious*
199	.37	149	Read *rhinoceros; surveillance; hierarchy*
199	.36	151	Read *streptomycin; Massachusetts Episcopal*
199	.41	176	Phonetic analysis; e.g., what is the second letter in *cat;* first letter in *match?*
199	.37	177	Copy *B, L, ℒ, 𝒟, ℬ*
199	.40	179	Write words from memory after visual presentation
199	.44	185	Write words and phrases
199	.37	186	Grammar, spelling, and content in sentence written on specified topic
199	.38	204	Write 27, 34, 158, 396, 9845
199	.38	208	Read 27, 34, 158, 396, 9845
199	.41	256	Verbal analogies
200	.42	22	Tap your right hand twice and your left hand once
200	.42	23	Same as #22 but reverse order of hands
200	.44	144	Read *sp, th, pl, str, awk*
200	.45	151	Read *streptomycin; Massachusetts Episcopal*
200	.49	176	Phonetic analogies; e.g., what is the second letter in *cat;* first letter in *match?*
200	.41	179	Write words from memory after visual presentation
200	.41	183	Write *wren; knife*
200	.55	185	Write words and phrases
200	.40	186	Grammar, spelling, and content in sentence written on specified topic
200	.40	204	Write 27, 34, 158, 396, 9845
200	.40	207	Read IV, VI, IX, XI; 17, 71, 69, 96

*r = correlation

Table 8.2: **Reading Scale Item Intercorrelations**   *Continued*

Item	r*	Item	Description
200	.42	219	What number is missing? 12 − ( ) = 8; 12 + ( ) = 19
200	.42	223	Memory for seven words scored for errors
200	.41	230	Write words from memory after visual presentation

*r = correlation

we noted above, lesions in this area can interfere with spatial abilities and the use of arithmetic skills (Kinsbourne & Warrington, 1964; Benson & Wier, 1972; Luria, 1966).

Items 190, 191, and 192 require simple reading skills (letters and simple words). Disruption of these skills implicates the temporooccipital area of the brain or the temporoparietal region of the left hemisphere (Golden, Purisch, & Hammeke, 1979). These three items demonstrate significant correlations with items involving somesthetic and motor feedback, spatial-organizational skills, writing skills, and arithmetic abilities. These intercorrelations further implicate the left temporoparietooccipital area in the region of the angular gyrus in simple reading skills.

Tasks requiring visual memory and visual decoding are also highly correlated with this section of the Reading scale (items 190-192) as well as with other Reading scale items. Damage to the secondary area of the right temporal lobe also may lead to difficulty with these and other items, since the right temporal lobe has been associated with visual memory and visual decoding (Hebb, 1959). If parietal injuries are deep enough, performance on these items may be disrupted owing to interference with the visual tracts from the thalamus to the occipital lobes (Golden, 1978).

For items 193-196, the patient is asked to read increasingly difficult words. These items demonstrate significant correlations with Luria-Nebraska items requiring concept formation, arithmetic skills, writing proficiency, and memory skills—functions that, again, are localizable to the temporoparietooccipital region.

The final items of the scale (items 196–200) examine complex reading ability (sentences and paragraphs). Writing skills, visual memory, audioverbal memory, phonetic analysis, motor skills, and arithmetic abilities all correlate highly with these final items. Not surprisingly, this implicates the same region referred to previously, left temporoparietooccipital area. If the patient can read simple words but not entire sentences or paragraphs, a possible site of dysfunction is the tertiary parietal zone, responsible for the analysis of grammatical structure (Golden, Purisch, & Hammeke, 1979). Injuries to the secondary occipital region can disrupt visual scanning (Bender, Postel, & Krieger, 1957; Cumming, Hurwitz, & Perl, 1970).

As is suggested by the correlation of Reading scale items with Motor scale items, frontal lobe dysfunction may also result in reading disorders, particularly if the injury occurs in the secondary areas just anterior to the precentral motor cortex. Brodmann's area 8, the frontal eye field, controls oculomotor activity (Golden, 1978). Inability to control eye movements will make it difficult for patients to read more than one or two words in sequence without losing the place. Patients with tertiary frontal disorders may have trouble paying attention (Luria, 1966) and thus may appear much worse than they actually are on these tasks owing to distractibility.

Like the Writing scale, the Reading scale is highly sensitive to left posterior injury. Dysfunction in the region of the left angular gyrus (temporoparietooccipital zone) will apparently be manifested on a variety of tasks. Interpretation of deficits arising on these two scales therefore must be done carefully to obtain a complete picture of the extent and nature of a given injury.

Factor Analysis

WRITING SCALE

The Writing scale breaks down into two major factors (Table 8.3) when analyzed (Golden, Osmon, Sweet, Purisch, & Hammeke, 1980). The items on the first factor (Table 8.4) include simple and complex tasks that require analysis and synthesis of basic speech sounds or phonemes. The items on the second factor (Table 8.5) consist exclusively of copying and dictation tasks in which the primary component is motor behavior. The task in these items is to translate visually and aurally presented information such as letters, syllables, words, and phrases into written form.

These two factors appear to fit Luria's notions of the two components in the functional system for writing. Luria (1966) notes that phonemic analysis and synthesis constitute the basic ability that allows one to comprehend the verbal structure of the words to be written. Second, the ability to translate verbal symbols into written symbols depends on motor and sensory processes that convert auditorily coded verbal information into motor acts, resulting in writing.

Different performance relations between these two factors have various diagnostic implications. "Pure" cases in which there is poor performance on the phonemic analysis and synthesis factor in conjunction with good performance on the motor execution factor suggest left

Table 8.3: **Writing: Factor Structure**

Item	Factor 1	Factor 2
175	52	37
176	72	35
177	39	85
178	54	77
179	67	31
180	35	63
181	28	50
182	51	50
183	69	41
184	54	19
185	73	50
186	56	34
187	45	35

Table 8.4: **Items on Writing Factor 1**

Loading	Item	Description
.52	175	How many letters are there in the following words?
.72	176	Tell me the second letter in *cat,* etc.
.54	178	Copy these in your own handwriting.
.67	179	I am going to show you a card with three words. After I do, write them down.
.51	182	Write these sounds (dictate).
.69	183	Write these words (dictate).
.54	184	Write (dictate).
.73	185	Write these words or phrases (dictate).
.56	186	Write a few sentences about bringing up children (scored for grammar, spelling, and coherency).

Table 8.5: **Items on Writing Factor 2**

Loading	Item	Description
.85	177	Copy these letters.
.77	178	Copy these in your own handwriting.
.63	180	Write your first and last name.
.50	181	Write these letters (dictate).
.50	182	Write these sounds (dictate).
.41	183	Write these words (dictate).
.50	185	Write these groups of words or phrases (dictate).

Table 8.6: **Reading: Rotated Factor Matrix**

Item	Factor 1	Factor 2
188	43	31
189	47	45
190	12	70
191	13	40
192	57	22
193	43	50
194	09	54
195	68	30
196	47	05
197	33	52
198	43	41
199	65	18
200	71	20

Table 8.7: **Items on Reading Factor 1**

Loading	Item	Description
.45	189	What word is made by these letters: *s–t–o–n–e; k–n–i–g–h–t?*
.70	190	Tell me what you see here: *K, S, W, R, T.*
.40	191	Which of these letters, *B, J,* or *S,* stands for *John?*
.50	193	Read these words: *juice; bread; bonfire; cloakroom; fertilizer.*
.54	194	Read these letters: *U.N., U.S.A., U.S.S.R.*
.52	197	Read these sentences: The man went out for a walk. There are flowers in the garden.
.41	198	Read these sentences: The sun rises in the west. The boy went to bed because she was ill.

temporal lobe dysfunction. In this case the patient cannot distinguish between phonemes.

The reverse in which motor performance is poor and phonemic analysis and synthesis are adequate indicates a posterior left frontal lobe or left parietal disorder. More complicated relations between the two factors naturally require more detailed qualitative analysis of individual items to reveal their diagnostic significance. The complexity of brain function does not allow pure psychometric measures of any one function. For example, phonemic discrimination is represented in both factors, since analysis and synthesis of speech sounds are necessary before one can write. Left temporal lobe damage therefore may not be uniquely associated with poor performance on only the first factor.

READING SCALE

Two primary factors emerged from a factor analysis of the

Table 8.8: **Items on Reading Factor 2**

Loading	Item	Description
.43	188	What sound is made by these letters: *g–r–o; p–l–y*?
.47	189	What word is made by these letters: *s–t–o–n–e; k–n–i–g–h–t*?
.57	192	Read these sounds: *po, cor, cra, spro, prot.*
.43	193	Read these words: *juice; bread; bonfire; cloakroom; fertilizer.*
.68	195	Read these words: *insubordination; indistinguishable.*
.47	196	Read these words: *astrocytoma; hemopoiesis.*
.43	198	Read these sentences: The sun rises in the west. The boy went to bed because she was ill.
.65	199	Read this out loud. Scoring: errors.
.71	200	Scoring: time.

Reading scale (Table 8.6). Interpretation of these two factors follows from an understanding of the reading process. Simply described, reading requires the breakdown of printed speech into its relevant acoustic components, which are combined into meaningful units. Letters are combined into sounds, sounds into words, words into phrases, and so forth. If the words or phrases are habitually used, the process is greatly contracted, and the entire word or phrase is recognized as a unit with little or no deliberate or conscious breakdown and combination of the sounds. However, much of what we read is not familiar or sufficiently habitual to permit this type of automatic recognition. When material is unfamiliar or acoustically complex, a more conscious and deliberate process replaces automatic and direct recognition. It is this automatic recognition versus deliberate processing of written material that defines the two factors of this scale.

Factor 1 (Table 8.7) consists of seven items. Each item presents letters, words, or phrases that are easily recognized, familiar, and rather automatically read with minimal conscious processing. Therefore this factor has been labeled automatic reading.

Factor 2 (Table 8.8) presents items that are less familiar and more acoustically complex than factor 1 items. These types of items generally are not automatically recognized but require a more conscious and deliberate reading process. Thus, factor 2 has been named deliberate reading.

Three items are shared by both factors (items 189, 193, 198). In each of these items, features are present that account for either automatic recognition or deliberate processing. For example, item 198 consists of five words that become progressively less familiar and more acoustically complex. The first two words, *juice* and *bread,* are relatively familiar and might be automatically recognized. Later words such as *fertilizer* are less readily recognized and require a greater degree of deliberate processing.

It should be noted that breakdown of reading into two factors, one for automatic recognition and the other for deliberate processing, appears to be a theoretically and clinically relevant distinction. It is frequently observed with a variety of brain lesions that more automatic or habitual behaviors are preserved; for example, the ability to directly echo words said by another, the ability to speak habitually spoken words or phrases and, in the case of reading, to recognize directly familiar and habitually read words. However, impairment is often noted when cognitive processes need to assume a more active, conscious, and deliberate character; for example, during the organization of deliberate speech or, in reading, while actively analyzing and synthesizing the acoustic content of printed material.

Summary

Reading and writing are complex, multidetermined functional systems of language. These skills may exist at a variety of levels according to training. These varying levels, though producing the same overt behavior, represent different functional units and employ different neuropsychological processes.

Appropriate interpretation of the Reading and Writing

scales requires careful consideration of the patient's premorbid educational status and level of functioning. This will affect the degree of automatization of skills that can be expected. A significant consideration in patients with poor premorbid educational functioning is the possibility that early childhood or prenatal brain injury made learning difficult. One cannot dismiss an elevated score on the Reading or Writing scale as purely the result of lack of education. Lack of opportunity may produce elevated levels in the absence of early or later cortical damage, but in patients who had opportunity to learn to read and write but failed to do so the examiner must develop alternative hypotheses to account for disturbances, such as early injury or mental retardation.

The pattern of performance on the Reading and Writing scales must be interpreted in conjunction with performance on the remainder of the battery, as described in this chapter. It should be clear that reading and writing are highly complex functions, as is further evidenced by intercorrelation analysis. Although the aphasic syndromes can theoretically be described as pure clusters of expected behavior, in practice this is often not the case. Deficits in reading and writing reflect a disturbance in the functional system of language. Adequate interpretation requires the recognition that the basic syndromes may be seen in various combinations.

The multiple cortical units necessary for proficient learning and automatization of writing and reading make these skills especially vulnerable to disturbance, especially when they are not overlearned. Lowering of general cortical tone level may be reflected in performance on these scales. Sensitive interpretation of the Reading and Writing scales requires awareness of inter- and intrascale patterns of performance, awareness of the patient's premorbid educational status, and a thorough understanding of the complexity of these language-based skills.

9. The Arithmetic Scale

Arithmetic represents one of the most basic abilities necessary for survival in our modern, number-oriented society. Despite this, however, performance on arithmetic items differs widely among normal people, with "mathematics phobia" a common finding. This large variance among normal people is complicated by the ease with which arithmetic processes can be affected by a wide range of injuries to both the right and the left hemispheres. Compared with basic reading skills, arithmetic requires much more attention, concentration, memory, and ability to follow sequential rules, along with the ability to decipher written material and to convert oral material into its written equivalent. In addition, arithmetic requires that one translate from the verbal system to numbers in a logical manner, a skill measured on the Intellectual scale of the Luria-Nebraska. As a result of these considerations, performance on the Arithmetic scale requires close evaluation of an individual's errors and the way he or she goes about attempting to solve a problem. With proper evaluation, this scale can yield a wealth of insight into the patient's condition.

This scale consists of 22 items (201–222) intended to assess impairment of arithmetic ability. Prerequisite to actual arithmetic calculations is the ability to recognize and comprehend the relative value of numbers. This ability is assessed by items 201–211, which require the written and oral identification (reading) of several numbers. Items proceed from simple to complex numbers, first written from dictation and then read. Complexity is determined by the increasing need for true appreciation of the relative value of each of the component digits in a number according to its place—that is, units, tens, hundreds, and so forth. Comparison of the relative values of pairs of numbers ends this subsection, a task that relies greatly upon conscious rather than automatic appreciation of numerical significance.

Beyond the ability to recognize and appreciate numerical values is the ability to perform arithmetic operations, assessed by the remaining items of this scale (212–222). In many instances this is no more difficult than recognizing numbers. These operations are based upon rather automatic and memorized answers to simple problems provided by early items of this section. However, later items in the section become increasingly difficult and thus preclude the possibility of prelearning. In these one needs the ability to consciously manipulate numbers according to the required operations.

Comprehension of Number Structure

The ability to comprehend number structure and relative numerical values is assessed through visual and auditory presentation. Disorders of reading and writing such as those caused by visual perceptual impairment may cause problems in identifying numbers without actual inability to understand numerical structure and value. Primary impairment of reading or writing must be ruled out before one assumes a deficit in comprehension of number structure. Factors affecting reading and writing are discussed in detail elsewhere (see Chapter 6).

Other secondary disorders also may result in difficulties on these items. For example, impairment of acoustic analysis will result in difficulty in writing numbers from dictation. In fact, a multitude of receptive or expressive speech difficulties will affect the comprehension or reading of the required numbers.

Although many language and visually related disorders can result in mathematical difficulties, disorders of these types represent secondary systemic impairment. On the other hand, a disruption of the visual-spatial synthetic process creates a primary disturbance in the comprehension of number structure. The primary symptom of dyscalculia is typically observed when a lesion is present in the tertiary parieto-occipital area of the left (dominant) hemisphere (Luria, 1966).

The comprehension of numerical values based upon visual-spatial ability is easily understood if one looks at the development of numerical comprehension. Initially the child understands numerical values and arithmetic operations by manipulating objects in a concrete visual-spatial plane. Eventually these concrete representations and manipulative operations become internalized through visual imagery. Later these visual images are replaced by abstract verbal-numerical labels, and operations are performed linguistically. However, even as this process becomes contracted and automatized, it always remains based upon the system of spatial coordinates into which the numbers are placed.

A lesion of the parieto-occipital region disturbs the ability to integrate visual-spatial information. The ability to categorize numbers along the spatial dimension of units, tens, and so forth, thus loses its specificity. The recognition of single-digit numbers, however, remains unimpaired, since there is only the units category to spatially apprehend. Thus the writing and reading of single-digit numbers, as measured by items 201 and 206, remains unimpaired. Difficulties that do occur on these items result not from a visual-spatial synthesis impairment resulting in dyscalculia, but rather from a lesion elsewhere causing a secondary systemic disturbance.

Subsequent items require the writing and reading of multidigit numbers. For these items a lack of spatial appreciation causes problems in correctly recognizing the numerical categories. Items 202, 203, and 207, which require the writing and reading of visually complementary numbers, provide a particularly sensitive measure of this ability. For example, the roman numerals IV and VI and the arabic numbers 17 and 71 are to be read in item 207. Without the ability to appreciate the spatial positions that determine the value of each constituent digit, these visually complementary numbers are easily confused. Thus a person with a parieto-occipital lesion may read or write 17 as 71 or IV as VI.

Items 204 and 208 require writing and reading non-complementary multidigit numbers. The comprehension of these numbers depends on the ability to categorize the value of each component digit based upon its position in the sequence. For example, the number farthest right represents units, the second to the right tens, and so forth.

Five numbers are presented in these items, proceeding from a two-digit number (27) to a more spatially complex four-digit number (9845).

Item 205 requires writing a special series of multidigit numbers chosen because they are not written as they sound. The patient is required to write the numbers 14, 17, 19, 109, 1023 from dictation. This is a sensitive variant of the preceding multidigit items for detecting comprehension deficits of number structure owing to spatial impairment. In each case the value of each component digit must be appreciated solely by spatial placement. One cannot compensate by merely sequencing the digits the way they are spoken.

Lesions of the parieto-occipital region resulting in spatial impairment disturb the ability to recode the spoken number in accordance with the appropriate system of categorical values. Without this categorical structure the digits in the integer quickly lose their relation to each other. This is especially true for numbers including zeros (item 205). Thus, in writing the number 1023, the relation of 1000 to 23 is easily lost, and the two separate numbers, 1000 and 23, may be written instead of the one whole number.

Item 209 is another variant of the multidigit presentation. In this item numbers to be read are presented vertically rather than in the usual horizontal placement. Latent spatial disorders often are detected in this manner when horizontal placement reveals no such difficulties. Reading numbers presented vertically precludes success owing to automatic recognition, which is possible only with horizontal presentation. Rather, the vertical placement demands conscious and deliberate analysis of the categorical structure of the number.

The final part of the assessment of comprehension of the categorical structure of numbers is accomplished by items 210 and 211. Both require identification of the larger of a pair of numbers. Item 210 requires verbal identification, while 211 asks for a pointing response, thereby circumventing assessment difficulties in patients with expressive disorders.

The ability to determine the numerical difference in these items directly depends on assessment of the relative values of the digits in corresponding positions in each number being compared. For example, to determine the larger of the two numbers 17 and 68 (item 210) only the first digit, the tens place, need be compared. Obviously, without appreciation of the spatial position of each digit one cannot assess numerical differences.

Item 211 introduces a further factor in comprehension of numerical differences. For each of the number pairs, presented visually, the smaller of the two numbers consists of digits relatively greater than the corresponding digits of the larger of the two numbers, with the exception of the first and most important digit. For example, in the comparison between 189 and 201 the tens and units digits of the smaller number are greater than those of the larger number. Once again, without the ability to recognize the numerical category that distinguishes the relative magnitude of the two numbers (in this case, the hundreds place) there can be no meaningful comparison. In this example the appearance of larger numbers whose categorical significance is incorrectly evaluated can easily lead to an incorrect response.

As we mentioned earlier, a variety of functional disorders of visual, auditory, and speech processes can result in secondary disturbances of number recognition. Each of these systemic difficulties presents qualitatively different symptom clusters that differentiate them from primary number comprehension problems that are due to impairment of spatial synthesis. For example, dyslexia resulting from visual difficulties might preclude accurate reading of the numbers. But accurate comprehension of structure is verified by the ability to write the same numbers. Similarly, a disturbance in auditory phonemic perception will cause difficulty in writing numbers from dictation. However, in the absence of secondary expressive difficulties created by the phonemic imperception, the numbers are easily read when presented visually.

Another secondary disturbance of number recognition occurs in lesions of the frontal lobes that result in a disintegration of active analysis and critical evaluation. Symptoms of this disorder are most apparent on items in which a conflict must be analyzed and resolved. An example is item 205, which requires writing multidigit numbers whose digits are not arranged in the order they are spoken. Thus, writing the number 14, in which the number 4 is enunciated first but written second, requires the ability to critically analyze and rearrange the numbers instead of echolalically writing the digit 4 first.

Item 211 also is difficult for patients with the frontal syndrome. In many cases an impulsive, noncritical reaction is given to the larger digits in the smaller numbers, which are thereby identified as the larger of the pair. In cases like this it is hard to distinguish the cause of the ostensible numerical comprehension difficulties when critical evaluation and active analysis are replaced by an automatic impulsive or echolalic response. On the surface, the responses of a patient with the frontal syndrome appear similar to those described for spatial integration impairment owing to parieto-occipital damage. However, careful prompting and external guidance typically reveal that the frontally involved patient can recognize numerical differences and appreciate the categorical structure of numbers.

In severe frontal injuries a differential assessment may be impossible on the basis of response to external prompting and guidance. However, in these cases the frontal syndrome of aspontaneity and adynamia across all behaviors will be obvious. On the other hand, the patient with a lesion confined to the parieto-occipital region will exhibit only symptoms related to spatial impairment and will not show deficient spontaneity or initiative as is common with frontally injured patients.

Arithmetic Operations

The second half of the Arithmetic scale is intended to assess overall ability to perform arithmetic operations. This section comprises items 212–222, which become increasingly demanding in the underlying neuropsychological processes required. One such process is the comprehension of the categorical structure of numbers, measured by the previous section, an obvious prerequisite for arithmetic operations. A disorder of spatial synthesis profound enough to disturb comprehension of number structure will therefore make it impossible to perform most arithmetic operations.

In this section the items become progressively more demanding, moving through simple automatic calculations, complex calculations, identification of arithmetic operations, and serial arithmetic operations. Later items are to be done mentally, without the aid of writing, taxing the stability of visual-spatial synthesis as well as adding a mnestic component.

The first three items, 212–214, are intended to assess the ability to perform simple, automatic operations, including the multiplication of numbers typically memorized from multiplication tables (212), and the addition (213) and subtraction (214) of single-digit numbers. Little demand is placed upon spatial synthesis, disintegration of which results in primary acalculia at this level. Typically, a spatial disorder must be profound enough to disrupt the comprehension of number structure before it causes poor performance on these items.

Some patients have relatively good comprehension of number structure yet still make errors on these items. This is especially true with the multiplication items, where there may be disruption of the system allowing automatic retrieval of values from the multiplication table, usually the result of a rather pronounced deficit affecting simple and automatic functions across many areas. Errors may also result from language deficits that interfere with the processing of any verbal information, including numerical data. Regardless of the source of error, poor performance on items 214–216 forewarns of problems with subsequent, more complex arithmetic operations.

Relatively more complex and nonautomatic arithmetic operations are introduced in item 215. This item presents addition and subtraction problems requiring that one either carry over the sum of the units to the tens place (addition) or borrow from the tens to the units place (subtraction). This type of operation takes place on a more deliberate and conscious level than the previous automatic operations and requires a true appreciation of the numerical categories involved. A latent instability of spatial synthesis often is revealed in carrying over or borrowing beyond simple numerical comprehension.

Greater complexity is added on item 216, the addition of 5, 9, and 7. This item requires adding three, rather than two, numbers, thus entailing two separate operations. Each addition also requires carrying over, which compounds the difficulty. Finally, unlike previous problems, this is to be performed mentally rather than in writing. Multiple operations require the ability to keep the digits properly aligned to maintain their categorical significance. Carrying over further taxes this ability. Thus, this problem is quantitatively more demanding than the previous items.

Mental rather than written computation requires an additional memory component. The three numbers are presented visually, which precludes forgetting the three digits. But the sum of the first two numbers, 5 plus 9, must be remembered as the basis for performing the second operation, 14 plus 7, in which the 14 is not recorded. Patients with lesions of the medial and inferior portions of the left temporal cortex will be especially susceptible to forgetting the sum of the first operation and will have trouble remembering what value to carry over owing to instability of acoustic traces.

The task is even more complicated in item 217, which visually presents the number 18 directly above the number 24 and asks the patient to "subtract the number above from the number below." The normal conditions of subtraction are thus spatially reversed, and greater demands are made upon accurate number comprehension. Without adequate spatial synthesis the categorical structure of the two numbers will not be maintained, and the tendency will be to revert to subtracting the smaller single digits from the larger. For example, if 18 is to be subtracted from 24, with

18 being the top number, the operation may proceed as follows: $8 - 4 = 4$, $2 - 1 = 1$, answer, 14. Similar difficulties may occur, as discussed above, even when the original conditions of the problem, $24 - 18$, are maintained—that is, breakdown of categorical comprehension when borrowing from the tens to the units place.

An interesting complication is introduced into the visual presentation of item 217, besides the superior position of the subtrahend. A division symbol ($\div$) is placed to the left of the numbers although the instructions specify subtraction. This presents a distraction for patients who have trouble directing attention to appropriate stimuli and screening out irrelevant ones. This condition is often found with injuries of the frontal or medial regions of the cerebral hemispheres. In these instances the patient very well may convert the problem into one of division rather than subtraction or may become so confused as to be unable to answer the problem at all. It should be noted that the distracting division sign is considered a subtraction sign in some countries. It was retained for the reasons noted above, rather than substituting an American minus sign.

A variant of the procedures above is presented in items 218 and 219. Item 218 requires the patient to supply the appropriate operation sign when provided all the numbers, including the answer—for example, $2 ( ) 5 = 10$. Item 219 uses the same presentation except that a number rather than a sign is to be supplied—for example, $12 - ( ) = 8$. Both these variants may be considered more difficult than previous items, since they demand conscious and deliberate simultaneous consideration of all the numerical relations involved. For example, to determine that the operation in $2 ( ) 5 = 10$ is multiplication, the relations among multiplier, multiplicand, and product must all be considered.

Luria (1966) intended these items to preclude the possibility of "dissociation" (p. 437), in which operations are performed automatically without true conscious appreciation of the numerical relations involved, resulting in a false positive assessment of arithmetic ability when prior items are correctly answered. In fact, it is not rare to see a patient correctly answer all the prior items but be unable to determine the appropriate operation (218) or supply the missing number (219), since it is impossible to arrive at an accurate answer without consciously appreciating the numerical relations among all the elements. A high degree of spatial synthesis is required for this task, and latent disorders are often revealed when conditions become this complex.

Item 220 also presents a variant of the typical arithmetic problem. Unlike several earlier items, the two addition problems are to be solved mentally rather than with the aid of writing. The problems also are relatively more difficult, since the first (27 + 34 + 14) presents three two-digit numbers and the second presents two three-digit numbers to be added. In addition to its great difficulty, however, this item in unique because the numbers are presented horizontally rather than in the usual vertical alignment. Without the aid of the usual columnar alignment of digits from corresponding spatial categories, a true appreciation of number structure is required.

A task common on mental-status examinations is presented on items 221 and 222, the last two items of the Arithmetic scale. Item 221 presents a task of subtracting serial sevens, counting backward from one hundred, and item 222 makes the process relatively more complex, requiring serial 13 subtraction. The serial subtraction problem is a highly demanding task that requires the functional integrity of several underlying neuropsychological abilities. As with all other problems in this section, an accurate comprehension of categorical number structure is necessary, especially when borrowing from tens to units is required. This has been discussed at length already, and no further comment will be made here.

Another very important prerequisite for serial operations is a high degree of dynamic flexibility and regulation of the mental processes. Many steps are performed during a serial operation, such as the initial subtraction, carrying over from tens to units, using the remainder from the previous step as the minuend of the subsequent one, keeping the intention of using either 7 or 13 as the subtrahend for each step, and so forth. Several operations must be performed simultaneously, and even with an adequate comprehension of number structure the entire process may quickly disintegrate.

The flexibility and regulation of mental processes are disrupted by lesions of the frontal regions of the cortex, which produce an adynamic state in which neuroprocesses become inert. A task such as serial subtraction that, as stated, requires the continual shifting of the role of the same number from remainder to minuend may be impossible when cognitive processes become inflexible, even after, for example, correctly subtracting 7 from 100 to arrive at 93 as the starting point of the next subtraction.

The regulatory function also is disrupted by lesions of the frontal regions. Thus there may be an inability to maintain the self-regulating instructions or intention of the task, for example, ''continue to subtract seven.'' Difficulties of this type often are reflected in confusion about the task instructions after each subtraction, even when the patient is given remainders at each juncture. Another reflection of this trouble might be the replacement of the original task or intention with a simpler, perseverative response (e.g., 100, 87, 77, 67, etc.).

The effects of frontal lobe lesions are typically observed on earlier items as well, especially when active and flexible processing is required. Difficulties may be manifested, for example, whenever numbers are to be carried over or borrowed between numerical categories. These difficulties may be superficially similar to those observed when there is a disintegration of spatial synthesis with left parieto-occipital lesions. In both instances a breakdown of comprehension of categorical structure is responsible for digit transfers. As previously discussed for parieto-occipital lesions, there is no problem in this regard with frontal lesions. In fact, frontally injured patients often show good ability to recognize complex and multidigit numbers and to assign appropriate values to component digits even when numbers are displayed in an unusual manner, as in the vertical presentation of item 209. The problem lies, rather, in the lack of mobility of cognitive processes, so that it becomes difficult to transfer the same number from smaller to larger categories (addition) or from larger to smaller categories (subtraction).

A disturbance in self-regulation may cause errors even when cognitive inflexibility is not severe. Thus the patient may be flexibile enough to recognize equivalent representations of the same number under different categories (e.g., 23 = 23 units or two tens and three units), but still have trouble transferring values from one category to the next because of a disturbance of self-regulation. This type of problem is revealed by the loss of the intention to transfer values. For example, when adding 158 and 396 (item 220) the patient will be able to add 8 + 6 from the units column to arrive at 14, mark the 4 in the answer place, but then lose the self-instruction to carry the 1 over to the tens column.

Another necessary condition for many arithmetic operations is stability of the mental processes. Instability of acoustic traces resulting from medial temporal cortex lesions or as a condition of generalized disturbance of neurodynamics seriously impairs mnestic processes. These difficulties are most evident when items require that operations be performed mentally rather than by writing. Thus, performance on items 216, 217, 220, 221, and 222 may suffer because of memory lapses. For example, when adding 27 + 34 + 14 in a column (i.e., first units, then tens), the sum of the units is 15, from which 5 is placed in the units column and 1 is carried over to the tens column. Next the sum of the tens column is computed to be 70. However, with unstable acoustic traces, the patient forgets the 5 originally obtained for the units column and is forced to start again. Similarly, serial subtraction demands that the previous remainder be remembered and used as the minuend of the subsequent operation.

Another important prerequisite for arithmetic operations is adequate language ability. Arithmetic operations are verbally based, and dysphasia will affect facility in numeric language as it affects speech abilities (See Chapters 6 and 7 on receptive and expressive speech). For example, lesions of Wernicke's area resulting in disintegration of phonemic analysis and synthesis may make it impossible to understand number sounds, producing confusion and extinction of meaning. While actual ability to perform arithmetic operations remains intact in this instance, the patient who can no longer acoustically understand numbers is unable to use them.

Finally, certain lesions of the right hemisphere, notably frontal and parieto-occipital injuries, result in generalized spatial perceptual disturbances that may cause secondary difficulties with arithmetic operations. These are different from spatial synthesis disturbances resulting from parieto-occipital lesions of the left hemisphere, which specifically affect verbal-spatial synthesis and the ability to integrate a number into a comprehensible whole. The former disturbs nonverbal perception of visual-spatial stimuli, so that visual elements such as direction, placement, and slope of numbers may be misperceived. No primary difficulty in categorical comprehension is apparent in these right hemisphere spatial disturbances; only accurate perception of visual-spatial relations in a number or a problem is impaired. A typical difficulty may be inability to line up the columns when writing a problem down.

The assessment of arithmetic operations in this section concludes with serial subtraction. However, serial operations do not present the most demanding conditions possible in arithmetic operations. While great mobility and stability of mental processes are required in serial operations, the strategy is relatively simple and the execution is repetitive. Arithmetic word problems represent a more demanding task. These problems require the active formation of strategies and intermediate operations aimed at achieving an end goal. Because of the complexity of the various processes and the great cognitive flexibility and self-regulation needed, arithmetic word problems are considered ideal for assessing intellectual reasoning. As such, these problems have been included in the Intellectual scale chapter, where they are discussed in depth.

Item Intercorrelations

Intercorrelation of items of the Arithmetic scale with all other items on the Luria-Nebraska Neuropsychological Battery reveals a number of significant correlations ($r > .35$; $p < .0001$) that can aid in the interpretation of poor performance on the items of this scale (Table 9.1). The Arithmetic scale is the most sensitive of all Luria scales to educational deficits. Even in normally educated adults, this is the scale most likely to indicate severe pathology when there is, in fact, no problem with the patient. Some patients may view as impossible the comparatively simple items that compose the Arithmetic scale. This appears highly related to an individual's general reaction to mathematics. Therefore, performance on this scale must always be interpreted with caution to avoid false diagnosis of brain injury.

The first section of the scale (items 201 through 209) has been designed to investigate spatial function as well as the ability to comprehend number structure and relative numerical values. As the numbers increase in complexity, it is not unusual for patients with spatial deficits owing to right hemisphere or left parieto-occipital dysfunction to write the numbers out of sequence (Golden, Purisch, & Hammeke, 1979).

This series of items correlates with items requiring reading and writing skills as well as spatial, naming, memory, concept-formation, comparison, and somatosensory abilities. The item intercorrelations suggest that the aspect of arithmetic ability involving reading and writing of numbers could be disrupted by injury to virtually any area of the brain. However, it appears that lesions to the temporoparieto-occipital area would have the greatest effect. Patients with alexia and agraphia for numbers have been found to demonstrate parietal lobe

Table 9.1: **Item Intercorrelations with Arithmetic Scale**

Item	$r*$	Item	Description
201	.44	12	Left hand fingers extended in sagittal plane touching chin
201	.42	73	Determine whether stimulus is moving up or down left arm
201	.48	86	Name visually presented objects
201	.47	113	Point to the picture that shows: typewriting; mealtime; summer
201	.40	136	Repeat *house; table; apple*
201	.42	147	Read *house; table; apple*
201	.43	158	Name body parts from pictures
201	.40	159	Name objects from description
201	.41	162	Tell me the days of the week
201	.51	177	Copy *B, L, ℒ, 𝒟, ℬ*
201	.44	178	Copy *pa, an, pro, pre, sti*
201	.47	180	Write your first and last names
201	.48	181	Write *ba; da; back; pack*
201	.59	258	Discursive reasoning—elementary arithmetic problems
202	.38	21	Clench your right hand and extend fingers of left hand, then reverse
202	.36	59	How many beeps in all groups together?
202	.41	82	Stereognosis—right hand errors
202	.37	144	Read *sp, th, pl, str, awk*
202	.44	183	Write *wren; knife*
202	.42	223	Memory for seven words scored for errors
202	.38	235	Logical memory—recalling by visual aid
202	.40	252	Concept formation—logical relationships
202	.45	254	Concept formation—logical relationships
202	.44	256	Verbal analogies
202	.41	268	Discursive reasoning—elementary arithmetic problems
203	.41	19	Point to your left eye with your right hand
203	.40	73	Determine whether stimulus is moving up or down left arm
203	.42	74	Identify shapes drawn on right wrist
203	.40	95	Draw hands on blank clockface at: 12:50, 4:35, 11:10

$*r = correlation$

Table 9.1: **Item Intercorrelations with Arithmetic Scale**   *Continued*

Item	r*	Item	Description
203	.45	108	Point to eye; nose; ear
203	.46	121	Show, by pointing, who is the daughter's mother
203	.45	124	Which is correct: Spring comes before summer, or Summer comes before spring?
203	.45	142	Repeat *house-ball-chair; ball-chair-house*
203	.44	146	Read *cat; dog; man*
203	.43	147	Read *house; table; apple*
203	.44	159	Name objects from description
203	.44	178	Write words from memory after visual presentation
203	.45	181	Write *f, t, h, l*
203	.45	182	Write *ba; da; back; pack*
203	.44	190	Tell me what you see here: *K, S, W, R, T*
203	.41	194	Read *U.N.; U.S.A.; U.S.S.R.*
204	.45	19	Point to your left eye with your right hand
204	.45	86	Name visually presented objects
204	.45	110	Identify objects from pictures by pointing
204	.49	145	Read *see-seen; tree-trick*
204	.45	147	Read *house; table; apple*
204	.45	163	Say the days of the week backward starting with Sunday
204	.47	176	Phonetic analysis; e.g., what is the second letter in *cat;* first letter in *match?*
204	.53	182	Write *ba; da; back; pack*
204	.44	185	Write words and phrases
204	.44	189	What word is made by these letters: *s-t-o-n-e; k-n-i-g-h-t?*
204	.47	193	Read *juice; bread; bonfire; cloakroom; fertilizer*
204	.43	256	Verbal analogies
204	.43	258	Discursive reasoning—elementary arithmetic problems
205	.51	86	Name visually presented objects
205	.44	90	Name overlapping objects in pictures
205	.48	95	Draw hands on blank clockface at: 12:50, 4:35, 11:10

Table 9.1: **Item Intercorrelations with Arithmetic Scale**   *Continued*

Item	r*	Item	Description
205	.50	110	Identify objects from pictures by pointing
205	.46	112	What do *cat, bat, pat* mean?
205	.48	124	Which is correct: Spring comes before summer, or Summer comes before spring?
205	.44	142	Repeat *house-ball-chair; ball-chair-house*
205	.45	147	Read *house; table; apple*
205	.45	154	Repeat sentences
205	.46	159	Name objects from description
205	.45	177	Copy *B, L, ℒ, 𝒟, ℬ*
205	.45	178	Copy *pa, an, pro, pre, sti*
205	.46	181	Write *f, t, h, l*
205	.50	182	Write *ba; da; back; pack*
205	.44	185	Write words and phrases
205	.53	260	Discursive reasoning—elementary arithmetic problems
206	.52	73	Determine whether stimulus is moving up or down left arm
206	.51	108	Point to eye; nose; ear
206	.45	112	What do *cat, bat, pat* mean?
206	.53	113	Point to the picture that shows: typewriting; mealtime; summer
206	.46	115	Whose watch is this (examiner's)? Whose is this (patient's)?
206	.48	146	Read *cat; dog; man*
206	.51	147	Read *house; table; apple*
207	.40	112	What do *cat, bat, pat* mean?
207	.41	156	Repeat sentences
207	.40	163	Say the days of the week backward starting with Sunday
207	.40	176	Phonetic analysis; e.g., what is the second letter in *cat;* first letter in *match?*
207	.44	185	Write words and phrases
207	.40	195	Read *insubordination; indistinguishable*
207	.40	200	Time taken to read paragraph
207	.40	223	Memory for words
207	.47	251	Concept formation—logical relationships

*r = correlation

Table 9.1: **Item Intercorrelations with Arithmetic Scale**   *Continued*

Item	r*	Item	Description
207	.43	261	Discursive reasoning—elementary arithmetic problems
208	.40	51	If I knock hard, you knock gently; if I knock gently, you knock hard
208	.40	90	Name overlapping objects in pictures
208	.42	91	Name overlapping objects in pictures
208	.42	110	Identify objects from pictures by pointing
208	.44	112	What do *cat, bat, pat* mean?
208	.43	113	Point to the picture that shows: typewriting; mealtime; summer
208	.45	124	Which is correct: Spring comes before summer, or Summer comes before spring?
208	.43	146	Read *cat; dog; man*
208	.43	147	Read *house; table; apple*
208	.45	150	Read *cat–hat–bat*
208	.45	163	Tell me the days of the week backward starting with Sunday
208	.53	177	Copy *B, L, ℒ, 𝒟, ℬ*
208	.46	178	Copy *pa, an, pro, pre, sti*
208	.43	182	Write *ba, da, back, pack*
208	.55	190	Tell me what you see here: *K, S, W, R, T*
208	.47	193	Read *juice; bread; bonfire; cloakroom; fertilizer*
208	.44	258	Discursive reasoning—elementary arithmetic problems
208	.45	150	Read *cat–hat–bat*
208	.45	162	Tell me the days of the week
208	.46	163	Say the days of the week backward starting with Sunday
208	.53	177	Copy *B, L, ℒ, 𝒟, ℬ*
208	.46	178	Copy *pa, an, pro, pre, sti*
208	.43	182	Write *ba; da; back; pack*
208	.55	190	Tell me what you see here: *K, S, W, R, T*
208	.47	193	Read *juice; bread; bonfire; cloakroom; fertilizer*
208	.44	258	Discursive reasoning—elementary arithmetic problems

*r = correlation

Table 9.1: **Item Intercorrelations with Arithmetic Scale**   *Continued*

Item	r*	Item	Description
209	.41	12	Left hand fingers extended in sagittal plane touching chin
209	.42	95	Draw hands on blank clockfaces at 12:50, 4:35; 11:10
209	.43	119	Point with key toward pencil; point with pencil toward key
209	.41	129	If Arnie hit Tom, which boy was the victim?
209	.41	145	Read *see–seen; tree–trick*
209	.45	163	Say the days of the week backward starting with Sunday
209	.42	178	Copy *pa, an, pro, pre, sti*
210	.46	19	Point to your left eye with your right hand
210	.43	72	Determine whether stimulus is moving up or down right arm
210	.42	73	Same as #72 with left arm
210	.42	90	Name overlapping objects in pictures
210	.42	106	Phonetic hearing—conditioned reflex
210	.46	108	Point to eye; nose; ear
210	.46	110	Identify objects from pictures by pointing
210	.58	112	What do *cat, bat, pat* mean?
210	.47	113	Point to the picture that shows: typewriting; mealtime; summer
210	.44	115	Whose watch is this (examiner's)? Whose is this (patient's)?
210	.43	123	Draw a cross beneath a circle; draw a circle to the right of a cross
210	.57	124	Which is correct: Spring comes before summer, or Summer comes before spring?
210	.43	126	Which is correct: A fly is bigger than an elephant, or An elephant is bigger than a fly?
210	.44	129	If Arnie hit Tom, which boy was the victim?
210	.57	137	Repeat *hairbrush; screwdriver; laborious*
210	.52	142	Repeat *house–ball–chair*
210	.46	145	Read *see–seen; tree–trick*
210	.53	147	Read *house; table; apple*
210	.48	153	Read *house–ball–chair*
210	.51	159	Name objects from description

*r = correlation

Table 9.1: **Item Intercorrelations with Arithmetic Scale** *Continued*

Item	r*	Item	Description
210	.57	258	Discursive reasoning—elementary arithmetic problems
211	.36	112	What do *cat, bat, pat* mean?
211	.44	146	Read *cat; dog; man*
211	.35	260	Discursive reasoning—elementary arithmetic problems
212	.37	19	Point to your left eye with your right hand
212	.36	135	Repeat *see-seen; tree-trick*
212	.38	147	Read *house; table; apple*
212	.41	175	How many letters are there in: *cat; trap; banana; hedge*?
212	.42	176	Phonetic analysis; e.g., what is the second letter in *cat;* first letter in *match*?
212	.39	260	Discursive reasoning—elementary arithmetic problems
212	.35	268	Discursive reasoning—complex arithmetic problems
213	.35	16	Raise the same hand I do (left hand)
213	.36	51	If I knock hard, you knock gently; if I knock gently, you knock hard
213	.36	53	Determine which of two tones is higher
213	.41	159	Name objects from description
213	.42	176	Phonetic analysis; e.g., what is second letter in *cat;* first letter in *match*?
213	.44	188	What sound is made by these letters: *g–r–o; p–l–y*?
213	.38	189	What word is made by these letters: *s–t–o–n–e; k–n–i–g–h–t*?
213	.42	193	Read *juice; bread; bonfire; cloakroom; fertilizer*
213	.38	252	Concept formation—logical relationships
213	.37	260	Discursive reasoning—elementary arithmetic problems
213	.37	261	Time taken to solve item 260
214	.43	86	Name visually presented objects
214	.42	129	If Arnie hit Tom, which boy was the victim?
214	.42	146	Read *cat; dog; man*
214	.44	147	Read *house; table; apple*
214	.45	163	Say the days of the week backward starting with Sunday
214	.40	253	Concept formation—logical relationships
214	.41	258	Discursive reasoning—elementary arithmetic problems
214	.46	260	Discursive reasoning—elementary arithmetic problems
215	.38	59	How many beeps in all groups together?
215	.38	84	Stereognosis—left hand errors
215	.39	91	Name overlapping objects in pictures
215	.38	94	Tell me exactly what time these clocks tell: 7:53, 5:09, 1:25, 10:35
215	.42	95	Draw hands on blank clockface at: 12:50, 4:35, 11:10
215	.42	176	Phonetic analysis; e.g., what is the second letter in *cat;* first letter in *match*?
215	.45	178	Copy *pa, an, pro, pre, sti*
215	.44	223	Memory for seven words scored for errors
215	.40	236	Understanding of thematic pictures
215	.45	256	Verbal analogies
216	.37	59	How many beeps in all groups together?
216	.37	62	Reproduce rhythm
216	.37	90	Name overlapping objects in pictures
216	.38	129	If Arnie hit Tom, which boy was the victim?
216	.39	251	Concept formation—logical relationships
216	.36	252	Concept formation—logical relationships
216	.36	259	Discursive reasoning—elementary arithmetic problems
216	.38	260	Discursive reasoning—elementary arithmetic problems
216	.42	261	Discursive reasoning—elementary arithmetic problems
217	.36	10	Do as I do (place left hand under chin with fingers bent)
217	.37	94	Tell me exactly what time these clocks tell: 7:53, 5:09, 1:25, 10:35
217	.39	97	Intellectual operations in space

*r = correlation

Table 9.1: Item Intercorrelations with Arithmetic Scale   *Continued*

Item	r*	Item Description
217	.37	195 Read *insubordination; indistinguishable*
217	.39	264 Discursive reasoning—complex arithmetic problems
217	.38	268 Discursive reasoning—complex arithmetic problems
218	.39	21 Clench your right hand and extend fingers of left hand, then reverse
218	.42	84 Stereognosis—left hand errors
218	.44	92 Number of errors on tasks from Raven's Matrices
218	.45	95 Draw hands on blank clockface at: 12:50, 4:35, 11:10
218	.40	104 Repeat of sound triplets
218	.49	157 Name objects from pictures
218	.41	185 Write words and phrases
218	.47	223 Memory for seven words scored for error
218	.44	227 Draw geometric shapes from memory
218	.40	236 Understanding of thematic pictures
218	.46	254 Concept formation—logical relationships
218	.45	256 Concept formation—logical relationships
218	.46	257 Verbal analogies
218	.45	262 Discursive reasoning—elementary arithmetic problems
218	.43	268 Discursive reasoning—complex arithmetic problems
219	.42	84 Stereognosis—left hand errors
219	.43	90 Name overlapping objects in pictures
219	.43	91 Name overlapping objects in pictures
219	.44	95 Draw hands on blank clockface at: 12:50, 4:35, 11:10
219	.42	112 What do *cat, bat, hat* mean?
219	.43	113 Point to the picture that shows: typewriting; mealtime; summer
219	.42	159 Name objects from description
219	.44	163 Say the days of the week backward starting with Sunday
219	.44	189 What word is made by these letters: *s–t–o–n–e; k–n–i–g–h–t*?

Table 9.1: Item Intercorrelations with Arithmetic Scale   *Continued*

Item	r*	Item Description
219	.41	248 Concept formation—definition
219	.41	255 Concept formation—opposites
219	.47	257 Verbal analogies
219	.42	268 Discursive reasoning—complex arithmetic problems
220	.41	62 Reproduce rhythm
220	.40	63 Make series of taps of varying length and intensity
220	.42	95 Draw hands on blank clockface at: 12:50, 4:35, 11:10
220	.41	256 Verbal analogies
220	.36	261 Discursive reasoning—elementary arithmetic problems
220	.36	258 Discursive reasoning—complex arithmetic problems
221	.37	62 Reproduce rhythm
221	.40	94 Tell me exactly what time these clocks tell: 7:35, 5:09, 1:25, 10:35
221	.41	97 Intellectual operations in space
221	.40	99 Intellectual operations in space
221	.41	112 What do *cat, bat, pat* mean?
221	.41	175 How many letters are there in: *cat; trap; banana; hedge*?
221	.42	195 Read *insubordination; indistinguishable*
221	.44	223 Memory for seven words scored for errors
221	.42	230 Write words from memory after visual presentation
221	.41	234 Retention and retrieval—paragraphs
221	.41	247 Understanding of thematic texts
221	.43	248 Concept formation—definition
221	.41	250 Concept formation—comparison and differentiation
221	.49	256 Verbal analogies
221	.42	257 Verbal analogies
221	.46	264 Discursive reasoning—complex arithmetic problems
221	.49	268 Discursive reasoning—complex arithmetic problems

*r = correlation

Table 9.1: **Item Intercorrelations with Arithmetic Scale** *Continued*

Item	r*		Item Description
222	.42	94	Tell me exactly what time these clocks tell: 7:53, 5:09, 1:25, 10:35
222	.39	97	Intellectual operations in space
222	.38	175	How many letters are there in: *cat; trap; banana; hedge*?
222	.42	223	Memory for seven words scored for errors
222	.39	246	Understanding of thematic texts
222	.41	248	Concept formation—definition
222	.41	251	Concept formation—logical relationships.
222	.44	256	Verbal analogies
222	.41	264	Discursive reasoning—complex arithmetic problems
222	.43	268	Discursive reasoning—complex arithmetic problems

r = correlation

dysfunction bilaterally as often as in the left hemisphere only (Levin, 1979). Consequently, an inability to read or write numbers that is not an artifact of a neglected visual field strongly suggests a left parietal lesion but does not exclude involvement of the right hemisphere.

In the next section of the Arithmetic scale (items 210, 211), patients are asked to compare numbers with each other, an operation basic to the left parietal area. These items are significantly correlated with tasks involving other parietal as well as temporoparietooccipital functions, such as somatosensory abilities, visual identification, and spatial and reading skills. The tertiary parietal area disorders have been shown to significantly impair the understanding of relational words as well as arithmetic operations (McFie, 1969).

Dysfunction on items 212–214, problems most patients can do from memory, suggests either serious inability to understand what is being asked or severe left hemisphere damage, especially in the parietal area. Again, these items demonstrate significant correlations with items requiring phonetic analysis, visual-spatial

abilities, naming skills, and reading, receptive, and expressive speech skills, as well as complex discursive reasoning abilities. Parieto-occipital deficits, while not interfering with the ability to do well-practiced arithmetic problems requiring only memory and not arithmetic skill, do interfere with the ability to understand and manipulate arithmetic skills and processes (Benson & Wier, 1972; Luria, 1966, 1973). Severe attentional difficulties may also hamper performance on these items, which suggests left frontal involvement (Golden, 1978; Luria, 1973).

Items 215–217 involve more complex arithmetic problems that cannot be done from memory. They are closely associated with items requiring spatial skills, discursive reasoning abilities, concept formation, and somatosensory functioning. The parieto-occipital region of the left hemisphere is involved with the comprehending and manipulating of arithmetic concepts (Benson & Wier, 1972). Additionally, Cohn (1961) has noted that the tertiary right parietal zone is involved with arithmetic done mentally as well as with more basic spatial abilities. Therefore impaired performance on these items may reflect bilateral parietal lobe injury rather than simply left parietal damage.

Items 218, 219, and 220 require somewhat more difficult manipulations. Deficits here are often seen in people with limited education and are not considered as serious as deficits in other parts of the test (Golden, Purisch, & Hammeke, 1979). However, individuals with higher educational levels should be able to do them. Often a left parietal dysfunction in a highly educated patient will not be manifested until this section. The item intercorrelations suggest that performance of these items depends on intact visual analysis, concept formation, discursive reasoning, spatial abilities, stereognosis, and audioverbal and visual memory, as well as expressive and receptive language functions. That such items correlate highly with this section of the Arithmetic scale strongly suggests the potential involvement of all areas of the brain in arithmetic computations.

The last section of this scale (items 221, 222) involves

typical subtraction of serial sevens and serial thirteens. Extremely poor performance is usually connected with brain dysfunction, especially if the rest of the items on the Arithmetic scale have been performed relatively well and basic arithmetic skills appear to be intact. These two items correlate most highly with memory, concept formation, discursive reasoning, and spatial skills implicating involvement of temporoparieto-occipital regions (Benson & Wier, 1972; Golden, 1978; Luria, 1966, 1973; Warrington, Logue, & Pratt, 1971). Note that concentration difficulties may show up on these items even in the presence of normal arithmetic skills, which suggests left frontal lobe dysfunction (Golden, 1978; Luria, 1973).

Several localization studies for functional asymmetry imply that arithmetic skills are primarily served by the left hemisphere (e.g., Henschen, 1925; Hecaen, Angelergues, & Hocillier, 1961; Kinsbourne & Warrington, 1963; Sperry, 1968). The item intercorrelations seem to support this contention.

Factor Analysis

Factor analysis of the Arithmetic scale of the Luria-Nebraska reveals two emergent factors, as is seen in Table 9.2 (Golden, Purisch, & Hammeke, 1980). The first factor (Table 9.3) involves tasks that require the ability to do simple arithmetic calculations such as 27 + 8 or serial sevens. This factor represents basic arithmetic operations and may be so named.

The second factor (Table 9.4) largely involves items that test the patient's ability to write and read multidigit numbers. This factor loads heavily on two items, 204 and 205. Errors on these two items occur almost exclusively because the patient is unable to write 9845, 109, and 1023 correctly. The numbers are written 9 0 0 0 8 4 5 or 1 0 0 9 or 1 0 0 0 23 because their categorical structure is incorrectly comprehended. The other items loading on this factor are either tasks that require spatial abilities, such as item 203, in which the columns are reversed, or simple tasks like

Table 9.2: **Arithmetic Factor Structure**

Item	Factor 1	Factor 2
201	33	−72
202	62	−45
203	37	−77
204	60	−81
205	57	−60
206	31	−51
207	67	−50
208	51	−65
209	60	−69
210	50	−71
211	39	−50
212	55	−45
213	56	−44
214	56	−62
215	69	−45
216	54	−42
217	61	−34
218	66	−41
219	70	−53
220	59	−34
221	71	−36
222	69	−32

Table 9.3: **Items on Arithmetic Factor 1**

Loading	Item	Description
.62	202	Write the following roman numerals.
.60	204	Write these numbers.
.67	207	Read these numbers.
.60	209	There are three numbers on this card arranged from top to bottom. Read each number as a whole number.
.69	215	Solve these problems.
.61	217	Subtract the number above from the one below.
.66	218	What is the missing sign in these equations?
.70	219	What is the missing number in these equations?
.71	221	Serial sevens.
.69	222	Serial thirteens.

Table 9.4: **Items on Arithmetic Factor 2**

Loading	Item	Description
.72	201	Write these numbers.
.77	203	Write these numbers.
.81	204	Write these numbers.
.80	205	Write these numbers.
.65	208	Read the numbers on this card.
.69	209	There are three numbers on this card, arranged from top to bottom. Read each number as a whole number
.71	210	Tell me which number is larger.

item 201 that are missed only by those with severe mathematical deficits. The resultant factor, then, involves very basic comprehension of number meaning and structure.

Luria's theory of neuropsychological structure of arithmetic ability helps explain the factor structure of this section. The two predominant features of the arithmetic functional system that distinguish it from other functional systems are the ability to do arithmetic operations and the

ability to comprehend the meaning and structure of numbers.

These two factors have important localizing significance. The first, as a measure of basic arithmetic ability, represents left posterior parietal function. The second, as a test of basic spatial ability, is largely associated with the function of both hemispheres.

Summary

As can be seen from this chapter, the Arithmetic scale can be highly useful in localizing brain dysfunction in the left parietal and parieto-occipital areas. There are, however, indications that both the frontal and the temporal lobes, as well the right hemisphere, are involved in performance of these items. Additionally, as noted above, educational level and the patient's anxiety about mathematics can confound performance on this scale. It is clear that interpretation of deficits on the Arithmetic scale is not a simple matter. It can, however, be clarified to some degree by using information from other Luria scales to yield a more complete picture of the extent and nature of a deficit.

10. Memory

Memory constitutes one of the most thoroughly studied branches of the whole field of clinical psychology, and particularly of neuropsychology, yet there remains much we do not know about it. However, this chapter must be limited to the items on the Memory scale and the brain processes they appear to tap.

Recent work has suggested that memorizing is a complex process consisting of a series of stages that differ in their psychological structure, in the "volume" of memory traces capable of fixation, and in the duration of their storage. It has been suggested that memorization begins with the imprinting of multiple sensory cues. The process emphasizes the cues that are appropriate. Imprinting is thought to be very narrow in scope and to involve a very short duration of the imprinted traces.

The next step in the mnestic process is thought to be the transfer of stimuli to the stage of image memory, that is, perceptions are converted into visual images. However, this conversion is never simple, but requires that one select an appropriate image from all possible ones. This is the process of coding the stimuli. Luria (1973) notes that this is generally thought to be an intermediate stage, quickly followed by a final stage referred to as the complex coding of traces, or their inclusion in a system of categories. This system of categories forms multidimensional matrices in which the individual must place the memory. Such an approach demonstrates that memory is not passive but an active, ongoing process. A person wishing to recall information must employ a strategy that involves choosing the necessary means, differentiating between relevant and irrelevant information, selecting the appropriate sensory or logical components of the imprinted material, and ultimately fitting them into the appropriate systems (Luria, 1973).

In man, the highly organized process of recall is based on a complete system of mechanisms in the cortex and subcortex, each of which makes its own specific contribution to memory. Therefore the destruction or alteration of any one of these mechanisms may lead to a disturbance of the memory, but the exact symptoms will vary depending on which area of the brain is involved.

Investigation of the Learning Process

The Memory scale consists of 13 items (items 223–235) intended to assess a variety of aspects of memory.

In items 223–235 the patient is read a list of seven words and then asked to repeat as many as possible. After the first trial the patient is told how many of the seven words were remembered. Before repeating the procedure with the same words, the patient is asked to predict how many words will be remembered on this trial. This procedure is continued until the patient reaches the criterion of two consecutive perfect trials or until five trials have been performed.

A disturbance of higher cortical functions in individuals with localized brain injury may lead to significant changes in the process of learning, affecting both the quality and the character of the results obtained (Luria, 1966). Individuals with generalized, diffuse cerebral dysfunction and patients with injuries in the posterior half of the brain perform normally. When predicting the number of words they will remember, they consider their prior performance. In general their initial predictions are higher than their performance; later they become more accurate. But the amount of material they are capable of learning is less than for normal individuals.

Patients with frontal lesions can demonstrate grosser errors of prediction. Asked to predict the number of elements of the series they will memorize, they may reply without considering their abilities and prior performance. Such prediction may be static, never changing, or random. They will continue to repeat a mistake, making no corrections. They may also say the same word twice in a series, again with no apparent awareness of their error (Luria, 1966).

Retention and Retrieval

Item 226, the beginning of the second section of the scale, is a measure of visual, nonverbal memory with interference. The patient is to remember the distinguishing characteristic of a card after counting aloud to 100 between stimulus and retrieval.

Items 227–230 deal with immediate sensory trace recall. For item 227 the patient is briefly (7 seconds) shown a card with simple geometric figures on it and is then asked to reproduce as much of the design as possible from memory. The next item (228) involves reproducing a series of rhythmic taps. The patient is next asked to reproduce a series of three hand positions (item 229). In the last item of this series (230), the patient is shown a card with five words on it and asked to repeat the words after the card is removed.

Patients with deep lesions of the hemispheres involving the brainstem, thalamic nuclei, and pathways from the hypothalamus, mammillary bodies, and hippocampus perform poorly on such tasks (Christensen, 1975). Additionally, individuals with frontal lobe dysfunction will have difficulty and may seem confused and disoriented. These patients may be completely unaware of memory deficits. Their attention is easily distracted, which adds to their problems, since impressions are easily lost.

Luria (1973) notes that a fundamental condition for the "imprinting" of memory traces is maintenance of necessary cortical tone or excitation. Lowering of cortical tone can be a major factor interfering with memory. The work of Scoville, Milner, and Penfield (e.g., Scoville & Milner, 1957; Penfield & Milner, 1958) has demonstrated that, although bilateral hippocampal lesions do not interfere with higher memory functions, they do interfere with a patient's general ability to retain current experience in the face of interference, a disorder similar to the classic Korsakov's syndrome (Luria, 1973).

Studies of the brainstem and thalamic portions of the reticular formation have shown that the limbic areas of the brain are structures with an essential role in the regulation of cortical excitation. Thus dysfunction of these areas will lead to disturbance of memory (Luria, 1966).

The hippocampus does not respond to specific modalities but acts to compare current stimuli with traces of "past experience" (Luria, 1973). This area of the brain (medial zones of the cortex) therefore appears to play an important role in the retention of memory traces.

Luria (1973) describes three distinct features of memory dysfunction in the subcortex. First, the loss is not confined to any particular modality. Second, these disturbances affect the ability to sustain memory traces. Patients with mild problems often compensate for the deficit, such as by making notes of things to do. This is characteristic of patients with bilateral hippocampal lesions (Milner, 1958a, 1958b). The third feature is forgetfulness. This may be slight in mild cases, but in massive lesions it may lead to severe disturbances of consciousness that are never found with focal disorders of the cortex.

Retention and Retrieval of Words, Sentences, and Paragraphs

Disturbances of memory in patients with lesions of the lateral cortical areas differ from those found in patients with lesions of the medial zones of the cortex. These are never global and rarely lead to general disorders of consciousness. As a rule these disturbances tend to be limited to one modality or to impair goal-directed behavior (Luria, 1966).

A number of items on the Memory scale investigate the effect on memory functioning of this form of cortical lesion. In item 231 patients are asked to remember a set of three words and repeat them after an interval filled by heterogeneous activity (describing a picture). On item 232, patients are read two sets of three words. After hearing the second set of words they are asked to repeat the first set and then the second set (proactive and retroactive interference). They next are asked to retrieve the first and then

the second of two short sentences read to them in succession (item 233). On the final item of this section of the scale, patients are to reproduce a short story immediately after hearing it.

Patients with cerebral dysfunction that involves the deep parts of the hemispheres will have difficulty with these items. They typically are aware of their memory defects and function reasonably well in ordinary circumstances. However, difficulties arise when they are faced with interference.

In normal individuals, interference has little or no effect on recall. Patients with lesions of the deep zones of the brain will perform differently on each type of interference task. Such patients can easily recall three words, but the distraction of an interfering activity will result in memory impairment. If, after memorizing a group of three words, a second, similar group of words is memorized, such patients will be completely unable to recall the first set (Luria, 1973).

Specific disturbances of what Luria (1966) refers to as audiovisual memory are typical of lesions of the temporal cortex of the dominant hemisphere. Lesions of the left temporal or temporoparietal regions tend to cause difficulties in the retrieval of verbal-acoustic information (Luria, 1966). Patients can remember figures, but they have trouble with words presented auditorily. They may be able to understand the general meaning of a sentence and they are able to search memory normally, but they may substitute words (e.g., *Plymouth* for *Dodge*) (Luria, 1966).

Failure on these items may also arise owing to lesions of the "speech area," especially the tertiary temporoparietooccipital zone of the dominant hemisphere. Luria (1966, 1973) refers to such disturbances as amnestic aphasia. Here, the patient can easily retain nonverbal stimuli, even after interference but has trouble remembering specific words.

Memory disturbances also arise from lesions of the left parietal or left parieto-occipital region and are likely to become most obvious when a person tries to remember sentences and paragraphs (items 233, 234). Here the patient reproduces the general meaning of the story, but the grammatical structures are incorrect. This form of disorder is clearly manifested in literal and verbal paraphasias (Luria, 1973).

Memory deficits also result from dysfunction of the frontal lobes. Such patients may retain the initial part of a story but later may confabulate or complete the story incorrectly.

Logical Memorizing

In evaluating logical, or indirect, memorizing, which involves both memory and intellectual processes, one attempts to describe and define the active aids invoked in memorizing logical material.

Item 235, the final item on the Memory scale, evaluates logical memory through recall by visual aid. The patient is to retain seven orally presented words. As each word is presented, the patient is shown a picture. After all seven words and pictures have been presented, the patient is shown only the pictures, one at a time, and is asked to say the word that was paired with each.

Patients with localized cerebral dysfunction have no trouble doing this. With the aid of the picture, they easily remember the associated word. Aids like this can be used extensively in reeducation. It is only in patients with severe forms of generalized dementia and general disturbances of the memory processes that the selective logical connection may be lost (Luria, 1966).

Patients with injuries to the frontal lobes cannot select and use logical connections to aid them in memorization. The patient may associate the words with pictures that have nothing to do with them, even when the word and picture are clearly related. Direct description of picture content may also occur. Thus presenting the picture the second time does not remind the patient of the word. This logical relationship process is an important aspect of intellectual aids to memory.

Item Intercorrelations

As Table 10.1 shows, item intercorrelations between the items composing the Memory scale and all other Luria-Nebraska items yield several significant correlations, $r \geq .35$; $p < .0001$ (Golden and Berg, in press). Such information allows for a better and more specific understanding of the specific dysfunction represented by the inability to perform a given test item.

The first items on the scale (items 223-225) look at the patient's ability to both memorize a list of seven words and predict performance on this task. The ability to predict is, as noted earlier, a frontal lobe function. Not surprisingly, therefore, the items that correlate highly with this section of the Memory scale represent a number of frontal lobe functions, including motor movements and attention, as well as a variety of temporoparietal area functions such as spatial organization, arithmetic skills, and concept formation. Patients with tertiary frontal lobe dysfunction may have difficulty attending. They are often distracted by small noises or events that others can easily ignore (Luria, 1966). Consequently, performance may actually appear worse owing to distractibility (Golden, 1978).

Item 226, the second section of the scale, is a measure of visual, nonverbal memory with interference. This item demonstrates no significant correlations with items not on the Memory scale. As such, it may represent a fairly "pure" measure of nonverbal visual memory. Poor performance on this item may reflect a variety of disturbances. Patients with right temporal dysfunction have been found to be impaired on tasks requiring retention of nonverbal materials (Butters, 1979). Losses in the secondary area of the right temporal lobe may disturb analysis of visual patterns (Meier & French, 1965). Such a memory disturbance may also be a function of right occipital lobe injury, which may cause inattention as well as inability to appreciate unfamiliar visual patterns (Golden, 1978).

The hippocampal areas have been associated with memory acquisition (Corkin, 1965; DeJong, Itabashi, & Olson, 1969; Douglas & Pribram, 1966; Isaacson, 1972;

Table 10.1: **Item Intercorrelations with Memory Scale**

Item	r*	Item	Description
223	.43	1	Using your right hand, touch your fingers in turn with your thumb while you count them
223	.42	2	Same as #1 with left hand
223	.42	33	Rapid, repeated oral movements
223	.43	92	Number of errors on tasks from Raven's Matrices
223	.45	99	Intellectual operations in space
223	.46	155	Repeat sentences
223	.43	156	Repeat sentences
223	.42	200	Time taken to read paragraph
223	.44	215	How much is: 27 + 8; 44 + 57; 31 − 7; 44 − 14?
223	.47	218	What sign is missing? 10 ( ) 2 = 20; 10( )2 = 12; 10( )2 = 8; 10( )2 = 5
223	.42	222	Serial 13 subtraction from 100
223	.42	246	Understanding of thematic texts
223	.51	251	Concept formation—logical relationships
223	.44	254	Concept formation—logical relationships
223	.44	256	Verbal analogies
224	—		No correlations ≥.35 with items from other scales
225	.36	33	Rapid, repeated oral movements
225	.36	92	Number of errors on tasks from Raven's Matrices
225	.36	200	Time taken to read paragraph
225	.36	220	Mental computation
225	.38	221	Serial seven subtraction from 100
225	.39	251	Concept formation—logical relationships
226	—		No correlations ≥.35 with items from other scales
227	.45	1	Using your right hand, touch your fingers in turn with your thumb while you count them
227	.42	2	Same as #1 with left hand
227	.48	92	Number of errors on tasks from Raven's Matrices
227	.43	99	Intellectual operations in space
227	.40	105	Write speech sounds
227	.42	157	Name visually presented objects

Table 10.1: **Item Intercorrelations with Memory Scale**   *Continued*

Item	r*	Item	Description
227	.41	215	How much is: 27 + 8; 44 + 57; 31 − 7; 44 − 14?
227	.44	218	What sign is missing? 10 ( ) 2 = 20; 10( )2 = 12; 10( )2 = 8; 10( )2 = 5
227	.51	256	Verbal analogies
228	.37	33	Rapid, repeated oral movements
228	.35	48	Time taken to copy triangle
228	.39	62	Reproduce rhythm
228	.35	221	Serial seven subtraction from 100
228	.37	256	Verbal analogies
229	.36	92	Number of errors on tasks from Raven's Matrices
229	.38	99	Intellectual operations in space
229	.35	157	Name visually presented objects
229	.35	251	Concept formation—logical relationships
229	.38	256	Concept formation—verbal analogies
229	.36	257	Verbal analogies
230	.39	57	If I knock hard, you knock gently; if I knock gently, you knock hard
230	.40	112	What do *cat, bat, pat* mean?
230	.40	113	Point to the picture that shows: typewriting; mealtime; summer
230	.46	123	Draw a cross beneath a circle; draw a circle to the right of a cross
230	.38	137	Repeat *hairbrush; screwdriver; laborious*
230	.42	140	Repeat *streptomycin; Massachusetts Episcopal*
230	.39	159	Name objects from description
230	.38	185	Write words and phrases
230	.42	205	Write 14, 17, 19, 109, 1023
230	.42	210	Which is larger: 17 or 68; 23 or 56; 189 or 201?
230	.42	221	Serial seven subtraction from 100
230	.41	247	Understanding of thematic texts
230	.43	252	Concept formation—logical relationships
230	.42	256	Concept formation—verbal analogies
231	—		No correlations ≥.35 with items from other scales

*r = correlation

Table 10.1: **Item Intercorrelations with Memory Scale**   *Continued*

Item	r*	Item	Description
232	.40	54	Determine whether two groups of tones are same or different
232	.35	55	Reproduce pitch relationships
232	.35	92	Number of errors on tasks from Raven's Matrices
232	.38	137	Repeat *hairbrush; screwdriver; laborious*
232	.36	149	Read *rhinoceros; surveillance; hierarchy*
232	.35	176	Phonetic analysis; e.g., what is the second letter in *cat;* first letter in *match?*
232	.37	251	Concept formation—logical relationships
232	.35	256	Verbal analogies
233	.42	117	Conflicting instructions
233	.40	137	Repeat *hairbrush; screwdriver; laborious*
233	.38	142	Repeat *house–ball–chair; ball–chair–house*
233	.48	148	Read *hairbrush; screwdriver; laborious*
233	.43	221	Serial seven subtraction from 100
233	.38	222	Serial 13 subtraction from 100
233	.40	246	Understanding of thematic texts
233	.40	247	Understanding of thematic texts
233	.42	248	Concept formation—definition
233	.39	251	Concept formation—logical relationships
233	.41	256	Verbal analogies
234	.36	62	Reproduce rhythm
234	.36	90	Name overlapping objects in pictures
234	.45	92	Number of errors on tasks from Raven's Matrices
234	.39	117	Conflicting instructions
234	.36	218	What sign is missing? 10 ( ) 2 = 20; 10( )2 = 12; 10( )2 = 8; 10( )2 = 5
234	.41	221	Serial seven subtraction from 100
234	.43	244	Understanding of thematic texts
234	.38	245	Understanding of thematic texts
234	.37	246	Understanding of thematic texts
234	.39	247	Understanding of thematic texts
234	.40	248	Concept formation—definition
234	.38	249	Concept formation—comparison and differentiation

*r = correlation

Table 10.1: **Item Intercorrelations with Memory Scale**   *Continued*

Item	r*	Item	Description
234	.38	250	Concept formation—comparison and differentiation
234	.41	254	Concept formation—logical relationships
234	.38	256	Verbal analogies
234	.37	264	Discursive reasoning—complex arithmetic problems
235	.36	62	Motoric reproduction of rhythmic groups
235	.38	92	Number of errors on tasks from Raven's Matrices
235	.36	99	Intellectual operations in space
235	.38	149	Read *rhinoceros; surveillance; hierarchy*
235	.35	187	Number of words written in 60 seconds on a specific topic
235	.39	218	What sign is missing? 10 ( ) 2 = 20; 10( )2 = 12; 10( )2 = 8; 10( )2 = 5
235	.35	236	Understanding of thematic pictures
235	.38	241	Understanding of thematic pictures
235	.35	249	Concept formation—comparison and differentiation
235	.35	250	Concept formation—comparison and differentiation
235	.35	251	Concept formation—logical relationships
235	.39	254	Concept formation—logical relationships
235	.39	256	Verbal analogies

*r = correlation

Penfield & Milner, 1958). Bilateral hippocampal injury primarily results in deficits in the acquisition of new long-term memories (Penfield & Mathieson, 1974; Scoville & Milner, 1957). Such patients have trouble retaining new information. Although short-term memory remains intact if there is no interference, mental activity between learning and recall with no chance for rehearsal produces deficits (Drachman & Arbit, 1966; Drachman & Ommaya, 1964; Luria, 1971; Milner, 1968). These efforts are minimal when only one hippocamal gyrus is involved (McLardy, 1970). Left hippocampal lesions produce verbal memory deficits (Russell & Espir, 1961), while lesions of the right hippocampal zones can lead to impaired nonverbal spatial memory (Corkin, 1965; Milner, 1965).

Items 227–230 involve immediate sensory trace recall, examining visual memory, rhythmic memory, and tactile-visual memory. These items can be affected by both left and right hemisphere dysfunction but are more sensitive to right hemisphere dysfunction (Golden, Purisch, & Hammeke, 1979). This is especially true if these items are missed while the more verbal items on the scale are performed without difficulty. As would be expected, these items (227–230) demonstrated significant relationship with items requiring motor movements, spatial organization, visual naming, and writing and copying skills, as well as concept formation, arithmetic skills, and both expressive and receptive language skills. As a consequence, items 227–230 are probably best used as indicators of general level of sensory trace memory. However, the items appear to involve such diffuse aspects of brain functioning that they should not be heavily relied upon for localization or lateralization of cerebral dysfunction.

Items 231–234 measure verbal memory under varying forms of interference. Several difficulties in short-term memory, especially owing to injuries in the left hemisphere, are seen in those items (Golden, Purisch, & Hammeke, 1979). Injuries to the bilateral hippocampal areas, which cause losses in long-term memory coding, will also show problems on items that involve interference. The items within this section of the Memory scale demonstrate a strong relationship with motor abilities, the ability to analyze pitch and rhythmic series, spatial-organizational abilities, and arithmetic skills, as well as with higher-order abilities including the understanding of thematic texts, concept formation, and discursive reasoning. These abilities all require the capacity to concentrate, plan, and evaluate voluntary behavior. As such, they represent frontal lobe functions. The tertiary area of the frontal lobes is responsible for planning, structuring, and evaluating behavior (Golden, 1978). In adding, attentional deficits are frequently noted in patients with left frontal dysfunction,

as are extreme memory deficits, especially for verbal material (Luria, 1966).

The final item of the scale, item 235, measures the ability to associate a verbal stimulus with a picture. Performance here can be disrupted by either right or left hemisphere dysfunction and is sensitive to high-level disturbance in memory skills. This item correlates significantly with spatial organizational skills, motor skills, arithmetic skills, and the higher-level skills of understanding thematic texts and concept formation. All the tasks, as well as item 235, require attention, concentration, and some degree of mental flexibility. Frontal lobe injury can therefore affect performance on them all. The patient with left frontal damage may not be able to act on verbal instructions. Disorders of the tertiary right frontal areas may also hinder performance on like items, since such disorders can lead to impairment on complex spatial tasks (Teuber, 1963) and tasks requiring some aspects of nonverbal visual memory.

Factor Analysis

The Memory scale breaks down into two factors (Golden, Osmon, Sweet, Purisch, & Hammeke, 1980), as is seen in Table 10.2. The first factor (Table 10.3) represents immediate memory and tests the strength of memory trace impressions. The items loading on this factor all require rote repetition of the stimulus material within five seconds of presentation. The second factor (Table 10.4) consists of items that are more complicated in that the information must be organized or otherwise cognitively transformed upon recall. While two of the items require only simple repetition of the presented material, the recall is more elaborate than the simple verbal rote repetition of the first factor and necessitates higher-order cognitive abilities to reconstruct the information presented. If one looks at items 227 and 228, it can be seen that they constitute a neuropsychologically more demanding task, since the memory traces must be retained while the informa-

Table 10.2: **Memory Rotated Factor Matrix**

Item	Factor 1	Factor 2
223	77	41
224	22	26
225	62	37
226	13	17
227	44	51
228	35	31
229	11	67
230	56	27
231	38	34
232	60	24
233	63	19
234	43	52
235	38	60

Table 10.3: **Items on Memory Factor 1**

Loading	Item	Description
.77	223	Errors in learning list of seven words.
.62	225	Trials to learn list of seven words.
.56	230	Memorize words from card.
.60	232	Memory with retroactive and proactive inhibition.
.63	233	Sentence memory.

Table 10.4: **Items on Memory Factor 2**

Loading	Item	Description
.41	233	Errors in memorizing list of seven words.
.51	227	Match card in memory with present card.
.67	229	Memory for three finger positions.
.52	234	Memorize short story (logical memory).
.60	235	Memorize word-picture combinations.

tion is physically reconstructed. This is far more difficult than the repetition item in the first factor. For items 234 and 235, the information to be recalled must be interpreted and organized before being repeated.

Comparing performance of these two factors can provide important inferences about the intactness of the temporolimbic areas of the brain in reference to the rest of the cortex. Performance on the trace impression factor (factor 1) is directly related to the function of the temporolimbic areas of the brain, especially in the left hemisphere (Golden, Osmon, Sweet, Purisch, & Hammeke, 1980). When deficits occur, an unstable memory trace must be suspected. By contrast, the reconstructive factor (factor 2) appears to represent higher cortical functions. Thus, deficient performance on this factor and good performance on the first factor suggest more complex cognitive deficits arising from lesions of the cerebral cortical convexity. Such information can be particularly useful in evaluating dementia and other diffuse disorders that may have subcortical effects.

Summary

Overall, the Memory scale is most sensitive to impairments of verbal function because of its importance in a majority of the items. However, nonverbal dysfunction caused by right hemisphere injury shows up in a moderately elevated score on the Memory scale. Extremely high elevations are generally associated with either left hemisphere or bilateral dysfunction. Therefore it is important to look for the pattern of items missed before hypothesizing a possible lesion location. The item intercorrelations and factor analysis of the Memory scale help point out the complexity of memory functioning and underscore the need to look at the individual pattern of performance when interpreting deficits on this scale.

11. Intellectual Processes

Evaluating intellectual activity in individuals with cerebral dysfunction is one of the most complex tasks in clinical neuropsychology. Lesions in different cerebral locations may cause completely different forms of intellectual disturbance.

Intellectual activity is a particularly complex form of mental activity that occurs only where solving a task requires preliminary analysis and synthesis of the situation as well as special auxiliary operations. To investigate intellectual processes we must therefore create situations in which the individual has no ready-made or automatic, previously established means of responding. The patient must be made to analyze the situation, picking out its essential components and correlating them with each other, to formulate hypotheses, to develop a "strategy," and finally to select definite operations for dealing with (responding to) the situation.

Such tasks may be constructive in nature and take place in the concrete or "practical" plane, or they may be devised within a verbal system and take place as complex, discursive speech activity. In each instance, however, the task must be constructed in such a way that a significant portion of the process carried out by the individual is "clearly manifested" and is hence open to objective examination and qualitative analysis. A thorough investigation of the process by which problems are solved, achieved by presenting problems that offer the greatest mobility of change in the particular process, will yield a valid analysis of the factors underlying clinically observable disturbances.

Understanding of Thematic Pictures

Investigating a patient's comprehension of a topic expressed pictorially or verbally has long been widely used as a clinical method for studying intellectual processes. It has been employed extensively in psychiatric practice and under certain conditions may be used for the topical diagnosis of brain lesions. In this section of the Luria test (items 236–247) the patient is shown a picture or series of pictures illustrating a certain subject or is read a short story (parable) dealing with a general theme. Despite their different forms (pictorial vs. verbal), both tasks require analysis of the subject, identification of its essential elements, and synthesis of these elements to elicit the basic theme of the picture or story. To prevent the process of comprehension from deteriorating into the direct recognition of familiar material, the picture or story is structured so the patient cannot interpret it directly or by guessing from any one fragment. The themes of the pictures and stories used are of necessity relatively complex, with their meaning becoming clear only through special analytic-synthetic activity.

To test comprehension of thematic pictures, the patient is first shown pictures with simple and complicated themes (items 236, 237), and then is asked to describe what is occurring in each picture. The response is scored for inclusion of all essential details and actions. In items 238–240 the patient is given a series of pictures that illustrate the development of a certain event, then asked to arrange them in correct order so the theme conveyed makes sense. The last items of this section of the scale (242, 243) require the patient to view a picture or series of pictures and determine what is "comical" about them.

Poor performance on these items can yield evidence of general intellectual deterioration. It is well known that when patients with general intellectual dysfunction and organic dementia are asked to identify the theme of a picture, they typically can do no more than describe the directly perceived connection or the individual objects illustrated; they cannot express the deeper logical relationships brought out by the theme (Luria, 1966). Analysis of the general theme of a series of pictures is beyond them and is usually replaced by simple descriptions of the individual picture(s), each considered apart from the others (Luria, 1966).

Individuals with latent forms of visual agnosia (particularly simultaneous agnosia), arising in association with lesions of the occipital regions, may have consider-

able trouble understanding thematic pictures though they have no true intellectual deterioration (Luria, 1966). They will be unable to grasp the whole situation illustrated in the picture at a glance or to carry out visual synthesis. Such individuals thus may be unable to see all the objects in a picture together or to establish the associations depicted visually (Luria, 1966).

Some patients can understand the details of a picture but not evaluate its theme. This is sometimes encountered with lesions of the right hemisphere, but Luria (1966, 1973) notes that the precise nature of such lesions has not yet been clarified.

Patients with various aphasic disorders also typically have trouble understanding thematic pictures. Gross disturbances in the comprehension of thematic pictures also may be found in individuals with frontal lobe lesions. These patients cannot analyze the picture or subsequently synthesize its details, and so they reach impulsive conclusions based solely on perception and identification of fragments of the picture (Luria, 1966).

The ability to analyze a series of pictures that develop a specific theme is usually impaired severely in patients with frontal lobe lesions (Luria, 1966). Luria further notes that these individuals are particularly likely to consider each aspect of the picture separately. They may personalize what they see ("This is my mother"). Distinguishing features are the confidence with which they reach their false conclusions and the difficulty of making them doubt them (Luria, 1966, 1973). This is an important indicator of intent and result, characteristic of the frontal syndrome (Golden, 1978).

Understanding of Thematic Texts

Items designed to investigate the comprehension of thematic texts are similar in nature and importance to those used for thematic pictures. The patient is asked to "analyze" passages in various ways. The items typically contain a number of essential as well as nonessential details.

Thus the patient must identify and synthesize the essential parts in order to understand the principal theme. These items (244–247) are also entirely verbal.

The first item in this series (item 244) examines the patient's understanding of complete texts. The text used is relatively short and is simple in grammatical structure, but the meaning to be determined is fairly subtle. The patient is asked to identify essential components of the text, to synthesize them, to inhibit or delay premature conclusions, and to deduce the general meaning of the text.

In the next items (245, 246), the individual is asked to explain the meaning of well-known metaphors ("iron hand," "green thumb") and proverbs ("Don't count your chickens before they have hatched"). The final item of this section of the scale (item 247) allows a somewhat closer inspection of the individual's ability to analyze metaphors. The item uses a proverb and several phrases, of which some contain words that sound like those of the proverb but have a different meaning and one expresses the meaning of the proverb using different words. Here the patient is asked to select the phrase closest in meaning to the proverb.

Individuals with generalized organic defects of the brain cannot perform the necessary analysis or do more than understand the meaning of each separate fragment. Luria (1966) notes that as a rule these patients simply relate the fragments, showing no appreciation of the general theme.

Disturbances like those noted above are found in patients with generalized lesions that give rise to an acute hypertensive-hydrocephalic syndrome (Luria, 1966), but these patients do not exhibit a fixed lowering of intellectual functioning. Frequently they have difficulty in retaining any type of material, which becomes increasingly evident as the passage to be read becomes longer.

Considerable difficulties in textual understanding may be experienced by patients with semantic aphasia or other amnestic-aphasic disorders (Luria, 1966). The limitations to understanding are naturally influenced by the length of the passage, the number of details it contains, and the complexity of the logical-grammatical relations involved. A patient who has a limited range of operations or has trouble grasping logical and grammatical relations is unable to grasp the fundamental theme of the text. Generally, however, individuals with semantic aphasia attempt to compensate by making a prolonged and systematic analysis of the text. Since they have no primary difficulty in comprehending metaphors, they can understand both the general theme of the text and any subsidiary themes. By contrast, any complex logical-grammatical constructions present immense difficulties for them (Luria, 1966).

In amnestic-aphasic disturbances, the problems with relating the components of any long passage are made worse by loss of word comprehension or by a general inability to remember a series of phrases. Attempts to comprehend a given text can be successful only when the patient is able to adjust for his basic defect, but the process is tedious and prolonged. The patient can, in the long run, understand both the general theme of a text and its emotional tone.

Those who have sustained frontal lobe dysfunction are incapable of the sustained activity required for these intellectual tasks. A patient with marked frontal lobe dysfunction replaces systematic analysis of a text with impulsive guesses. Very often, uncontrollable, irrelevant associations are superimposed on such guesses. As a result, a series of irrelevant associations and perseverations replaces analysis, making understanding impossible. These individuals can understand a metaphor only if the corresponding associations are firmly established by experience.

Investigation of Concept Formation

The process by which abstract ideas are formed has been studied extensively. Luria (1966) notes that for a time it was felt that, because of the complexity of intellectual operations, they are disturbed by any brain lesions, the assumption being that a cerebral lesion impairs all complex forms of cortical activity. While it is difficult to object to this as a general concept, the inference that intellectual activity is disturbed by every brain lesion is not at all true and detracts from the correct analysis of the mechanisms underlying such disturbance (Luria, 1966).

It is known that, though a general failure in cerebral process impairs abstract intellectual activity, most cases of focal brain damage may cause such deficits secondarily. In general, disturbance of an individual's intellectual activity cannot arise directly from subcortical lesions or from lesions localized to the sensorimotor, auditory, or visual cortex. When such difficulties do occur, they must be regarded as a consequence of other damage from these lesions (Luria, 1966).

In the Luria-Nebraska test, a variety of the more abstract intellectual operations are examined. Items 248–257 investigate various aspects of concept formation. In item 248, the patient is asked to define words that denote various ideas. Of interest here is the patient's ability to use abstract categories. It is noteworthy when definitions are framed only in terms of particular objects and concrete situations.

Other items investigating mental activity involve comparison and differentiation of ideas (items 249, 250). In these items the patient is to compare two ideas, finding their commonalities, then to designate them by a single word (e.g., table and sofa are both furniture). Or the difference between them may have to be discerned (e.g., a fox is a wild animal, a dog is a domestic animal). Particular attention must be paid to the extent of generalization in the patient's classification.

The next group of items in this scale involve logical relationships. In item 251 the patient must relate each word in a given series to a more general category (e.g., a trout is a fish); conversely, in item 252 a general term must be related to a more particular idea (e.g., an animal might be a cow).

Similar operations are required in items 253 and 254, where the patient is to find the parts of a whole and to construct the whole from its parts. Next, the patient is

given a word and must state its opposite (e.g., *high–low*). In these items it is important to determine whether the patient performs the operations easily, whether random associations appear, and whether there is perseveration across items.

The final items of this section of the scale (256, 257) concern analogies. Along with a pair of words bearing a definite relationship to each other, the patient is given a third word and must find a fourth bearing the same relationship to it as the second bears to the first (e.g., *high–low; good–?*). The examiner observes the extent to which the patient grasps the necessary principle, transfers it to the solution of the new problems, and, particularly important, changes from one task to another without reproducing a relationship previously established. Item 257 requires the patient to determine which of four words does not belong (bears no relationship) with the other three. The examiner notices how well the patient grasps the instruction and is able to make a true classification of objects on the basis of their relation to a definite category.

Various forms of organic deterioration of mental processes may be revealed by the items used to investigate the formation of concepts. These deficiencies may appear as a deficit in abstract skills or as a lowering of intellectual level to the simplest and most concrete types of functioning.

Highly characteristic disturbances in operations involving abstract relationships are seen in patients with frontal lobe lesions. The basic feature of the intellectual disorder in such patients is the loss of selectivity and the prevalence of irrelevant associations or stereotypes. Patients with marked frontal lobe dysfunction may briefly exhibit apparent integrity of the processes involved in the establishment of fundamental abstract relationships; when it fails, these relationships are replaced by past learning, random associations, or perseverations from previous items (Luria, 1966).

Impairments in abstract intellectual activity that are based on speech often occur secondary to sensory and motor aphasia. Luria (1966) has observed that patients with these forms of aphasia are unable to operate with complex systems of speech associations, so that intellectual operations that are purely verbal in nature cannot be investigated. When these restrictions are removed, however, such individuals regain their ability to abstract. Within the limits of their ability, they can grasp logical relationships that, though developed on the basis of speech, have required some degree of speech independence.

The final items of the Intellectual Processes scale (items 258–269) deal with discursive reasoning that requires inhibition of all digressions and subordination of all operations to the final goal. This section consists of arithmetic problems, beginning at an elementary level (258–263) and concluding with complex tasks (items 264–269). The items at the elementary level can be solved either by simple addition and subtraction or by a simple intermediate operation. The complex arithmetic items, which are initially easy, requires that the individual adhere to the propositions and carry out sequential analysis. The final items of the section are complex tasks in which the patient must formulate and solve a series of intermediate problems.

Lesions of the left inferoparietal and parieto-occipital regions of the cortex, accompanied by simultaneous agnosia, construction difficulty, and semantic aphasia, may affect arithmetic operations and interfere with the patient's ability to survey all the conditions of the problem at the same time. Such an individual therefore cannot grasp the conditions at once but studies them piecemeal for a long time. If allowed to write the problem out so it can be broken up into its component parts, the patient may be able to solve it, but he or she cannot perform the problem mentally (Luria, 1966).

Different defects are observed during solution in patients with lesions of the temporal lobes and those with manifestations of acoustic aphasia. The instability of word meanings, with their meaning easily lost, and quick memory loss are the main difficulties. For this reason, the required sequence of analysis remains beyond the patient's grasp. If a patient with what Luria (1966) refers to as the amnestic variant of temporal aphasia is given a short enough problem, or if its components are reinforced by concrete aids, powers of solution are far greater than would normally be expected (Luria, 1966).

A different picture is seen in individuals with frontal lobe dysfunction. They generally are able to repeat the elements of a problem rather easily, but the elements cannot be analyzed properly and may give rise to irrelevant associations and processes. Although there is typically no appreciable defect in simple arithmetic operations, such patients generally focus on one aspect of the problem, calculating on the basis of this limited inference. Thus, while they may solve the simplest problems, they have great difficulty with those incorporating an intermediate operation not specified in the instructions. They do not solve the problem correctly, but simply add or subtract the numbers it contains. Even if the solution is explained a number of times, these patients continue to approach a problem in the same fashion. This inability to profit by instruction is a characteristic sign of disintegration of the general behavior pattern in patients with frontal lobe damage (Luria, 1966).

Diffuse brain lesions associated with acutely increased intracranial pressure or vascular insufficiency may lead to appreciable difficulties in discursive reasoning. However, these disturbances tend to be unstable and vary significantly with the patient's general condition.

Item Intercorrelations

A series of item intercorrelations between the Intellectual Processes scale and all other Luria-Nebraska items yields numerous significant correlations ($r \geq .35; p < .0001$), as can be seen in Table 11.1. The intercorrelations demonstrate that the items that constitute the Intellectual Processes scale tap a wide variety of cerebral functions.

All items on this scale have been selected because they are able to discriminate between brain-injured and normal

Table 11.1: **Item Intercorrelations with Intellectual Scale**

Item	r*	Item	Description
236	.43	87	Name objects from pictures
236	.36	90	Name overlapping objects in pictures
236	.36	112	What do *cat; bat; pat* mean?
236	.35	113	Point to the picture that shows: typewriting; mealtime; summer
236	.36	157	Name objects from pictures
236	.40	215	How much is: 27 + 8; 44 + 57; 31 − 7; 44 − 14?
236	.40	218	What sign is missing? 10 ( ) 2 = 20; 10 ( ) 2 = 12; 10 ( ) 2 = 8; 10 ( ) 2 = 5
236	.38	223	Memory for words
236	.35	235	Logical memory—recalling by visual aid
237	—		No correlations ≥.35 with items from other scales
238	.35	232	Retention and retrieval—homogeneous interference
238	.35	235	Logical memory—recalling by visual aid
239	.35	85	Stereognosis—left hand time
239	.40	157	Name objects from pictures
239	.35	235	Logical memory—recalling by visual aid
240	—		No correlations ≥.35 with items from other scales
241	.38	84	Stereognosis—left hand errors
241	.35	85	Stereognosis—left hand time
241	.36	99	Intellectual operations in space
241	.44	157	Name objects from pictures
241	.37	235	Logical memory—recalling by visual aid
242	—		No correlations ≥.35 with items from other scales
243	—		No correlations ≥.35 with items from other scales
244	.37	90	Name objects from pictures
244	.35	126	Which is correct: A fly is bigger than an elephant, or An elephant is bigger than a fly?
244	.35	129	If Arnie hit Tom, which boy was the victim?
244	.36	132	Logical grammatical structure—complex structures
244	.36	179	Write words from memory after visual presentation
244	.35	196	Read *astrocytoma; hemopoiesis*
244	.36	199	Read paragraph—score for errors
244	.37	233	Retention and retrieval—sentences
244	.43	234	Retention and retrieval—paragraphs
245	.35	199	Read paragraph—score for errors
245	.35	200	Read paragraph—score for time
245	.36	202	Write IV and VI; IX and XI
245	.35	207	Read IV, VI, IX, XI; 17, 71, 69, 96
245	.36	222	Serial 13 subtraction from 100
245	.32	223	Memory for seven words scored for errors
245	.39	233	Retention and retrieval—sentences
245	.38	234	Retention and retrieval—paragraphs
246	.39	222	Serial 13 subtraction from 100
246	.42	223	Memory for seven words scored for errors
246	.39	233	Retention and retrieval—sentences
246	.37	234	Retention and retrieval—paragraphs
247	.37	52	Determine whether two tones are same or different
247	.38	53	Determine which of two tones is higher
247	.37	59	How many beeps in all groups together?
247	.40	63	Reproduce rhythm
247	.37	90	Name overlapping objects in pictures
247	.36	92	Number of errors on tasks from Raven's Matrices
247	.38	123	Draw a cross beneath a circle; draw a circle to the right of a cross
247	.37	129	If Arnie hit Tom, which boy was the victim?
247	.39	148	Read *hairbrush; screwdriver; laborious*
247	.41	151	Read *streptomycin; Massachusetts Episcopal*
247	.39	156	Reflective speech—sentences
247	.39	159	Name objects from description
247	.38	178	Copy *pa, an, pro, pre, sti*
247	.43	195	Read *insubordination; indistinguishable*

*r = correlation

Table 11.1: **Item Intercorrelations with Intellectual Scale**

Item	r*	Item	Description
247	.38	219	What number is missing? 12 − ( ) = 8; 12 + ( ) = 19
247	.41	221	Serial seven subtraction from 100
247	.41	223	Memory for words
247	.41	230	Write words from memory after visual presentation
247	.40	233	Retention and retrieval—sentences
247	.39	234	Retention and retrieval—paragraphs
248	.38	59	How many beeps in all groups together?
248	.41	123	Draw a cross beneath a circle; draw a circle to the right of a cross
248	.39	202	Write IV and VI; XI and IX
248	.42	207	Read IV, VI, IX, XI; 17, 71, 69, 96
248	.39	215	How much is: 27 + 8; 44 + 57; 31 − 7; 44 − 14?
248	.41	219	What is the missing number? 12 − ( ) = 8; 12 + ( ) = 19
248	.44	221	Serial seven subtraction from 100
248	.41	222	Serial 13 subtraction from 100
248	.41	223	Memory for words
248	.42	233	Retention and retrieval—sentences
248	.40	234	Retention and retrieval—paragraphs
249	.37	219	What number is missing? 12 − ( ) = 8; 12 + ( ) = 19
249	.37	223	Memory for seven words scored for errors
249	.37	234	Retention and retrieval—paragraphs
249	.35	235	Logical memory—recalling by visual aid
250	.36	207	Read IV, VI, IX, XI; 17, 71, 69, 96
250	.37	218	What sign is missing? 10 ( ) 2 = 20; 10 ( ) 2 = 20; 10 ( ) 2 = 8; 10 ( ) 2 = 5
250	.41	221	Serial seven subtraction from 100
250	.41	222	Serial 13 subtraction from 100
250	.41	223	Memory for seven words scored for errors
250	.37	234	Retention and retrieval—paragraphs
251	.37	40	Draw a triangle
251	.40	58	Tell me how many beeps you hear
251	.45	82	Stereognosis—right hand errors
251	.42	112	What do *cat, bat, pat* mean?
251	.41	117	Simple sentences—conflicting instructions
251	.43	159	Name objects from description
251	.41	176	Phonetic analysis; e.g., what is the second letter in *cat;* first letter in *match*?
251	.43	185	Write words and phrases
251	.42	205	Write 14, 17, 19, 109, 1023
251	.47	207	Read IV, VI, IX, XI; 17, 71, 69, 96
252	.37	48	If I knock once, you knock twice; if I knock twice, you knock once
252	.37	82	Stereognosis—right hand errors
252	.40	129	If Arnie hit Tom, which boy was the victim?
252	.43	159	Name objects from pictures
252	.41	204	Write 27, 34, 158, 396, 9845
252	.41	205	Write 14, 17, 19, 109, 1023
252	.40	223	Memory for words
253	.36	58	Determine number of beeps in each group
253	.35	71	Two-point tactile discrimination—left hand
253	.37	92	Number of errors on tasks from Raven's Matrices
253	.39	138	Repeat *rhinoceros; surveillance; hierarchy*
253	.38	195	Read *insubordination; indistinguishable*
253	.41	204	Write 27, 34, 158, 396, 9845
253	.38	205	Write 14, 17, 19, 109, 1023
253	.40	214	How much is: 7 − 4; 8 − 5?
253	.40	234	Retention and retrieval—paragraphs
254	.35	117	Simple sentences—conflicting instructions
254	.36	132	Logical grammatical structure—complex structure
254	.40	144	Read *sp, th, pl, str, awk*
254	.40	148	Read *hairbrush; screwdriver; laborious*
254	.39	151	Read *streptomycin; Massachusetts Episcopal*
254	.38	189	What word is made by these letters: *s–t–o–n–e; k–n–i–g–h–t*?

*r = correlation

Table 11.1: **Item Intercorrelations with Intellectual Scale**

Item	r*	Item	Description
254	.39	195	Read *insubordination; indistinguishable*
254	.45	202	Write IV and VI; IX and XI
254	.40	215	How much is: 27 + 8; 44 + 57; 31 − 7; 44 − 14?
254	.45	218	What sign is missing? 10 ( ) 2 = 20; 10( )2 = 12; 10( )2 = 8; 10( )2 = 5
254	.44	223	Memory for words
254	.41	234	Retention and retrieval—paragraphs
254	.39	235	Logical memorizing—recalling by visual aid
255	.41	72	Determine whether stimulus is moving up or down right arm
255	.40	90	Name overlapping objects in pictures
255	.42	113	Point to the picture that shows: typewriting; mealtime; summer
255	.42	138	Repeat *rhinoceros; surveillance; hierarchy*
255	.50	159	Name objects from description
255	.40	205	Write 14, 17, 19, 109, 1023
255	.41	219	What number is missing? 12 − ( ) = 8; 12 + ( ) = 19
256	.41	21	Clench your right hand and extend fingers of left hand, then reverse
256	.41	22	Tap your right hand twice and your left hand once as quickly as you can
256	.42	59	How many beeps in all groups together?
256	.40	62	Reproduce rhythms
256	.41	99	Intellectual operations in space
256	.42	123	Draw a cross beneath a circle; draw a circle to the right of a cross
256	.46	144	Read *sp, th, pl, str, awk*
256	.41	157	Name objects from pictures
256	.41	173	Rearrange words on card to make a meaningful sentence
256	.41	176	Phonetic analysis; e.g., what is the second letter in *cat*; first letter in *match*?
256	.41	199	Read paragraph—score for errors
256	.40	200	Read paragraph—score for time
256	.43	204	Write 27, 34, 158, 396, 9845
256	.45	219	What number is missing? 12 − ( ) = 8; 12 + ( ) = 19
256	.41	220	How much is 27 + 34 + 14; 158 + 396?
256	.50	221	Serial seven subtraction from 100
256	.44	222	Serial 13 subtraction from 100
256	.44	223	Memory for seven words scored for errors
256	.41	233	Retention and retrieval—sentences
257	.41	60	How many beeps in each group
257	.41	107	Determine whether two letters you hear are the same or different
257	.40	157	Name objects from pictures
257	.46	18	What sign is missing? 10 ( ) 2 = 20; 10( )2 = 12; 10( )2 = 8; 10( )2 = 5
257	.48	219	What number is missing? 12 − ( ) = 8; 12 + ( ) = 19
257	.42	221	Serial seven subtraction from 100
258	.45	72	Determine whether stimulus is moving up or down right arm
258	.47	73	Same as #72 with left arm
258	.47	108	Point to eye; nose; ear
258	.44	110	Identify objects from pictures by pointing
258	.45	112	What do *cat; bat; pat* mean?
258	.46	113	Point to the picture that shows: typewriting; mealtime; summer
258	.44	136	Repeat *house; table; apple*
258	.47	162	Tell me the days of the week
258	.50	201	Write 7-9-3; 3-5-7
258	.51	203	Write 17 and 71; 69 and 96
258	.43	204	Write 27, 34, 158, 396, 9845
258	.43	205	Write 14, 17, 19, 109, 1023
258	.59	206	Read 7-9-3; 3-5-7
258	.44	208	Read 27, 34, 158, 396, 9845
259	.37	86	Name visually presented objects
259	.38	129	If Arnie hit Tom, which boy was the victim?
259	.42	205	Write 14, 17, 19, 109, 1023
259	.40	207	Read IV, VI, IX, XI; 17, 71, 69, 96

*r = correlation

Table 11.1: **Item Intercorrelations with Intellectual Scale**

Item	r*	Item	Description
259	.40	208	Read 27, 34, 158, 396, 9845
260	.48	72	Determine whether stimulus is moving up or down right arm
260	.43	73	Same as #72 with left arm
260	.36	147	Read *house; table; apple*
260	.42	210	Which is larger: 17 or 68; 23 or 56; 189 or 201?
260	.39	212	How much is: 3×3; 5×4; 7×8?
260	.45	214	How much is: $7 - 4$; $8 - 5$?
260	.39	216	On this card the numbers are arranged up and down. Add them in your head: $5 + 9 + 7$
261	.36	25	Pretend you are holding a teapot; show me how to pour and stir tea
261	.38	59	How many beeps in all groups together?
261	.41	90	Name overlapping objects in pictures
261	.37	106	Phonetic hearing—conditioned reflex
261	.39	112	What do *cat, bat, pat* mean?
261	.39	128	Logical grammatical structures—comparative constructions
261	.42	129	If Arnie hit Tom, which boy was the victim?
261	.46	159	Name objects from description
261	.39	204	Write 27, 34, 158, 396, 9845
261	.43	205	Write 14, 17, 19, 109, 1023
261	.43	207	Read IV, VI, IX, XI; 17, 71, 69, 96
261	.42	210	Which is larger: 17 or 68; 23 or 56; 189 or 201?
261	.42	216	On this card the numbers are arranged up and down. Add them in your head: $5 + 9 + 7$
262	.41	99	Intellectual operations in space
262	.45	218	What sign is missing? 10 ( ) 2 = 20; 10( )2 = 12; 10( )2 = 8; 10( )2 = 5
262	.39	227	Draw geometric shapes from memory after visual presentation
262	.39	234	Retention and retrieval—paragraphs
263	—		No correlations ≥.35 with items from other scales
264	.36	215	How much is: 27 + 8; 44 + 57; 31 − 7; 44 − 14?

Table 11.1: **Item Intercorrelations with Intellectual Scale**

Item	r*	Item	Description
264	.39	220	How much is: 27 + 34 + 14; 158 + 396?
264	.46	221	Serial seven subtraction from 100
264	.41	222	Serial 13 subtraction from 100
264	.38	223	Memory for seven words scored for errors
264	.38	233	Retention and retrieval—sentences
264	.37	234	Retention and retrieval—paragraphs
265	.39	221	Serial seven subtraction from 100
265	.37	222	Serial 13 subtraction from 100
266	.36	218	What sign is missing? 10 ( ) 2 = 20; 10( )2 = 12; 10( )2 = 8; 10( )2 = 5
266	.40	221	Serial seven subtraction from 100
266	.46	222	Serial 13 subtraction from 100
267	—		No correlations ≥.35 with items from other scales
268	.35	58	Tell me how many beeps you hear
268	.42	97	Intellectual operations in space
268	.39	99	Intellectual operations in space
268	.35	175	How many letters are in: *cat; trap; banana; hedge*?
268	.39	176	Phonetic analysis; e.g., what is the second letter in *cat;* first letter in *match*?
268	.36	198	Read sentences
268	.41	202	Write IV and VI; IX and XI
268	.39	207	Read IV, VI, IX, XI; 17, 71, 69, 96
268	.45	215	How much is: 27 + 8; 44 + 57; 31 − 7; 44 − 14?
268	.43	218	What sign is missing? 10 ( ) 2 = 20; 10( )2 = 12; 10( )2 = 8; 10( )2 = 5
268	.42	219	What number is missing? 12 − ( ) = 8; 12 + ( ) = 19
268	.49	221	Serial seven subtraction from 100
268	.43	22	Serial 13 subtraction from 100
269	.36	83	Stereognosis—right hand time
269	.36	86	Name visually presented objects
269	.37	210	Which is larger: 17 or 68; 23 or 56; 189 or 201?

*r = correlation

*r = correlation

Table 11.1: **Item Intercorrelations with Intellectual Scale**

Item	r*	Item	Description
269	.38	218	What sign is missing? 10 ( ) 2 = 20; 10 ( ) 2 = 12; 10 ( ) 2 = 8; 10 ( ) 2 = 5
269	.39	219	What number is missing? 12 − ( ) = 8; 12 + ( ) = 19
269	.38	227	Draw geometric shapes from memory after visual presentation

*r = correlation

patients. This differentiates the items on this scale from items on a test such as the Wechsler Adult Intelligence Scale (WAIS), in which many of the items are not sensitive to the presence of brain dysfunction. Thus, rather than giving a level of intelligence that can be associated with a person's learning history, the items on the Intellectual Processes scale tend to assess the person's functional intelligence. In general, the functional level at which the brain-injured patient is currently performing is probably less than his or her intelligence as measured by the WAIS. In the person without brain injury, the estimates of intelligence by the two tests seem approximately equal below an IQ of about 120 (the upper limit for the Luria-Nebraska).

The initial items in the Intellectual Processes scale (items 236–243) involve understanding of thematic pictures. These items are often missed in full by patients with frontal lobe dysfunction that interferes with interpretation of verbal schemes (Golden, Purisch, & Hammeke, 1979). Deficits in visual scanning also can be seen, in which patients cannot appreciate the complexity of a picture and thus tend to focus on one area. Luria (1966) presents a detailed analysis of the type of visual movements present in various types of brain disorders, such as injuries to the premotor areas of the frontal lobes and injuries to the occipital cortex.

The items of this section (236–243) correlate with a number of other Luria items that tap both left and right hemisphere functions, including visual naming, mental arithmetic skills, audioverbal and visual memory,

stereognosis, and visual-spatial organization. The tertiary right parietal area plays a major role in basic spatial abilities (DeRenzi & Faglioni, 1967; Piercy & Smyth, 1962; Warrington & James, 1967). It is also involved with arithmetic done mentally, in which numbers must be spatially aligned (Cohn, 1961). Disorders of the left occipital lobe may cause inability to appreciate a complex figure or picture because only one part of the stimulus material can be seen. Also, injuries to this area may disrupt motor movements of the eyes, so the patient has trouble scanning the visual field or directing attention to important details (Bender, Postel, & Krieger, 1957; Cumming, Hurwitz, & Perl, 1970). Injuries to the right frontal areas have reportedly resulted in impairment on spatial tasks (Teuber, 1963; Corkin, 1965; Milner, 1971).

Items 244–247 require an understanding of thematic texts. This section of the scale is quite similar to the initial section except that it is more verbal. Again, these items are closely related to items reflecting both left and right hemispheric function, including both expressive and receptive speech functions, writing skills, reading skills, visual naming, audioverbal and visual memory, arithmetic skills, spatial organization, and acoustic analysis. The left temporoparietal area in the region of the angular gyrus plays an important role in many speech processes. As we noted earlier, this area acts as an "integration center" for information from multiple sensory modalities. Disorders here may result in a loss of reading and writing skills as well as impairment of the ability to associate names to objects (Butters & Brody, 1969). Lesions in this area also interfere with verbal memory (Warrington, Logue, & Pratt, 1971). Lesions of the tertiary frontal areas of the left hemisphere may cause speech difficulties (Zangwill, 1966). Both left and right parieto-occipital dysfunction can impair spatial skills.

Items 248–257 deal with various aspects of concept formation. All these items are highly dependent upon intact language functioning and are thus susceptible to posterior left hemisphere disorders. Left frontal lobe injury will also cause difficulty on these items, not only because they depend on speech but also because of the frontal lobes' general involvement in all forms of higher behavior. Luria (1966) has suggested that frontal lobe injuries, particularly those on the left, may result in thinking disorders because they interfere with internal speech, which he believes is the basis for thought. The tertiary area of the frontal lobes is responsible for planning, structuring, and evaluating voluntary behavior, and severe damage will cause volitional behavior in general to disintegrate. It is not surprising, therefore, that the significant intercorrelations with items 248–257 reflect virtually the entire spectrum of brain functioning: motor skills, acoustic analysis, tactile functions, visual-spatial organization, receptive and expressive speech, attention, concentration, writing and reading skills, arithmetic abilities, and audioverbal and visual memory.

The final items on the scale, items 258–269, all involve arithmetic word problems of increasing difficulty very similar to those seen in the WAIS Arithmetic subtest. These items tend to be more sensitive to left hemisphere injury in the frontal and parietal regions. They correlate highly with items requiring a wide variety of abilities and functions, including simple mental and written arithmetic skills, sequencing, motor abilities, and tactile and stereognostic functions as well as phonetic analysis, visual-spatial organization, and receptive and expressive speech functions. A pattern of correlations like this suggests that this section of the Intellectual Processes scale is sensitive to both left and right hemisphere dysfunction.

Factor Analysis

Factor analysis of the Intellectual Processes scale results in the emergence of four factors (Golden, Hammeke, Osmon, Sweet, Purisch, & Graber, 1980), as is shown in Table 11.2. The first intelligence factor (Table 11.3) most closely resembles a verbal intelligence factor. It consists of items similar to those found on the Comprehension, Vocabulary, Similarities, and Arithmetic sections of the

WAIS. In addition, the patient must also make simple generalizations and deductions, as well as verbally analyze complex pictorial stimuli, tasks not found on the WAIS. This factor is clearly related to functioning of the left hemisphere, and it is likely that it is specifically responsible for the high correlation (−0.84) between this scale and verbal IQ (Golden, Hammeke, & Purisch,

Table 11.2: **Intelligence: Factor Structure**

Item	Factor 1	Factor 2	Factor 3	Factor 4
236	51	26	34	44
237	45	16	33	35
238	36	15	13	63
239	16	19	24	73
240	37	34	22	47
241	29	34	30	59
242	48	14	13	16
243	56	06	17	16
244	60	31	40	39
245	62	26	30	27
246	50	32	30	34
247	51	34	40	28
248	68	28	38	22
249	55	28	25	45
250	59	38	33	32
251	61	25	56	39
252	53	24	63	30
253	49	33	45	24
254	66	36	45	37
255	53	22	54	27
256	65	43	43	35
257	55	33	39	36
258	17	26	56	18
259	30	22	63	33
260	30	21	50	13
261	41	23	73	16
262	46	34	34	28
263	17	30	48	33
264	46	57	24	28
265	26	59	40	32
266	40	72	13	26
267	02	52	19	16
268	50	56	37	16
269	36	61	48	37

Table 11.3: **Items on Intelligence Factor 1**

Loading	Item	Description
.51	236	Describe this picture.
.45	237	Describe second picture.
.48	242	Describe what is comical in pictures.
.56	243	Describe what is comical in pictures.
.60	244	Analyze story (hen that laid golden eggs).
.62	245	Define "iron hand"; "green thumb."
.50	246	Interpret proverb.
.51	247	Interpret proverb.
.68	248	Define words.
.55	249	Find similarities between objects.
.59	250	Find differences between objects.
.61	251	Go from specific to general.
.53	252	Go from general to specific.
.49	253	Go from whole to part.
.66	254	Go from part to whole.
.53	255	Define opposites.
.65	256	Logical relationships.
.55	257	Find word that does not belong in series.
.41	261	Easy arithmetic item (time).
.46	262	Easy arithmetic item (correct answer).
.46	264	Moderate arithmetic item (correct answer).
.50	268	Difficult arithmetic item (correct answer).

1980). Like the WAIS Verbal scale it is expected that this factor would more closely reflect temporoparietal functioning than frontal lobe skills.

Intelligence factor 2 (Table 11.4) is quite clearly an arithmetic factor, featuring items of moderate to great difficulty. These items differ from the easy arithmetic items, which require little arithmetic but do require verbal understanding of the problem, for they require both verbal comprehension and arithmetic skill. Not surprisingly, several of these items also load on verbal comprehension, factor 1 of this scale.

Intelligence factor 3 (Table 11.5) generally involves many of the same items as factor 1. The major difference is that these items tend to be more difficult or abstract than the items loading on factor 1. Thus this factor is tentatively labeled advanced verbal comprehension to contrast it with factor 1. These items often show higher frontal lobe loadings upon item analysis of the Luria, reflecting an important difference in interpretation. Whereas parietal lesions may affect all factors on the scale, frontal lobe injuries (depending on size and side) will confine their effects to this factor, along with factors 2 and 4. Thus this represents one subset of verbal comprehension items that probably indicate frontal as well as parietal involvement.

The final factor (Table 11.6) consists primarily of two picture-arrangement items. This is the purest Luria measure of right anterior functioning and often is elevated in right frontotemporal injuries.

Summary

The Intellectual Processes scale is highly sensitive to disorders in both hemispheres but, owing to the dependence of the items on speech and language functioning, is more sensitive to damage on the left. Injuries to either the frontal or the parietal lobes will likely cause maximum dysfunction.

Poor performance on this scale, with no significant psychiatric thought disorder, is generally associated with prefrontal lobe dysfunction. Laterality, however, must be determined by investigating the specific items to see if the initial items, which are right-hemisphere-oriented, suggest intact visual interpretation skills. If these skills appear to be intact, then there is likely to be left hemisphere dysfunction. Conversely, if these initial items are the only ones missed, there is a strong possibility of right frontal dysfunction.

The constant interaction of all areas of the brain cannot be overemphasized. Although each part of the brain plays a unique role in each behavioral configuration, no part can

Table 11.4: **Items on Intelligence Factor 2**

Loading	Item	Description
.57	264	Moderate arithmetic item (correct).
.59	265	Moderate arithmetic item (time).
.72	266	Hard arithmetic item (correct).
.52	267	Hard arithmetic item (time).
.56	268	Hard arithmetic item (correct).
.61	269	Hard arithmetic item (time).

Table 11.5: **Items on Intelligence Factor 3**

Loading	Item	Description
.56	251	Go from specific to general.
.63	252	Go from general to specific.
.45	253	Go from whole to part.
.45	254	Go from part to whole.
.54	255	Define opposites.
.43	256	Logical relationships.
.56	258	Easy arithmetic item (correct).
.63	259	Easy arithmetic item (time).
.50	260	Easy arithmetic item (correct).
.73	261	Easy arithmetic item (time).
.48	263	Moderate arithmetic item (correct).
.48	269	Hard arithmetic item (correct).

Table 11.6: **Items on Intelligence Factor 4**

Loading	Item	Description
.44	236	Describe picture.
.63	238	Picture arrangement, the seasons (order).
.73	239	Picture arrangement, the seasons (time).
.47	240	Picture arrangement, potato (order).
.59	241	Picture arrangement, potato (time).

operate effectively without the others. Even such an apparently simple task as looking at something involves the frontal, parietal, and occipital areas. By considering why a person missed a specific item as well as analyzing scale scores and the pattern of items missed, the examiner can achieve a more qualitative and intuitive understanding of the dysfunction. Often this will lead to many of the same conclusions that would have been reached by looking only at the patterns of test performance, but looking at specific items and at how each item relates to other parts of the test can give a fuller understanding of the individual.

Intellectual processes are so complex that their impairment in patients with brain lesions cannot always be used directly for localization. Not until the various aspects of the difficulties have been carefully analyzed is it possible either to identify the factors responsible for them or to use the assessment of intellectual processes to make a topical diagnosis of brain lesions.

12. Pathognomonic Scale and Right and Left Hemisphere Scales

In addition to the eleven basic scales already discussed, a number of others, derived from the 269 items, have been proposed. Most of these at present are new scales not yet in general use. However, three additional scales have been in regular use since the introduction of the test. These three scales—Pathognomonic, Right Hemisphere, and Left Hemisphere—will be discussed first in this chapter.

Pathognomonic Scale

The Pathognomonic scale was created to bring together items that are highly indicative of brain dysfunction. These items are significantly less often missed by non-neurological patients than by those with brain damage.

The scale consists of 34 items (Table 12.1) from the Luria-Nebraska battery that have been found to be particularly sensitive to the presence of brain damage. The interpretive significance of the items has been dealt with at length in previous chapters and will not be repeated here.

In a normal population, T scores greater than 60 on the Pathognomonic scale generally indicate brain dysfunction, and in a schizophrenic population scores above 65 typically do so. This scale can also measure the seriousness of brain dysfunction. In general, acute destructive lesions cause marked elevations of the Pathognomonic scale, whereas resolving injuries generally lower the score on this scale, often to a point below the cutoff indicating cerebral dysfunction. Since the scale is highly sensitive to brain dysfunction, mistakes on these items should be carefully investigated. Also, it is imperative that the items be correctly administered so as to avoid false positives.

The scale was developed from early studies in which these items appeared to provide maximum separation of normal controls, schizophrenics, and neurological patients. The items appear to be very basic ones rarely missed by normals, as well as the most difficult items on the test, which are very rarely done correctly by brain-

Table 12.1: **The Pathognomonic Scale**

Item	Description
8	With your eyes closed, place your left hand in the same position I place your right hand in. (Thumb and middle finger are placed against each other for 2 seconds.)
9	Do as I do. (Place the right hand under the chin with fingers bent.)
19	Point to your left eye with your right hand.
37	Draw a circle. Scoring: time.
39	Draw a square. Scoring: time.
42	Copy this figure as best you can without lifting your pencil from the paper (circle).
43	Scoring: time.
45	Copy this figure (square). Scoring: time.
64	Tell me where I am touching you. (Right hand.)
77	(On back of left wrist.) What number is this?
79	(On back of left wrist.) What letter is this?
82	Feel this object and tell me exactly what it is. Right hand.
83	Right hand time.
85	Left hand time.
89	What is this picture supposed to be?
101	Write b, p, m.
102	Repeat two sounds: m–p, p–s, d–t, k–g, r–l.
103	Write m–p, p–s, d–t, k–g, r–l.
108	Point to your: eye; nose; ear.
139	Repeat cat–hat–bat.
157	What objects do these pictures represent? (Guitar; table; can opener; candle; stapler.)
162	Tell me the days of the week.
166	I am going to read this short story out loud. Follow along carefully, because when I'm through I'm going to take the card away and then you'll have to tell the story back to me in your own words. Scoring: response time.
169	Please make up a short speech about the conflict between the generations. Scoring: words.
175	How many letters are there in: cat; trap; banana; hedge?
178	Copy these in your own handwriting: pa, an, pro, pre, sti.
184	Write physiology; probabilistic.
185	Now write these words and phrases: hat–sun–dog; all of a sudden; last year before Christmas.

Table 12.1: **The Pathognomonic Scale**   Continued

Item	Description
187	Write a few sentences about bringing up children. Scoring: number of words.
196	Read astrocytoma; hemopoiesis.
211	Look at this card and show me, by pointing, which of the top two numbers is the larger. Which of the bottom two is larger? 189 or 201; 1967 or 3002.
227	I am going to show you a card; look at it carefully, then draw as much as you can remember.
241	These pictures are in the wrong order. Put them in the right order so they make sense. Scoring: time.
267	There were 18 books on two shelves; there were twice as many on one shelf as on the other. How many books were there on each shelf? Scoring: time.

damaged patients. Thus the tasks appear to represent the extremes of the items in the Luria-Nebraska.

FACTOR ANALYSIS

Factor analysis of the Pathognomonic scale yields four factors, as is seen in Table 12.2 (Golden, Hammeke, Osmon, Sweet, Purisch, & Graber, 1980). The first factor (Table 12.3) loads primarily on items that are so simple that no normal person would be expected to miss them under ordinary conditions. Thus, repeating simple phonemes heads the list of items, followed by the ability to recognize objects placed in one's hand (stereognosis), the ability to remember simple shapes, and the ability to name common objects. In all cases, essentially perfect performance is expected from normals. In general the items emphasize simple receptive skills, allowing us to label the factor simple perceptual-expressive functions.

Factor 2 (Table 12.4) shows only five significant loadings. Four of these items assess how quickly a simple figure (e.g., square, circle) is drawn. Thus, this factor could most aptly be named simple construction speed. In practice, Golden and associates (1980) note that this factor has been found to be related to the functioning of the

Table 12.2: **Pathognomonic Factor Structure**

Item	Factor 1	Factor 2	Factor 3	Factor 4
8	33	20	44	−28
9	22	17	45	−24
19	27	10	56	−14
37	13	66	16	−03
39	17	74	20	−09
42	27	23	36	−17
43	20	83	22	−18
45	21	77	16	−27
64	35	09	52	−05
77	38	22	39	−24
79	43	21	40	−18
82	55	32	53	−35
83	51	42	41	−32
85	51	35	43	−30
89	35	26	32	−28
101	59	15	28	−14
102	79	15	22	−28
103	80	24	38	−32
108	21	10	42	−12
139	33	07	34	−23
157	56	33	48	−43
162	13	22	46	−22
166	13	04	14	−26
169	19	16	16	−09
175	23	08	39	−44
178	40	35	64	−46
184	19	13	15	−63
185	27	29	48	−61
187	38	20	38	−46
196	16	11	13	−59
211	10	16	37	−25
227	55	16	33	−48
241	39	30	26	−38
267	16	01	18	−17

Table 12.3: **Items on Pathognomonic Factor 1**

Loading	Item	Description
.43	79	Identify letter written on left hand.
.55	82	Stereognosis—right hand errors.
.51	83	Stereognosis—right hand time.
.51	85	Stereognosis—left hand time.
.59	101	Write dictated phonemes (single).
.79	102	Repeat dictated phonemes (two at a time).
.80	103	Write dictated phonemes (two at a time).
.56	157	Name simple objects.
.40	178	Copy nonsense syllables.
.50	227	Draw six simple shapes from visual memory.

Table 12.4: **Items on Pathognomonic Factor 2**

Loading	Item	Description
.66	37	Draw a circle. Scoring: time.
.74	39	Draw a square. Scoring: time.
.83	43	Copy a circle. Scoring: time.
.77	45	Copy a square. Scoring: time.
.42	83	Stereognosis—right hand time.

dominant hand and, to some degree, the nondominant parietal area.

Factor 3 consists of a wide variety of items, primarily from the Motor, Tactile, Receptive Speech, Expressive Speech, and Writing scales, as is shown in Table 12.5. With only a few exceptions, all the items involve spatial skills: reproducing a position from tactile feedback, from

verbal command, or from imitation; recognizing a letter or object on or in the hand; identifying visually presented objects; reverse counting; and copying nonsense syllables. Only item 185 requires no clear visual-spatial function. In addition, all except item 185 have a further quality in common: all are quite simple and would usually not be missed by a normal individual. Thus, in the first three factors on the Pathognomonic scale we have a series of simple items representing basic perceptual-expressive skills, basic motor skills, and visual-spatial skills.

Factor 4 (Table 12.6) is completely different from the previous three. The items it includes are generally some of the most difficult on the Luria-Nebraska and are most effective in discriminating between brain-injured and

Table 12.5: **Items on Pathognomonic Factor 3**

Loading	Item	Description
.44	8	With your eyes closed, place your left hand in the same position I place your right hand in (thumb against middle finger).
.45	9	Do as I do. (Place the right hand under the chin with fingers bent.)
.56	10	Same as #9 with left hand.
.52	64	Tell me where I am touching you. (Right hand.)
.40	79	(On back of left wrist.) What letter is this?
.53	82	Stereognosis—right hand errors.
.41	83	Stereognosis—right hand time.
.43	85	Stereognosis—left hand time.
.42	108	Point to eye; nose; ear.
.48	157	What objects do these pictures represent?
.46	162	Tell me the days of the week.
.64	178	Copy *pa, an, pro, pre, sti.*
.48	185	Write phrases (e.g., *all of a sudden*).

Table 12.6: **Items on Pathognomonic Factor 4**

Loading	Item	Description
−.46	178	Copy *pa, an, pro, pre, sti.*
−.63	184	Write *physiology; probilistic.*
−.61	185	Write phrases.
−.46	187	Write a few sentences about bringing up children. Scoring: number of words.
−.59	196	Read *astrocytoma; hemopoiesis.*
−.48	227	Draw six figures from memory.

normal people at high levels of education. Overall, these items tend to be missed by a significant number of normals; but they are missed by a much higher percentage of brain-damaged individuals (as much as 70% to 80%, making these items the most ''sensitive'' on the test in certain respects). All involve some aspect of expressive language skills, so the factor has been labeled complex expressive skills. This factor is thought to be responsible for the ability of the Pathognomonic scale to uncover subtle disorders in apparently normal profiles.

Right and Left Hemisphere Scales

These two scales were developed as initial measures of lateralization of cerebral dysfunction. The Right Hemisphere scale consists of all items reflecting left-hand motor or sensory performance, while the Left Hemisphere scale consists of all items reflecting right-hand motor or sensory

Table 12.7: **Item Numbers for Right and Left Hemisphere Scales**

Right Hemisphere	Left Hemisphere
2	1
4	3
6	5
8	7
10	9
12	11
14	13
16	15
18	17
20	19
65	64
67	66
69	68
71	70
73	72
75	74
77	76
79	78
81	80
84	82
85	83

performance (Table 12.7). These items are drawn from the Motor and Tactile scales, as indicated on the summary profile sheet used to record the data. The items on these scales are sensitive to lateralized disorders that involve the motor-sensory strip in the central part of the brain or those areas directly adjacent to the motor-sensory strip.

Lesions that do not affect the motor-sensory area may not show up as a lateralized discrepancy on the Right and Left Hemisphere scales. Thus lesions that are more posterior or more anterior tend to appear nonlateralized. Conversely, extreme differences between the Right and Left Hemisphere scales almost always indicate a lateralized disorder in which the motor-sensory areas of the brain are involved. In general, right hemisphere injuries involving the motor-sensory area will produce an elevation on the Right Hemisphere scale, but the Left Hemisphere scale will remain within normal limits, that is, generally a T score of less than 60. However, in left hemisphere injuries the Left Hemisphere scale will often be elevated above a score of 60, while the Right Hemisphere scale will show elevations of 5 to 20 points. However, the Left Hemisphere scale will be 10 to 20 or more points higher than the Right Hemisphere scale. Bilateral injuries, as a rule, will elevate both scales, but the two will be within 10 to 20 points of each other.

Overall, the Right and Left Hemisphere scales alone are about 75% accurate in lateralizing neurological disorders. However, the exact accuracy of the scale depends on the type of population involved. For example, on a stroke population in which middle cerebral artery problems are common the test is highly effective, whereas for dealing purely with lesions of the prefrontal areas of the frontal lobe the two scales would be rather useless in most instances (Golden, Purisch, & Hammeke, 1979). With these limitations in mind, however, the information offered by these two scales, if integrated with the analysis of the results on the rest of the test, permits a highly accurate determination of lateralized damage in most cases of localized neurological dysfunction.

FACTOR ANALYSIS

Factor analysis of both the Right Hemisphere and Left Hemisphere scales yielded only one general factor encompassing nearly all items on both scales (Golden, Hammeke, Osmon, Sweet, Purisch, & Graber, 1980), so the factor structure is not described in the text. Examining the scales suggests a possible explanation. The Left Hemisphere scale consists of the first 10 right-hand items of the Motor scale, which deal with simple motor skills (items 1, 3, 5, 7, 9, 11, 13, 15, 17, 19) and the 11 items on the Tactile scale that require right hand or right body side input (items 64, 66, 68, 70, 72, 74, 76, 78, 80, 82, 83). The Right Hemisphere scale consists of the same tasks except that these items use the left hand or body side rather than the right (items 2, 4, 6, 8, 10, 12, 14, 16, 18, 20, 65, 67, 69, 71, 73, 75, 77, 79, 81, 84, 85). Thus the two scales theoretically represent the left hemisphere motor-sensory area (the pre- and postcentral gyrus) and the right hemisphere motor-sensory area.

Luria (1973) argues that these areas should be considered a single unit, separate from the rest of the brain. Indeed, he indicates this clearly in the organization of *The Working Brain* by devoting a separate chapter to the sensorimotor region of the brain. Because of the heavy interconnections between these areas, the dependence of motor skills upon tactile feedback and the importance of motor feedback for tactile skills (also see Motor and Tactile scale item intercorrelations), and the presence of significant numbers of motor cells in the "sensory strip" (postcentral gyrus) and of tactile cells in the "motor strip" (precentral gyrus), Luria argues that these two areas of the brain are closely intertwined.

Factor analysis of these two scales clearly supports this contention, since the scales do not break up into separate motor and sensory components. It is unlikely that there could be a clearer demonstration of the strong interactions between these areas of the brain and their mutual dependence. Thus, as Golden et al. (1980) note, these results do support Luria's theory in this area.

Localization Scales

A particularly interesting area of research with the Luria-Nebraska battery is the empirical identification of specific test items that are highly discriminative of damage to specific areas of the brain. The Luria-Nebraska format allows for the design of specific scales so that dysfunction in specific areas of the brain can be pinpointed by determining which items are missed more frequently by individuals with lesions in those areas. A recent report by Lewis, Golden, Moses, Osmon, Purisch, & Hammeke (1979) has shown that the summary scales of the Luria-Nebraska battery can identify fairly stable patterns of performance in individuals with localized lesions.

McKay and Golden (1979b) have empirically derived a series of eight scales used to localize the site of a lesion. The localization scales were derived in the following manner. The Luria-Nebraska Neuropsychological Battery was administered to 77 normal subjects and 53 subjects with confirmed localized brain damage. The brain-damaged group comprised 5 right frontal, 3 right sensorimotor, 7 right parieto-occipital, 4 right temporal, 12 left frontal, 6 left sensorimotor, 10 left parieto-occipital, and 6 left temporal patients. Multiple t tests were performed comparing the performance of each brain-damaged group with normals on each Luria battery item. First, items that significantly discriminated only one brain-damaged group from normals were assigned to that group's scale. Next, items that significantly discriminated only two groups from normals were assigned to those two groups' scales. In the third step, items discriminating more than two groups were discarded unless they discriminated one or two groups much better than others, with a probability less than one-third that for the next most significant item. Thus, an item discriminating one group from normals at the .05 level, another group at the .015 level, and another group at the .01 level would be assigned to the last two groups. Finally, no item was assigned to more than two scales, and no two scales had more than two items in common; where items had to be eliminated to conform to this rule, the more significantly discriminating item was kept.

While these rules for item assignment involve some apparently arbitrary criteria, they were designed to allow for scales that efficiently discriminate each brain-damaged group from normals and from other brain-damaged groups. The score for each subject, as well as the mean and standard deviation for each group, was computed based upon the mean and standard deviation of the normal group on each scale.

CONTENTS OF THE LOCALIZATION SCALES

The *Left Frontal* (LF) scale includes 33 Luria items (1, 59, 62, 104, 105, 123, 125, 134, 138, 140, 143, 144, 148, 157, 161, 162, 164, 166, 168, 192, 196, 202, 207, 208, 219, 225, 230, 237, 248, 250, 257, 259, 261). Major groupings of items include fluency and articulation of expressive speech (12 items), latency of verbal responses (5 items), abstraction skills (3 items), and immediate verbal memory (2 items).

The *Left Sensorimotor* (LSM) scale includes 30 items (5, 11, 17, 21, 22, 38, 40, 41, 44, 46, 52, 56, 61, 70, 71, 78, 82, 86, 87, 88, 99, 145, 150, 221, 228, 229, 240, 242, 249, 258). Major groupings occur in motor skills, mainly in the upper right extremity (15 items), including correct positioning of hands, coordination of hand movements, drawing quality, integration of motor and rhythm skills, integration of visual and verbal skills (5 items) in naming objects and reading words, and tactile spatial perception (4 items). Tasks assessing mental flexibility, visual construction, and visual sequencing also appear.

The *Left Parieto-occipital* (LPO) scale includes 25 items (5, 7, 8, 90, 95, 96, 149, 151, 175, 179, 187, 191, 195, 199, 203, 204, 207, 215, 221, 222, 233, 243, 251, 255, 263). This scale includes items that combine visual and verbal skills, such as reading words and paragraphs (5 items), visualizing the letters in words (2 items), and visual discrimination and naming (1 item). Visual-spatial perception (2 items) and immediate visual memory item appear, as do arithmetic (4 items), concept formation (2 items), and correct positioning of the hands (3 items).

The *Left Temporal* (LT) scale includes 24 items (31, 63, 100, 101, 102, 103, 109, 120, 121, 122, 126, 129, 130, 131, 155, 156, 176, 183, 186, 199, 214, 232, 238, 239). These items emphasize grammar (9 items), verbal memory (4 items), and phonemic discrimination (4 items) as well as items assessing motor, rhythm, and visual analysis skills.

The *Right Frontal* (RF) scale includes 16 items (6, 7, 13, 33, 39, 40, 44, 45, 47, 53, 63, 93, 94, 117, 125, 169). These items emphasize motor speed and coordination skills (7 items), rhythm (2 items), positioning of hands (3 items), and visual-spatial perception (2 items).

The *Right Sensorimotor* (RSM) scale includes 16 items (4, 10, 14, 36, 46, 51, 54, 56, 84, 89, 92, 172, 175, 179, 202, 218). Major groupings represented here are motor skills (4 items), rhythm (2 items), spatial perception and position sense in the upper left extremity (3 items), and visual construction of verbal material (6 items).

The *Right Parieto-Occipital* (RPO) scale includes 27 items (10, 24, 39, 53, 59, 60, 65, 75, 77, 79, 81, 83, 84, 85, 87, 90, 91, 94, 97, 103, 158, 215, 225, 236, 239, 257, 265). These items feature tactile, spatial, and kinesthetic skills in the upper left extremity (9 items), visual skills (9 items) involving visual-spatial perception, identifying pictures of body parts, and visual discrimination; other items assess rhythm skills (3 items) and arithmetic operations (2 items).

The *Right Temporal* (RT) scale includes 25 items (29, 62, 66, 69, 95, 98, 117, 127, 157, 172, 173, 174, 184, 195, 217, 227, 233, 235, 237, 239, 247, 254, 256, 262, 264). Most involve some type of verbal task that is aided by visual constructive ability, visual analysis, or rhythm sense. Some motor, tactile, visual-spatial, and concept formation items also appear on this scale.

The results of this initial study were fairly impressive, promising considerable usefulness clinically and in theoretical investigation of localized brain function. One problem was the small number of subjects in some of the localized brain-damaged groups (as few as three or four in some cases). Recently, however, a cross-validation with more subjects per group (Golden, et al., 1981) essentially confirmed the findings of the initial localization scale study. The means and standard deviations of each of the groups are shown in Table 12.8.

Subjects were included in this study if they had identifiable, localized brain damage that had been confirmed by computed tomography (CT) scan, EEG, brain scan, or neurological tests. The type of cerebral damage was identified as one of the following: tumor, occlusion, laceration, aneurysm, hemorrhage, hematoma, contusion, or abscess. The controls were individuals with a normal neurological history. Overall, 71% of the subjects were male and 29% were female. The right frontal group had a mean age of 46.57 (SD = 7.76) and a mean education of 13.29 years (SD = 3.55). In primary occupational categories this group was divided between professionals and retired people. The right sensorimotor group had a mean age of 55.50 (SD = 20.56), a mean education of 11.44 years (SD = 1.33), and consisted of people with a variety of occupational backgrounds including professionals, business people, blue-collar workers, homemakers, and students. Individuals who made up the right parietal group had a mean age of 57.07 (SD = 9.41) and mean education of 12.40 years (SD = 2.03). They were primarily blue-collar workers. Those in the right temporal group had a mean age of 52.00 (SD = 8.09) and mean education of 13.00 years (SD = 2.65) and were mostly either business people or blue-collar workers. The mean age of the left frontal group was 47.08 (SD = 12.53), and the mean education level was 12.75 years (SD = 2.14). This group was fairly evenly divided among business people, blue-collar workers, and retired persons. For the left sensorimotor group there was a mean age of 59.50 (SD = 10.80), and all individuals had 12 years of education. The primary occupations of this group were business, blue-collar work, and farming. The left parietal group was overall the youngest (mean age = 45.82; SD = 14.63), among the most highly educated (mean education = 13.29 years; SD = 1.76), and included mostly professionals, business people, blue-collar workers, and homemakers. The final brain-injured group, left temporal, had a mean age of 50.36 years (SD = 19.63) and mean education of 11.21 years (SD = 3.33) and consisted largely of retired persons. Finally, the control subjects had a mean age of 47.70 years (SD = 11.62)

Table 12.8: **Means and Standard Deviations for Localization Scales by Group**

Group	Left Frontal		Left Sensorimotor		Left Parietal		Left Temporal	
	Mean	SD	Mean	SD	Mean	SD	Mean	SD
Entire population	63.74	17.83	58.53	13.30	62.74	17.90	59.59	17.50
Right frontal	65.57	14.77	61.57	14.79	64.28	17.83	63.42	20.07
Right sensorimotor	56.55	7.79	59.88	10.49	59.66	10.51	50.77	7.29
Right parietal	62.26	12.26	62.40	14.00	61.60	13.11	56.20	13.11
Right temporal	64.57	9.62	66.28	9.89	60.57	9.57	61.85	10.20
Left frontal	85.25	16.35	63.83	13.83	69.75	18.28	66.58	17.58
Left sensorimotor	76.16	36.59	76.33	16.26	72.00	23.17	66.33	17.61
Left parietal	73.23	9.80	60.70	7.59	81.52	12.31	66.00	11.04
Left temporal	67.42	15.90	57.64	12.54	66.28	18.27	78.92	22.81
Normal controls	47.83	7.55	47.16	7.61	47.43	11.50	45.73	9.18

Group	Right Frontal		Right Sensorimotor		Right Parietal		Right Temporal	
	Mean	SD	Mean	SD	Mean	SD	Mean	SD
Entire population	58.19	14.00	59.99	13.92	66.23	18.05	60.78	14.84
Right frontal	74.00	19.63	69.57	20.79	71.57	22.25	61.71	17.42
Right sensorimotor	59.11	9.54	69.11	9.85	69.88	17.38	49.55	12.99
Right parietal	62.00	14.55	66.40	14.51	83.00	13.59	63.46	11.03
Right temporal	60.28	11.01	66.71	11.68	75.14	14.67	72.28	12.17
Left frontal	64.16	14.64	61.75	15.39	72.75	18.92	68.83	13.23
Left sensorimotor	59.66	14.67	60.00	13.34	68.83	20.98	66.16	19.38
Left parietal	62.11	9.99	61.58	6.98	68.64	9.63	68.64	7.99
Left temporal	60.92	9.00	61.35	13.03	69.35	15.20	66.92	14.24
Normal controls	45.66	9.10	48.00	8.58	47.46	7.12	48.30	10.05

Table 12.9: **Success Rates by Groups for Presence, Lateralization, and Localization of Brain Dysfunction**

Group	Presence	Lateralization	Localization	
	Elevated Scores	Localization Scales	One-Point Code	Two-Point Code
Right frontal	7/7	6/7	3/7	5/7
Right sensorimotor	7/9	9/9	5/9	8/9
Right parietal	12/15	15/15	14/15	15/15
Right temporal	6/7	7/7	3/7	5/7
Left frontal	11/12	12/12	11/12	12/12
Left sensorimotor	4/6	5/6	4/6	5/6
Left parietal	17/17	16/17	13/17	16/17
Left temporal	13/14	13/14	11/14	11/14
Left-handed patients	9/9	9/9	5/9	8/9
Overall	77/87	81/87	64/87	77/87
Normal controls	24/30	—	—	—

and mean education of 13.00 years (*SD* = 3.91). The occupations of those in the control group ranged over the entire spectrum of employment, with professionals, business people, blue-collar workers, and homemakers in the majority.

Table 12.9 presents the success rates in discriminating brain-damaged groups for the presence, lateralization, and localization of brain damage. This table compares the effectiveness of a variety of techniques for identifying brain damage. As can be seen, elevation of three or more scales is highly indicative of brain damage, with an overall success rate of almost 87%. A given scale's *T* score is considered significantly elevated when the value obtained for that scale exceeds a critical value found by using the empirically derived formula: critical value = 68.8 − (1.47 × education) + (.214 × age).

It is of interest that when the localization scales are used to lateralize a lesion to the left or right side of the brain (by using the side of the highest scale), the scales are 93% effective for a given injury.

Although still experimental in nature, the localization scales empirically derived by McKay and Golden (1979b) appear to be highly effective in locating fairly circumscribed brain lesions. If we use a patient's single highest localization scale score (the one-point code; see Figure 12.1), there is an average success rate of approximately 73%. Such a success rate is significant, particularly considering that a 12.5% success rate is to be expected by chance. Using the two highest scales (two-point code), we achieve a success rate of 88%, calculated by assuming a "success" when either of the two highest scales identifies the area affected by a given brain lesion. The success rate of 88% is well above that expected by chance (25%). Thus it appears that the localization scales will be effective in clinical situations.

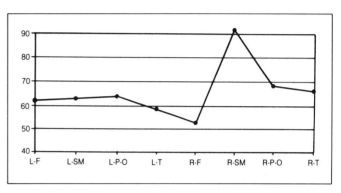

Figure 12.1.   Example of performance of a patient with a right sensorimotor dysfunction, using the Localization scales.

It must be reemphasized that these scales are still experimental and not in general use. Further research is necessary on larger samples of brain-injured patients with localized injuries. Such work will take time, since such localized injuries are the exception rather than the rule. However, such cross-validation is increasing the confidence that can be placed in these scales.

Summary

The Pathognomonic, Right and Left Hemisphere, and Localization scales can be quite useful in determining the chronicity, severity, and localization of a given brain injury, and can offer much information on lateralization. However, the reader is cautioned against relying too heavily on these scales, particularly when none are significantly elevated. Only a careful analysis of the patient's performance on all scales of the LNNB battery will enable one to accurately interpret it in terms of the presence, extent, and localization of brain injury.

13. Item Summary

Item analysis of the Luria-Nebraska is a complex process. This chapter provides a quick summary of selected aspects of items, including the input and output modalities, the skill to be assessed, and hypotheses concerning localization of the injury associated with deficits on clusters of items. These last are abstracted from previous chapters and are intended as a quick reference to these extended analyses.

Description of neuropsychological test items in terms of input and output modality stems directly from Luria's theories of brain function and assessment. Luria viewed the employment of a skill as a complex sequence beginning with the sensory stimulus and ending with the motor or verbal response. Successful completion of a task requires a series of operations organized by functional brain systems. A deficit on an individual neuropsychological item could therefore result from failure at any point along a sequential chain from input to output. This could involve peripheral sensory or motor deficits, problems at early stages of sensory analysis, failure of the target process, or impaired motor or verbal expression. Thus, although a neuropsychological task may be intended to evaluate a specific cognitive operation, any psychological test necessarily assesses a range of input and output functions not directly related to the more abstract cognitive process that is the target of evaluation. This is particularly true when the verbal instructions are complex and difficult to comprehend or when the motor output or verbal expression required to communicate the target skill is complex.

Luria-Nebraska items 42 and 43, in which the patient is asked to copy a circle, may be used as examples. The target skill is construction or visual-spatial-motor integration. The input involves a simple visual stimulus and a simple verbal instruction, so failure on these items is not likely to be due to deficits in sensory perception or analysis. However, the motor output is quite complex, and individuals with brain damage in the motor cortex contralateral to the dominant hand would find it difficult to draw an adequate circle.

Classifying Luria-Nebraska items in terms of sensory

and expressive modalities helps reveal the underlying structure of the test. Luria adopted an approach to neuropsychological assessment that emphasized reducing cognitive processes to their most elementary functions. This may be contrasted with the Halstead-Reitan battery, which employs highly complex test items that tap a large number of cognitive functions simultaneously.

On the Luria-Nebraska, most items are intended to assess some highly specific cognitive skill or process. However, careful analysis reveals considerable redundancy in the sense that disparate items are intended to tap the same skill. When the items are described in terms of input and output modalities, it becomes apparent that the same skill is being assessed while the sensory modality or method of expression is systematically varied. Examples of this are items 62 and 63 of the Rhythm scale, in which the patient is asked first to copy a rhythm, then to make new rhythms on verbal command. The input on the first item is a complex auditory stimulus, and impairment may reflect a deficit in rhythmic comprehension. In the second item, the focus is on the motor execution of the task and on verbal control over dynamic behavior. On the Expressive Speech scale, items 133-142 are presented orally, then these same items are presented in written form in items 143-156. This allows inferences concerning expressive articulation with an oral versus a written input modality. Therefore an effective item analysis requires close attention to the item's input modality, target skill or process, and motor or verbal mode of expression. Hypotheses concerning the deficit implied by failure on any cluster of items must consider the possibility of impairment in various aspects of the skills involved, including the input and output modalities. A cluster of failed items reflects a deficit in the target skill only if failure occurs in almost every sensory or response modality.

Another feature of this analysis is that input and output modalities are classified by complexity. The more complex the sensory stimulus or motor response, the more likely it is that failure on the item might reflect dysfunction in the brain areas associated with the input or the output.

On the motor and sensory scales, the reader will note that the sensory stimuli or motor requirements of the items become increasingly complex. This allows assessment of individuals at different performance levels and avoids "ceiling" or "floor" effects.

Finally, hypotheses are provided concerning localization of brain dysfunction associated with failure on each cluster of items. These hypotheses are necessarily brief, but they provide clues that may be pursued in comparison with other items or scale scores in the localization of brain dysfunction. In some cases localization hypotheses may relate more directly to the input or output modality of the item than to the target skill.

For many items, several possible areas of the brain are noted in the localization hypotheses, in approximate order of consideration. This reflects Luria's theoretical position that there is no one-to-one correspondence between failure on a neuropsychological task and dysfunction in a specific area of the brain. In no case is there an item which, if failed, invariably indicates a lesion in a specific area. The localization hypotheses are offered only as starting points for examining the pattern and severity of deficits on the entire test, including both scale interpretation and item analysis. In each case the reader is referred to the chapters on interpretation of each scale for a more complete discussion of the items and their interpretation in terms of brain dysfunction.

This summary also indicates which items are listed on the special scales (Localization, Lateralization, and Pathognomonic). This information is provided to suggest additional hypotheses concerning localization and to aid in the description of the types of processes involved in each item.

A complete Luria-Nebraska interpretation typically involves three stages: scale interpretation, evaluation of special scale elevations (Localization and Lateralization scales), and item analysis. The test interpreter frequently develops hypotheses in the first two stages, and these are confirmed or disconfirmed in the item analysis. This item summary may be useful in gaining further understanding of the basis for scale elevations and in doing a thorough item analysis. It is not uncommon that individuals who lack experience with the Luria-Nebraska tend to focus only upon item failures. However, equally important information can be obtained from noting successful completion of difficult items, particularly for disconfirming initial hypotheses.

For each significant scale elevation, item analysis should provide detailed information concerning the basis for it. As localization hypotheses are developed, they can be evaluated in terms of items failed or successfully completed. For example, a Visual scale elevation might alert the interpreter to a visual-spatial deficit. All items that employ a complex visual stimulus might then be examined to determine whether this hypothesis is borne out. This might include construction items on the Motor scale, photograph description items on the Expressive Speech and Intelligence scales, and nonverbal Memory scale items.

Another example would be the hypothesis of a kinesthetic deficit from a Tactile scale elevation. The test interpreter might then wish to determine whether a moderate Motor scale elevation was due to frontal involvement or was simply consistent with kinesthetic impairment of motor function. Item analysis would then focus on Motor scale items 5–8, 30 and 31, and construction items.

In other cases, item analysis might take the form of noting consistent failure on items associated with specific localization hypotheses. This would be done in conjunction with examining Localization scale patterns. This approach could be hazardous if undertaken without due consideration for consistencies in the psychological functions assessed by these items.

Explanation of Table

The following table presents this information in abbreviated form. The reader should be cautioned that the suggestions in this table are only tentative suggestions rather than final answers on what a given item can measure. As has been emphasized throughout this book, all items reflect functional systems and measure things other than their major focus.

This is especially important when one looks at the "localization hypotheses" presented with each section of the items. These reflect the areas most commonly associated with a given item on the test, but do not reflect all of the areas of the brain that may affect a given item. This particularly applies to the more complex items where the localization suggested is the hypothesis that would be generated if simpler skills which contribute to the task are intact. Thus, a spatial item may most generally reflect certain right hemisphere processes, but not if the patient misses the items because he or she fails to understand the instructions. In practice, this problem is overcome by attempting to measure some of the same skills in a different manner across the test as a whole. Thus, as noted above, final interpretive statements must take the test pattern as a whole into account: diagnosis or conclusions cannot be reached from single items.

It is also important to consider the qualitative aspects of the patient's performance. Was the patient's performance consistent with the type of error suggested in the table? By carefully observing the patient's behavior, the user of the test can increase the amount of information generated by the battery, taking advantage of the test's full potential.

Under lateralization in the table, four possibilities are listed. These listings indicate that the item is on the scale listed, and the absence of any indication in this column does not comment on the lateralizing significance of the item. L and R refer to the left and right hemisphere scales, respectively, as discussed in the previous chapter. FL and FR refer to empirically derived lateralization scales first presented by Golden and McKay (1979). These scales have not been discussed in detail, since we have not yet found a clear clinical application for them independent of the remaining scales of the battery. However, they are listed here for those interested in researching these scales.

Under localization, the eight localization scales are listed. A listing under this column indicates that the item is on that particular scale. The abbreviations used are those normally associated with these scales: Right Frontal (RF), Left Frontal (LF), Right Temporal (RT), Left Temporal (LT), Right Parietal (RPO), Left Parietal (LPO), Right Sensorimotor (RSM), and Left Sensorimotor (LSM).

A "P" under the Pathognomonic column indicates that the item is on the Pathognomonic scale as described in the previous chapter.

The remaining descriptions are generally self-explanatory within the context of the above introduction and the previous chapters.

Table 13.1: **Item Analysis: Motor Scale**

Item	Description	Localization	Lateralization	Pathognomonic	Analysis
1	Touch fingers (right hand)	LF	L, FL		Description: Simple movement, hands
2	Touch fingers (left hand)		R, FR		Input: Simple visual, simple verbal Processes: *Motor organization*
3	Clench fist (right hand)		L, FL		Output: Complex motor
4	Clench fist (left hand)	RSM	R		Localization hypotheses: Posterior frontal, motor cortex
5	Place fingers (right hand)	LSM, LPO	L, FL		Description: Kinesthetic basis of movement, hands
6	Place fingers (left hand)	RF	R, FR		Input: Tactile Processes: *Tactile-motor integration*
7	Place fingers (right hand)	LPO, RF	L, FL		Output: Simple motor
8	Place fingers	LPO	R	P	Localization hypotheses: Parietal, motor cortex
9	Place hand (right hand)		L	P	Description: Optic spatial organization, hands
10	Place hand (left hand)	RSM, RPO	R, FR		Input: Simple visual-spatial, simple verbal Processes: *Visual-motor integration*, right-left
11	Place hand (right hand)	LSM	L, FL		awareness, visual-spatial analysis
12	Place hand (left hand)		R		Output: Simple motor
13	Place hands	RF	L		Localization hypotheses: Frontal, right
14	Place hands	RSM	R		hemisphere
15	Raise hand (right hand)		L		
16	Raise hand (left hand)		R		
17	Point hand (right hand)	LSM	L, FL		
18	Point hand (left hand)		R, FR		
19	Point hand (right hand)		L	P	
20	Point hand (left hand)		R		
21	Alternate hand clenches	LSM	FL		Description: Dynamic organization, hands; complex praxis
22	Tap rhythm	LSM			Input: Simple verbal, simple visual-spatial
23	Tap rhythm		FR		Processes: *Motor organization*, bimanual coordination, construction apraxia
24	Draw pattern	RPO			

Table 13.1: **Item Analysis: Motor Scale**　*Continued*

Item	Description	Localization	Lateralization	Panthognomonic	Analysis
25	Show teapot				Output: Complex motor
26	Show thread				
27	Show scissors		FL		Localization hypotheses: Motor cortex, prefrontal, premotor
28	Puff cheeks				Description: Simple movement, oral; kinesthetic movement, oral
29	Stick out tongue	RT			
30	Roll tongue				Input: Simple verbal
31	Place tongue	LT			Processes: *Motor organization*
32	Mouth movements				Output: Simple and complex motor, oral
33	Mouth movements	RF	FR		
34	Show chewing				Localization hypotheses: Frontal, parietal, cranial nerve
35	Show whistling				
36	Draw circle	RSM			Description: Selectivity of motor act
37	Circle time			P	
38	Draw square	LSM			Input: Simple verbal
39	Square time	RF, RPO		P	Processes: *Visual-spatial-motor integration*
40	Draw triangle	LSM, FR			Output: Complex motor
41	Triangle time	LSM			Localization hypotheses: Right hemisphere, left parietal, motor cortex, prefrontal
42	Draw circle			P	Description: Selectivity of motor act
43	Circle time			P	
44	Draw square	LSM, RF	FL		Input: Simple visual-spatial
45	Square time	RF		P	Processes: *Visual-spatial-motor integration*
46	Draw triangle	LSM, RSM			Output: Complex motor
47	Triangle time	RF			Localization hypotheses: Right hemisphere, left parietal, motor cortex
48	Knock opposite				Description: Speech regulation of motor acts
49	Squeeze opposite				
50	Knock, raise hand				Input: Complex verbal
51	Knock opposite	RSM	FR		Processes: *Verbal-motor integration*
					Output: Simple motor
					Localization hypotheses: Left temporoparietal, frontal

Note.

LF = Left frontal scale
LSM = Left sensorimotor scale
LT = Left temporal scale
LPO = Left parieto-occipital scale

RF = Right frontal scale
RSM = Right sensorimotor scale
RT = Right temporal scale
RPO = Right parieto-occipital scale

R = Right scale
L = Left scale

FR = Functional right scale
FL = Functional left scale

P = Pathognomonic scale

"Target" process is italicized.

Table 13.2: **Item Analysis: Rhythm Scale**

Item	Description	Localization	Lateralization	Pathognomonic	Analysis
52	Tones, same–different	LSM			Description: Perception of pitch relationships
53	Tones, which higher	RF, RPO			Input: Auditory
54	Tone groups, same–different	RSM			Processes: *Pitch discrimination*, attention and concentration
					Output: Simple verbal
					Localization hypotheses: Right temporal, left temporal, subcortical
55	Hum tones				Description: Reproduction of pitch and melodies
56	Repeat melody	LSM, RSM			
57	Sing melody		FR		Input: Auditory
					Processes: *Pitch production*
					Output: Simple verbal
					Localization hypotheses: Left temporal, right frontal
58	Count beeps				Description: Perception of acoustic signals
59	Count groups	RPO, LF			
60	Count groups	RPO			Input: Simple and complex auditory
61	Count groups	LSM			Processes: *Evaluation of acoustic stimuli*, attention and concentration
					Output: Simple verbal
					Localization hypotheses: Left temporal, frontal, subcortical
62	Copy rhythm	RT, LF	FL		Description: Motor performance of rhythm
63	Make rhythm	LT, RF	FR		Input: Auditory, simple verbal
					Processes: *Auditory-motor integration*, attention and concentration
					Output: Complex motor
					Localization hypotheses: Right frontal, right temporal, subcortical

Note. For key to abbreviations, see note to Table 13.1.

Table 13.3: **Item Analysis: Tactile Scale**

Item	Description	Localization	Lateralization	Pathognomonic	Analysis
64	Where touching (right hand)		L	P	Description: Cutaneous sensation
65	Where touching (left hand)	RPO	R		Input: Simple tactile
					Processes: *Tactile recognition*
66	Pinpoint	RT	L		Output: Simple verbal

Table 13.2: **Item Analysis: Rhythm Scale**   *Continued*

Item	Description	Localization	Lateralization	Panthognomonic	Analysis
	(right hand)				
67	Pinpoint		R		Localization hypotheses: Anterior and midparietal
	(left hand)				
68	Pin pressure		L		
	(right hand)				
69	Pin pressure	RT	R		
	(left hand)				
70	Number points	LSM	L		
	(right hand)				
71	Number points	LSM	R, FR		
	(left hand)				
72	Moving up–down		L		
	(right arm)				
73	Moving up–down		R		
	(left arm)				
74	Trace figure		L, FL		Description: Cutaneous sensation
	(right hand)				
75	Trace figure	RPO	R, FR		Input: Complex tactile
	(left hand)				Processes: *Tactile recognition*, naming
76	Trace number		L		Output: Simple verbal
	(right hand)				
77	Trace number	RPO	R, FR	P	Localization hypotheses: Angular gyrus, left and right temporoparietal
	(left hand)				
78	Trace letter	LSM	L		
	(right hand)				
79	Trace letter	RPO	R, FR	P	
	(left hand)				
80	Place arm		L		Description: Muscle and joint sensation
	(right arm)				
81	Place arm	RPO	R, FR		Input: Simple kinesthetic
	(left arm)				Processes: *Kinesthetic-motor integration*
					Output: Simple motor
					Localization Hypotheses: Anterior and posterior parietal, angular gyrus
82	Palpate object	LSM	L	P	Description: Stereognosis
	(right hand)				
83	Time	RPO	L	P	Input: Complex tactile
	(right hand)				Processes: *Tactile recognition*, naming
84	Palpate object	RSM, RPO	R		Output: Simple verbal
	(left hand)				
85	Time	RPO	R, FR	P	Localization hypotheses: Parietal, left temporo-parietal
	(left hand)				

Note. For key to abbreviations, see note to Table 13.1.

Table 13.4: **Item Analysis: Visual Scale**

Item	Description	Localization	Lateralization	Pathognomonic	Analysis
86	Name object	LSM	FL		Description: Visual perception, objects
87	Name picture	LSM, RPO			
88	Blurred photo	LSM			Input: Simple and complex visual
89	Contrast photo	RSM	FR	P	Processes: *Naming,* visual recognition
90	Overlapping objects	RPO, LPO			Output: Simple verbal
91	Overlapping objects	RPO			Localization hypotheses: Right hemisphere, left temporoparietal, right parieto-occipital
92	Missing piece	RSM	FR		
93	Time	RF			
94	Tell time	RF, RPO	FR		Description: Spatial orientation
95	Draw hands on clock	RT, LPO			Input: Complex visual
96	Compass directions	LPO			Processes: *Visual-spatial,* spatial-analytic
					Output: Simple verbal, simple motor
					Localization hypotheses: Right hemisphere, left parieto-occipital
97	Count blocks	RPO			Description: Intellectual operations in space
98	Time	RT			
99	Rotate squares	LSM			Input: Complex visual
					Processes: *Visual-spatial,* visual imagery
					Output: Simple verbal, simple motor
					Localization hypotheses: Right hemisphere, right parieto-occipital

Note. For key to abbreviations, see note to Table 13.1.

Table 13.5: **Item Analysis: Receptive Speech Scale**

Item	Description	Localization	Lateralization	Pathognomonic	Analysis
100	Repeat sound	LT			Description: Phonemic hearing, repetition and writing
101	Write	LT		P	
102	Repeat sounds	LT		P	Input: Simple verbal
103	Write	LT, RPO		P	Processes: *Phonemic discrimination,* verbal memory
104	Repeat sounds	LF			
105	Write	LF	FL		Output: Simple verbal, simple writing
106	Raise hand				Localization hypotheses: Left temporal, left angular gyrus (writing items)
107	Letter sounds, different pitch				Description: Phonemic hearing, pitch
					Input: Simple verbal
					Processes: *Pitch discrimination*
					Output: Simple verbal
					Localization hypotheses: Right or left temporal

Table 13.4: **Item Analysis: Visual Scale**   *Continued*

Item	Description	Localization	Lateralization	Panthognomonic	Analysis
108	Point to eye			P	Description: Word comprehension
109	Point in order	LT			
110	Point at				Input: Simple verbal, simple visual
111	Point at				Processes: *Verbal comprehension*
112	Word meaning				Output: Simple motor
113	Point activity				Localization hypotheses: Left temporal parietal
114	Hand on head				Description: Simple sentences, instructions
115	Whose watch?				
116	Show me				Input: Simple verbal, simple visual
					Processes: *Verbal-motor integration,* verbal comprehension
					Output: Simple motor
					Localization hypotheses: Left hemisphere
117	Night now, gray card	RF, RT	FL		Description: Conflicting instructions
					Input: Complex verbal
					Processes: *Verbal comprehension,* verbal-motor integration
					Output: Simple motor
					Localization hypotheses: Left hemisphere
118	Point at				Description: Logical grammatical
119	Point with				
120	Point with	LT			Input: Complex verbal, simple visual
121	Daughter's mother	LT			Processes: *Grammatical comprehension*
					Output: Simple motor, simple verbal, simple
122	Father's brother	LT	FR		construction
123	Draw cross	LF			Localization hypotheses: Right hemisphere, left
124	Spring, summer				temporal, left parietal
125	Shorter	LF, RF			Description: Logical grammatical, structures
126	Fly, elephant	LT			
127	Lighter, darker	RT			Input: Complex verbal
128	Girl darkest				Processes: *Grammatical operations,* verbal
129	Arnie struck	LT			comprehension, verbal memory
130	Sawed wood	LT			Output: Simple verbal
131	Cleaned house	LT			
132	Mary studied				Localization hypotheses: Left parieto-occipital, left temporal, frontal

Note. For key to abbreviations, see note to Table 13.1.

Table 13.6: **Item Analysis: Expressive Speech Scale**

Item	Description	Localization	Lateralization	Pathognomonic	Analysis
133	Repeat vowel				Description: Articulation of speech sounds
134	Repeat sound	LF	FL		
135	See–seen				Input: Simple verbal
					Processes: *Verbal articulation*
					Output: Simple verbal
					Localization hypotheses: Left frontotemporal
136	Repeat house				Description: Reflected speech, words
137	Hairbrush				
138	Rhinoceros	LF			Input: Simple verbal
139	Cat–hat			P	Processes: *Word articulation*
140	Streptomycin	LF			Output: Simple verbal
141	Hat–sun				
142	House–ball				Localization hypotheses: Left frontotemporal, subcortical
143	Read sounds	LF			Description: Articulate speech, words
144	Read sounds	LF	FL		
145	Read words	LSM			Input: Simple written
146	Cat				Processes: *Verbal articulation*, reading comprehension
147	House				
148	Hairbrush	LF	FR		Output: Simple verbal
149	Rhinoceros	LPO			
150	Cat–hat	LSM			Localization hypotheses: Left frontotemporal, left angular gyrus
151	Streptomycin	LPO			
152	Hat–sun				
153	House–ball				
154	Read sentence				Description: Reflective speech, sentences
155	Read sentence	LT			
156	Read phrases	LT			Input: Complex written
					Processes: *Verbal articulation*, reading comprehension, verbal memory
					Output: Complex verbal
					Localization hypotheses: Left frontotemporal, left angular gyrus
157	Name objects	LF, RT	FR	P	Description: Nominative speech, naming objects
158	Name parts	RPO			
159	Name of item				Input: Simple visual, simple verbal
					Processes: *Naming*, visual-spatial recognition
					Output: Simple verbal
					Localization hypotheses: Left temporoparietal, right parietal

Table 13.6: **Item Analysis: Expressive Speech Scale**   *Continued*

Item	Description	Localization	Lateralization	Pathognomonic	Analysis
160	Count forward				Description: Automatization of speech
161	Count backward	LF			
162	Days of week	LF		P	Input: Simple verbal
163	Days backward				Processes: *Automatic speech,* verbal sequencing
					Output: Complex verbal
					Localization hypotheses: Left frontal
164	Describe photo	LF			Description: Predictive speech
165	Number of words				
166	Repeat story	LF		P	Input: Complex visual, complex verbal
167	Number of words		FR		Processes: *Verbal organization,* verbal
168	Make speech	LF			articulation
169	Number of words	RF	FR	P	Output: Complex verbal
					Localization hypotheses: Left frontal (or low IQ), right hemisphere
170	Omitted word		FR		Description: Complex grammatical expressions
171	Time		FR		
172	Make sentence	RT, RSM	FR		Input: Complex written
173	Arrange words	RT	FR		Processes: *Grammatical-spatial reasoning*
174	Time	RT			Output: Complex verbal
					Localization hypotheses: Right frontal, right temporal

Note. For key to abbreviations, see note to Table 13.1.

Table 13.7: **Item Analysis: Writing Scale**

Item	Description	Localization	Lateralization	Pathognomonic	Analysis
175	Number of letters	LPO, RSM		P	Description: Phonetic analysis
176	What letter	LT	FL		Input: Simple verbal
					Processes: *Visualizing words,* spelling apraxia
					Output: Simple verbal
					Localization hypotheses: Left angular gyrus
177	Copy letters				Description: Copying and writing, simple
178	Copy phonemes			P	
179	Write words	LPO, RSM			Input: Simple written
180	Write name				Processes: *Visual-motor symbolic integration*
					Output: Simple writing
					Localization hypotheses: Left angular gyrus
181	Write letters to dictation				Description: Copying and writing, complex

Table 13.6: **Item Analysis: Expressive Speech Scale**   *Continued*

Item	Description	Localization	Lateralization	Panthognomonic	Analysis
182	Write sounds		FL		
183	Write words	LT			Input: Simple verbal
184	Dictate	RT		P	Processes: *Visual-motor symbolic integration,*
185	Dictate		FL	P	verbal comprehension
186	Child-rearing	LT			Output: Complex writing
187	Time	LPO	FL	P	Localization hypotheses: Left angular gyrus, left temporal

Note. For key to abbreviations, see note to Table 13.1.

Table 13.8: **Item Analysis: Reading Scale**

Item	Description	Localization	Lateralization	Pathognomonic	Analysis
188	What sound?				Description: Phonetic synthesis, reading
189	What word?				
190	Read letters				Input: Complex verbal
191	Which letter?	LPO			Processes: *Letter organization,* spelling apraxia, verbal memory
					Output: Simple verbal
					Localization hypotheses: Temporal, parietal, left angular gyrus
192	Read sounds	LF			Description: Reading, syllables and words
193	Read words				
194	Read letters				Input: Complex written
195	Read words	LPO, RT			Processes: *Written-verbal integration*
196	Read words	LF		P	Output: Complex verbal
					Localization hypotheses: Left temporo-occipital, left temporoparietal
197	Read sentences				Description: Reading, complex
198	Read sentences				
199	Read paragraph	LPO, LT			Input: Complex written
200	Time				Processes: *Written-verbal integration,* verbal articulation
					Output: Complex verbal
					Localization hypotheses: Left angular gyrus, left frontotemporal

Note. For key to abbreviations, see note to Table 13.1.

Table 13.9: **Item Analysis: Arithmetic Scale**

Item	Description	Localization	Lateralization	Pathognomonic	Analysis
201	Write numbers				Description: Number comprehension
202	Write roman numbers	LF, RSM	FL		
203	Write numbers	LPO			Input: Simple written, simple verbal
204	Write numbers	LPO			Processes: *Number recognition*
205	Write numbers				Output: Simple written, simple verbal
206	Read numbers				
207	Read roman numbers	LF, LPO			Localization hypotheses: Left parieto-occipital
208	Read numbers	LF	FL		
209	Read down		FL		
210	Which larger		FL		Description: Numerical differences
211	Point larger			P	Input: Simple written
					Processes: *Numerical comparison*
					Output: Simple verbal, simple motor
					Localization hypotheses: Parietal
212	Solve multiplication				Description: Arithmetic operations, simple
213	Add				Input: Simple verbal
214	Subtract	LT	FL		Processes: *Arithmetic*
					Output: Simple verbal
					Localization hypotheses: Parietal
215	Add	LPO, RPO			Description: Arithmetic, complex
216	Add				
217	Subtract	RT	FR		Input: Simple verbal, simple written
					Processes: *Arithmetic,* memory, attention
					Output: Simple verbal
					Localization hypotheses: Parietal, frontal
218	Missing sign	RSM			Description: Arithmetic, signs
219	Missing number	LF	FL		
220	Compute		FL		Input: Simple visual
					Processes: *Arithmetic reasoning*
					Output: Simple verbal
					Localization hypotheses: Left parieto-occipital
221	Serial sevens	LPO, LSM			Description: Arithmetic, series
222	Serial thirteens	LPO			Input: Simple verbal
					Processes: *Repetitive arithmetic,* memory
					Output: Simple verbal
					Localization hypotheses: Frontal, left parietal

Note. For key to abbreviations, see note to Table 13.1.

Table 13.10: **Item Analysis: Memory Scale**

Item	Description	Localization	Lateralization	Pathognomonic	Analysis
223	Seven words		FL		Description: Learning unrelated words
224	Predicting				
225	Number of trials	RPO, LF	FL		Input: Simple verbal
					Processes: *Verbal memory*
					Output: Simple verbal
					Localization hypotheses: Frontal, temporal
226	Show card				Description: Retention and retrieval
227	Show card	RT	FR	P	Input: Complex visual-spatial
					Processes: *Visual-spatial,* sensory trace
					Output: Simple verbal, complex construction
					Localization hypotheses: Right hemisphere
228	Tap rhythm	LSM	FL		Description: Immediate sensory trace
229	Finger position	LSM			Input: Complex visual, complex auditory
230	Show card	LF			Processes: *Immediate recall,* nonverbal memory
					Output: Complex motor, simple verbal
					Localization hypotheses: Posterior right hemisphere
231	Words				Description: Retention and retrieval
232	Words	LT			
233	Sentences	LPO, RT			Input: Complex verbal, complex visual
234	Paragraph				Processes: *Verbal memory,* verbal-visual association, attention
235	Picture–words	RT			Output: Simple verbal
					Localization hypotheses: Diffuse dysfunction, left hemisphere

Note. For key to abbreviations, see note to Table 13.1.

Table 13.11: **Item Analysis: Intelligence Scale**

Item	Description	Localization	Lateralization	Pathognomonic	Analysis
236	Describe photo	RPO	FR		Description: Understanding pictures
237	Describe photo	LF, RT			
238	Picture arrangement	LT			Input: Complex visual
239	Time	LT, RT, RPO	FR		Processes: *Thematic,* sequential relations, abstraction
240	Picture arrangement	LSM	FL		

Table 13.10: **Item Analysis: Memory Scale**   *Continued*

Item	Description	Localization	Lateralization	Panthognomonic	Analysis
241	Time			P	Output: Complex verbal, simple motor
242	Why funny?	LSM			
243	Why funny?	LPO			Localization hypotheses: Diffuse dysfunction right hemisphere, frontal
244	Story				Description: Understanding text
245	Iron hand				
246	Proverb				Input: Complex verbal, complex written
247	Proverb	RT			Processes: *Abstraction,* verbal comprehension
					Output: Complex verbal
					Localization hypotheses: Diffuse dysfunction left temporal, frontal
248	Definition	LF	FL		Description: Concept formation, comparison and logical relationships
249	How alike?	LSM			
250	How different?	LF			Input: Complex verbal
251	What group?	LPO			Processes: *Verbal abstraction*
252	Group member				Output: Complex verbal
253	Whole, part				
254	Part, whole	RT			Localization hypotheses: Left hemisphere
255	Opposite	LPO			Description: Concept formation, opposites and analogies
256	Good, bad	RT			
257	What doesn't belong?	LF, RPO			Input: Complex verbal
					Processes: *Verbal abstraction,* verbal comprehension
					Output: Simple verbal
					Localization hypotheses: Left frontotemporal
258	Two apples	LSM	FL		Description: Discursive reasoning, arithmetic
259	Time	LF	FL		
260	Gave away				Input: Complex verbal
261	Time	LF	FL		Processes: *Abstract organization,* arithmetic, verbal comprehension, attention
262	Two more	RT			Output: Simple verbal
263	Time	LPO			
264	Ten acres	RT			
265	Time	RPO	FR		Localization hypotheses: Parieto-occipital, frontal, diffuse dysfunction
266	Books		FR		
267	Time			P	
268	Cyclist		FL		
269	Time		FL		

Note. For key to abbreviations, see note to Table 13.1.

14. Neuropsychological Evaluation of Neurosurgical Patients

The clinical neuropsychologist typically is required to study naturally occurring cerebral lesions such as those produced by neoplasm, cerebral metastasis, cerebrovascular accident, arteriovenous malformation, head trauma, or infectious or degenerative disease of the brain. Such lesions seldom are precise in their location or effect, and in the very great majority of cases it is not possible to obtain premorbid studies as a baseline against which to evaluate the course of the organic disorder. Neurosurgical patients provide a welcome alternative. They are very thoroughly studied with clinical neurological and radiographic examinations before surgery to precisely define the nature and location of the abnormal cerebral condition. The surgical procedures are explicitly operationalized, and postoperative clinical and radiographic evaluations are thorough. These physical findings can serve as excellent criteria for neuropsychological evaluations done pre- or postoperatively.

Here we present item analyses of performance by five patients who underwent neurosurgical treatment for correction of focal or generalized cerebral disorder. Two patients had left parietal arteriovenous malformations, two had hydrocephalus, and one underwent transcallosal removal of a tumor from the third ventricle and was found to have a recurrent tumor in the suprasellar region of the basal brain. All but the last patient were studied pre- and postoperatively with the Luria-Nebraska Neuropsychological Battery. Postoperative testing was done at intervals whenever there was some significant change in clinical status.

Patient 1

MEDICAL-SURGICAL BACKGROUND
Patient 1 is a 32-year-old right-handed Caucasian male with a 10th-grade education. He presented with pulsatile right/frontotemporal headache, right eye visual disturbances associated with headache, questionable loss of consciousness, progressive confusion, and memory loss.

The patient had been symptomatic for 32 months at the time of this examination. The neurologist's summary revealed that "the patient develops light and sound intolerance following the headache and then sees a halo of colors in the right eye with sparkling lights, and eventually kaleidoscopic visions." Radiographic tests showed no abnormality on skull films. A computed tomography (CT) scan revealed a calcified lesion in the left parietal area with a suggestion of increased blood flow in the distribution of the left middle cerebral artery. An arteriovenous malformation was suspected. Angiography demonstrated a "large left parietal arteriovenous malformation pointing to the left lateral ventricle, with major feeders from the middle cerebral, anterior cerebral, and posterior cerebral arteries and major drainage into the sagittal sinus." Amytal testing demonstrated dominance of the left cerebral hemisphere for speech.

The arteriovenous malformation was clipped and totally excised without complication. The postoperative course was benign. The only neurological deficit postoperatively was a right inferior quadrantanopsia that was associated with the surgical removal. Postoperative CT scanning and angiography showed complete obliteration of the lesion.

NEUROPSYCHOLOGICAL STUDIES

Patient 1 was examined with the Luria-Nebraska Neuropsychological Battery four times: two days preoperatively and three times postoperatively, at seven, 75, and 264 days. The importance of long-term follow-up is demonstrated by the progressive improvement in his performance during the postoperative course to a final point superior to the baseline performance. Examination with the Harris Tests of Lateral Dominance showed moderate right hand dominance. The patient had always shown preference for his right hand.

Motor Functions: Preoperatively the patient's fine manual dexterity was impaired. He could touch his fingertips to his thumb only slowly and deliberately. Fist clenching and extension of the fingers was slowed with the right

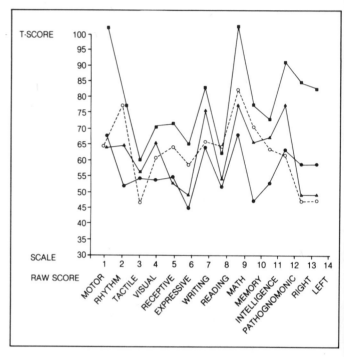

Figure 14.1. Age and education-corrected Luria-Nebraska Neuropsychological Battery scores for patient 1. The broken line with open circles shows the preoperative scores. The solid lines show postoperative scores, with values for seven, 75, and 264 postoperative days indicated by solid squares, solid triangles, and solid circles respectively.

hand but not with the left. Kinesthetic and optic-spatial organization were intact. Dynamic organization of the hands for alternating movements was impaired. If he attempted to repeatedly flex the right hand while extending the fingers of the left and vice versa, he could do the movements simultaneously only twice before he lost sequence and began to move one hand at a time. Rhythmic tapping of alternating beats (2R–1L or vice versa) was done slowly and laboriously. Minor inaccuracies of drawing detail occurred on freehand and copy reproductions of a circle, square, and triangle. The time to reproduce the figures was consistently slowed. Speech regulation of motor acts was intact. The other motor items, including complex forms of praxis, were performed normally.

At seven days postoperatively there was no change in

the impairment of fine motor dexterity. Consistent optic-spatial disorganization of the hands had developed, however, so that there was now consistent echopraxia. Errors on the more elementary items (9-12) had cleared by the ninth postoperative day, but the remainder of the items (13-20) showed persistent mirror-image imitation of the examiner's model. The dynamic organization of the hands was mildly improved but remained in the borderline impaired range. The tapping of alternating rhythms with the hands showed an echopractic variant. If the examiner demonstrated tapping twice with the right hand and once with the left, the patient imitated the model in mirror-image fashion and tapped twice with the left hand and once with the right. This continued when the rhythm was changed to two taps left and one tap right, to which the patient responded with two taps right and one tap left.

Kinesthetic oral movements was disturbed postoperatively. The patient did not protrude his tongue when told to stick it out and roll it up. He placed his tongue behind his upper teeth rather than between his upper teeth and upper lip. When asked to perform the sequence of showing his teeth, protruding his tongue, and then placing his tongue between his lower teeth and lower lip, he only clenched his teeth. He did not purse his lips to whistle, but blew air through his relaxed lips.

The mild construction difficulty in attempts to draw simple geometric figures spontaneously and from models was unchanged from the preoperative evaluation. Speech regulation of motor acts was intermittently disturbed postoperatively. On item 50 the patient performed correctly at first, raising his right hand for one tap and his left hand for two taps. On the third trial, when the examiner tapped once, the patient replied, "Do nothing, right?" On the fourth trial, when the examiner tapped twice, the patient tapped once. This was a perseveration from the instructions for item 48, where it would have been an appropriate response. On that item the patient imitated the examiner's example in one instance rather than giving the alternate response (if I knock once, you knock twice and vice versa). On item 51 a similar pattern was seen. The patient responded correctly at first (if I knock hard, you knock gently, and vice versa), but thereafter he began to imitate the examiner's model. Such attentional fatigue is understandable in the early postoperative period.

When the patient was examined at 75 days postoperatively the fine motor dexterity had reached a borderline (score of 1) level with both hands. The flexion-extension sequence with each hand separately was within normal limits. Kinesthetic basis of movement in the hands and optic-spatial organization of the hands was normal. There was no residual echopraxia. The difficulty with dynamic organization of the hands persisted unabated. The performance was slow, and the patient could not coordinate his hands to do the simultaneous flexion-extension or alternate tapping sequences of items 21-23. He remained slow but accurate in his reproduction of the figure in item 24, which had been too slow for credit since the postoperative course began. The kinesthetic basis for oral movement had returned to normal since the last evaluation. The patient could imitate the three-stage sequence of showing his teeth, protruding his tongue, and placing his tongue between his lower teeth and lower lip, but he could not perform the sequence spontaneously to verbal command. The mild construction difficulty on spontaneous drawing and copying persisted unchanged. Speech regulation of motor acts showed impairment only on item 50, where the patient made differential responses of raising the wrong hand in each instance.

The final examination at 264 days postoperatively showed residual mild impairment of finger dexterity and mild slowing of flexion-extension speed with the *left* hand only. An unexpected residual difficulty with optic-spatial organization reemerged at this examination. On items 11 and 12 the patient showed a 180° rotation of his hand in the sagittal plane. He also showed ipsilateral rather than contralateral imitation of the examiner's model on items 17 and 18 (e.g., examiner points with right hand to his left eye and patient points with his left hand to his left eye). Dynamic organization of the hands remained impaired at a level characteristic of brain-damage. The patient's performance on items 21–23 was slow, and he could not maintain the alternating synchrony for more than a few repetitions of the sequence. He made superfluous taps with the hand that made the multiple taps on items 22 and 23, a form of motor perseveration. The dynamic oral organization of item 33 that required the patient to show his teeth, protrude his tongue, and put his tongue between his lower teeth and lower lip was done adequately to imitation of the examiner's model but at a borderline level spontaneously because of slow execution. The mild construction difficulty was improved with respect to accuracy for freehand drawing and copying, but not for speed of execution, which remained very deliberate and exacting. The other motor functions were within normal limits.

Acoustic-Motor Organization (Rhythm): Preoperatively the patient had mild difficulty distinguishing whether pairs of tones were the same or different, but he had no trouble identifying the similarity or difference of groups of tones. He could not tell which of two tones was higher when they were presented in pairs. He was unable to hum pitch relationships or to sing a melodic line in imitation of a model, but he had no difficulty singing a melodic line spontaneously. He failed at more complex aural discriminations that were varied in speed, pitch, loudness, and number of items (items 60–61). Imitative tapping of the examiner's model of rhythmic groups was marginal on elementary items and consistently impaired on more difficult series that required tapping of loud and soft beats. The deficit was more pronounced when similar items were done to verbal command.

At seven days postoperatively the impairment in distinguishing tonal pairs was unchanged, but he had considerable difficulty with discrimination of groups of tones. Pairs of tones that varied in pitch were still misinterpreted in the range characteristic of brain dysfunction, but he made fewer errors than in the earlier postoperative period. Humming was adequate on the simplest item only, and the melodic intonation error patterns noted preoperatively were unchanged. Evaluation of brief rhythmic groups on item 58 was adequate, but an error was made on the first

portion of item 59, where a running total of sounds had to be determined. The reversal of these findings from the baseline workup appeared to be an attentional deficit variant. The more complex discrimination of pitch was impaired on item 60, but the more difficult item 61 discrimination was performed within normal limits. Auditory discrimination was improved postoperatively, but the effect this early in the postoperative course was still fluctuating as the patient's attention waxed and waned. Motor performance of rhythmic groups was still in the brain dysfunctional range, but errors were now confined to the more sophisticated items that emphasized accented tapping.

At 75 days postoperatively the patient still had mild difficulty with discrimination of pitch relationships. Groups of sounds to be discriminated on item 54 caused him more difficulty than single items. Items he missed were frequently described as sounding alike. His humming ability was improved to a borderline level. Melodic intonation in imitation of a model and in spontaneous singing were both impaired for the first time. Counting the number of items in smaller groups and maintaining a running total of sounds were performed adequately. The discrimination of faster accented beats on items 60 and 61 was improved to a borderline level. Motor performance of rhythmic groups continued to show impairment on the later taped items with accented beats because they were presented too quickly for the patient to grasp them. He performed errorlessly to verbal command on the similar tasks of item 63.

The final workup at 264 days showed borderline residual impairment in a number of areas of acoustic-motor organization. The patient still had difficulty discriminating pitch relationships and groups of sounds, humming pitch relationships, and counting the number of sounds per group in more complex series (item 60 only). Melodic intonation was adequate on a spontaneous and imitative basis. Motor performance of rhythmic groups showed substitution of a motor stereotype for the more complex accented items from a taped model. Spontaneous reproduction of rhythmic tapping patterns to verbal command showed mild impairment only when accented tapping was required.

Higher Cutaneous and Kinesthetic Functions (Tactile): Preoperatively the patient showed borderline ability to recognize pinprick pain to the dorsum of his right hand. He made one error on stereognostic recognition with the left hand, misidentifying a quarter as a nickel. The overall recognition time was borderline with the left hand for stereognostic items. The remainder of the sensory examination was within normal limits.

Seven days postoperatively there was confusion of some fingers of each hand in tactile identification. The patient misidentified the middle finger of the right hand as the ring finger, and he misidentified the ring finger as the index finger. He misidentified the middle finger of the left hand as the ring finger, and he identified his left forearm as his left shoulder. The letter *S* written on the back of the right wrist was misidentified as a *B,* and he could give no interpretation for the letter *S* written on the left wrist. The quarter was misidentified as a nickel with each hand separately, but with both hands stereognostic recognition times were within normal limits. The other sensory findings were normal.

The third workup at 75 days postoperatively revealed misidentification of the ring finger of the left hand as the middle finger. Graphesthesic difficulty persisted, with misidentification of the number 3 as an 8 when written on the back of the right wrist; the left-side performance was correct. The letter *S* was mistaken for a *G* when written on the back of each wrist. Stereognostic recognition time was slightly within the borderline range, but performance was errorless. The other sensory findings were noncontributory.

The final evaluation at 264 days postoperatively revealed borderline difficulty with interpretation of geometric figures drawn on the back of the left wrist. The number 3 was mistaken for an 8 when it was written on the right wrist. The patient could not distinguish numbers written on either wrist. The other sensory tasks were errorless.

Higher Visual Functions: Preoperatively, visual perception and naming of objects were accurate. On item 87, in which pictures of items are presented, the patient identified the nutcracker as tongs and the graduated cylinder as a metric scale. He identified the sunglasses in item 88 as glasses, but there was no perceptual difficulty. Overlapping figures were correctly identified, but the bowl in item 91 was omitted. The items from Raven's Progressive Matrices were performed marginally, both for accuracy and for speed of response.

Spatial disorientation was seen in misreading of a clockface set at 7:53 as 3:53, and one set at 10:35 as 9:35, and misdrawing of clock hands for 12:50 as 12:55. The patient could not tell cardinal directions on an unlabeled compass. He identified north as south and said there was "no way of telling" east and west. Perspective analysis of stacked block pictures was accurate on all items, but the first response was too slow to receive credit. The final plane rotation figure on item 99 was identified correctly in overtime, but the performance was otherwise errorless.

Seven days postoperatively, visual object naming remained intact, and errors on picture naming persisted. The nutcracker was identified as tweezers, and the graduated cylinder was called a ruler. The out-of-focus glasses could not be identified on the first, most blurred picture, but thereafter identifications were correct. The telephone in item 89 was perseveratively identified as an outline of glasses, since this had been the correct response for the previous three items. The glass in item 91's overlapping figures was identified as a cup, but this was not among the creditable alternatives. The Raven's Progressive Matrices items confused the patient. He said, "colors are wrong— none of 'em" for the first item, and he made the wrong choice for the second item.

Spatial orientation was more disturbed than previously. The clock set at 7:53 was read as 2:00, 5:09 was read as 5:00, and 10:35 was read as 2:10. The patient could not accurately set any clockfaces. He drew a line on an oblique axis from the 10–11 portion of the clockface to the 4–5 portion for all items. The cardinal directions north, east, and west were correctly identified on an unlabeled compass face. Perspective analysis was seriously impaired, with perseverative guessing as the rule. He was unable to perform the plane rotational task of item 99 because his attention wandered and he repeatedly lost track of the problem.

At 75 days postoperatively visual object-naming accuracy remained intact. Picture-naming errors were unchanged. Incomplete pictures were correctly identified, but the first item (telephone, item 89) required too much time to be credited. The overlapping figures of items 91 and 92 were perceptually recognized, but the patient identified the bowl as a "pan." The second Raven's Progressive Matrices item continued to be wrong, and recognition times continued to be in the borderline range.

Spatial disorganization was seen in difficulty with clock reading. Errors of varying degree were seen in the following responses: 7:53 read as 4:12; 5:09 read as 5:12; 1:25 read as 3:20; 10:35 read as 3:10. When the patient read the first two items he remarked "one of them is wrong," but he could not distinguish which item he had done in error. Clock setting was done slowly and meticulously, with counting around the clockface from the position of the number one each time to set each of the hands separately. Despite this procedure the patient drew 11:10 as 11:50. He correctly identified cardinal directions. All perspective analysis items were done wrong despite very slow and meticulous attempts. Item 99 was failed on the basis of excessive time, but the performance was 80% accurate at this administration; at the previous administration it was only 60% accurate.

The final evaluation at 264 days showed no change in visual perception integrity or picture-naming errors. Incomplete and overlapping figure identifications were fully correct for the first time. Raven's Progressive Matrices items were done at a borderline level for accuracy and speed. Clock reading showed continuing errors, with 7:53 read as 9:57 and 1:25 read as 2:25. Clock hands were drawn appropriately on blank clockfaces, but times to achieve correct performance were excessive. Cardinal di-

rections were correctly identified. Analysis of perspective was marginally impaired, with a minor error on the most difficult item and somewhat slow responses. One feature was missed on item 99, and the performance was within creditable time limits.

Receptive Speech Functions: Preoperatively the patient showed intact discrimination of phonemic units and consonant-vowel blends. He had trouble with phonemic discrimination associated with pitch change, as was expected given the difficulty with nonverbal pitch discrimination in the Rhythm scale. Sequencing was impaired on the pointing sequence of item 109. Identification of objects and concepts from pictorial arrays were errorless. Comprehension of simple sentence instructions was intact. Conflicting instructions on item 117 led to confusion and errors. Attributive grammatical relationships were disturbed. Although he identified the "mother's daughter" correctly, he could not tell whether the "father's brother" and the "brother's father" were the same person or two different people. He had difficulty with the complex three-person comparative analysis of item 128 and inverted grammatical structures, both of which confused him. Deficits in these higher-order, complexly organized linguistic structures that are dependent upon the tertiary left parieto-occipital association area were expected in view of the surgical resection.

Seven days postoperatively he had mild difficulty with auditory decoding of phonemes. Examples are the auditory misinterpretation of *b* as *p*, *k* as *h*, *g* as *c*, *b* as *m*, and *d* as *l*. Each item is read to the patient phonetically, rather than as a letter per se, so that the errors involve subtleties of interpretation. Much more dramatic was the patient's spatial disorientation in attempts to write letters. He asked "how does a *p* go?" He substituted the letter *d* for *b*, the sequence *b–p–b* was written as *r–b–l*, and the sequence *d–t–d* was written as *d–p–l*. Other similar errors could be cited, but these are illustrative. Conditioned hand-raising responses to phonemic cues were in the brain dysfunctional range; the patient substituted a single alternation sequence for the cued right–left–left–right sequence of item 106. The pointing sequence of item 109 continued to be impaired. Conflicting instructions of 117 continued to be carried out incorrectly.

Items involving spatially organized speech relationships were done incorrectly. The patient pointed to the key with the pencil when he was told to point to the pencil with the key. He recognized his error spontaneously. The "daughter's mother" was misidentified as the daughter. The "father's brother" was correctly identified as different from the "brother's father" at this testing. When asked to draw a cross beneath a circle, the patient drew a small circle beneath an oversized capital *A*. When asked to draw a circle to the right of a cross, he drew a horizontal line beneath a circle. The remainder of the receptive speech items were errorless.

The follow-up examination at 75 days showed improvement of phonemic hearing to the point that *m–p* was rendered as *m–b, b–p–b* was rendered as *b–p–d,* and *d–t–d* was rendered as *d–t–l.* The patient could not decode consonant-vowel blends on item 104. He reported that the sounds *bi–ba–bo* "don't sound right," by which he meant he could not discriminate one from another. The pointing sequence to verbal command on item 109 continued to be impaired. Spatial confusion persisted on the drawings to verbal command. The patient drew a circle to the left of a cross when asked to draw a cross beneath a circle. When asked to draw a circle to the right of a cross he drew the figures correctly. Some comparative constructions were done in error. He performed the three-person comparison of item 128 correctly for both comparisons. The double-negative comparative construction of item 131 was done incorrectly.

At the final workup, 264 days postoperatively, there was mild residual difficulty in phonemic decoding. Occasional errors were seen only on the three-item series. For example, *b–p–b* was rendered as *b–t–d,* and *d–t–d* was interpreted as *d–t–l.* These were the only errors of this kind. The deficit in phonemic hearing of pitch change persisted, as did the difficulty with sequential pointing. Conflicting instructions continued to be intermittently in-

correct. The three-person comparison of item 128 required more time than was allowed. The patient offered no solution to either part of the problem at this administration, though he had answered it correctly on the previous workup. Comprehension of most of these spatially organized grammatical structures had returned to normal.

Expressive Speech Functions: This section was relatively error-free preoperatively. The patient had some mild difficulty with phonemic and syllabic articulation, as in the errors *st* for *str* and *ark* for *awk*. He omitted a vowel from *laborious* and pronounced it *laborous,* and he misinterpreted *hierarchy* as *heresy.* He made minor errors of omission in reading simple sentences, and he was slightly slow in repeating days of the week in reversed order. Extemporaneous speech output and immediate story recall were limited by extended reaction time. More complex spatial analysis of language elements, such as the syntactical reorganization required on items 170–174, was beyond him.

At seven days postoperatively one noted occasional literal paraphasias. At the syllabic level, *pl* was repeated as *spl,* and *see–seen* was repeated as *seen–seen. Tree–trick* was rendered as *trick–tree–trick.* The sequence *ball–chair–house* was repeated as *wall–chair–house.* Attempting to count backward from 20 by ones produced "20, 11 . . . I goofed it up." He also could not say the days of the week in reversed order. Extemporaneous speech fluency had improved, but recall of a story was no more spontaneous than before. The syntactical speech organization deficit was unchanged from the preoperative level.

By the time of the 75-day follow-up evaluation there were isolated lexical misinterpretations (*heresy* for *hierarchy*) and persistent difficulty with spatially reordered sequences such as counting and reciting the days of the week in reversed order. Slowed reaction times for extemporaneous speech and immediate recall at paragraph level persisted unchanged, as did the more complex syntactical deficits. The paraphasic errors had resolved.

At the final workup 264 days postoperatively the patient continued to misread *hierarchy* as *heresy*, but his ability to perform automatic series in reversed order had resolved. The recitation of days of the week was a few seconds too slow to receive credit, but there were no errors. The complex syntactical grammatical expressions on items 170–171 and 173–174 persisted as problem areas at the final workup. This deficit parallels his spatial organization difficulty with linguistic material in other sections of the battery and is consistent with the site of the surgical resection.

Writing Functions: Preoperatively the patient had mild difficulty with phonemic analysis, as we have seen elsewhere on the battery. His copying of letters was slow and labored but consistently correct. His signature, an over-practiced motor stereotype, was fluid and legible. Spelling of unfamiliar words (*wren, physiology, probabilistic*) was incorrect, but more common words were written accurately from dictation. Extemporaneous writing on the topic of child rearing lacked necessary punctuation and was too brief to receive credit, but the limited content was relevant and logical.

Seven days postoperatively the phonemic analytic difficulty was somewhat more pronounced, and the speed of motor output for writing to dictation and copying was decreased. Reversals in this area were noted for the first time. For instance, the consonant-vowel blend *an* was written as *na*. A fine tremor was noted on all script writing, but the writing was legible. Subtitutions of letters occurred intermittently (*h* for *m*), and vertical inversions of letters occurred at literal (*f* and *l*) and lexical (*mren* for *wren*) levels. Writing at multiple-word, sentence, or paragraph levels was impossible.

By the time of the 75-day follow-up evaluation the letter inversions had resolved, but the patient's writing remained slavishly practiced and painstakingly slow. He was able to write letters in script from dictation, but these often lost credit because of slowness. Some sequencing errors also were noted. For example, the syllable *sti* was written as *sit*. The time taken to write his signature was too long to be creditable, but there was improved fine motor

control and fluidity to the reproduction that approximated the preoperative performance. The fine hand tremor had resolved. Longer series of words and extemporaneous writing at sentence level were gradually returning, but output was in the brain dysfunctional range on quantity of output. Spelling errors that were phonetic equivalents (e.g., *shoud* for *should*) were also noted.

At the final workup, 264 days postoperatively, the patient continued to write slowly but accurately at the literal and syllabic levels. Writing of unfamiliar words, word series, and sentences remained in the brain dysfunctional range, but the performance had improved from the previous workup.

Reading Functions: Preoperatively the patient had difficulty with phonetic synthesis of words from individual letters. He could not grasp the idea of an initial as an abbreviation for a given name, such as *J* standing for *John*. Reading aloud of syllables was slowed into the brain dysfunctional range, but reading of words up to the complexity level of *indistinguishable* was accurate. He had difficulty with phonemic analysis of more complex medical jargon such as *astrocytoma* and *hemopoiesis*, but he read commonplace sentences accurately. Reading at paragraph level was too slow to receive credit, since he analyzed each word individually rather than reading in larger, multiple-word units.

Seven days postoperatively one could note lexical approximations in reading syllables and words. The syllable *ply* was read as *play*, and the orally spelled word *k–n–i–g–h–t* was misinterpreted as *knife*. Similarly, *cor* was rendered as *crow*, and *prot* was interpreted as *pro*. The abbreviation *U.S.S.R.* was misread as *U.S.R.R.* An attempt to read *astrocytoma* produced *aristomatic*. Reading at brief paragraph level was unchanged.

The difficulty with phonetic synthesis had resolved by the 75-day follow-up evaluation. Some sequencing errors were noted intermittently (*cor* read as *cro*). The medical jargon terms of item 196 continued to perplex the patient. He continued to read slowly at brief-paragraph level. Errors were omissions, and these were all adjectives.

At the final workup, 264 days postoperatively, there were no further letter reversals. Attempts to phonetically analyze the medical jargon were more accurate than in previous workups (*hemopoiesis* read as *hemopophysis*). The difficulty in reading at the multiple-sentence level remained unresolved.

Arithmetic Skills: Preoperatively the patient was able to write single numbers in arabic and roman numerals accurately, but the latter were done very slowly and had to be analyzed in detail, so that none of them could be credited. Arabic numerals that are mirror images of each other (17 and 71; 69 and 96) also required extra time for detailed analysis and were written too slowly to receive credit. Numbers were written accurately up to two digits within creditable time limits, but three-digit numbers were written extremely slowly. The first breakdown of the categorical structure of number occurred at the four-digit level, when the patient wrote 9845 as 98045. At this relatively sophisticated level the idea of numerical place holders had become disturbed. In reading the earlier numbers that were mirror images of each other in roman or arabic numerals he was consistently overtime. Similarly, he was unable to read the four-digit number 9845 within the creditable period. He was able to read spatially reorganized multidigit numbers as integers when the place holders were written vertically instead of horizontally. Comprehension of number structure was disturbed at the higher level of comparison. The patient reported that 189 was larger than 201 after comparing the numbers piecemeal, since 189 has a set of digits that individually are larger than the elements of the number 201. When reading this comparison from a card, however, he was able to overcome the confusion and gave the correct answer. In simple calculations he made some multiplication-table errors, but very elementary addition and subtraction items were errorless. Two-place calculations were done too slowly to receive credit in some instances, and there were some "carrying" errors. The patient could not interpret an arithmetic equation with an addition sign omitted, such as 10 ( ) 2 = 12, though he solved similar items with omitted subtraction,

multiplication, and division signs. Serial sevens and thirteens were subtracted from 100 with borderline efficiency.

At the seven-day postoperative workup dramatic changes were readily apparent. Single numbers were confused with letters. The patient wrote the number 7 as 1 at first and then changed the 1 to a *P*. Analyzing the number 7 piecemeal led him to reproduce the vertical element, but the horizontal element was reversed from left to right, hence 7 was written as *P*. The numbers 3-5-7 were written as 3-*E*-*P,* all beyond the time limit. The roman numerals IV and VI were written correctly, but with great difficulty and constant cross-checking from one item to the other to analyze how one was different from the other; 69 was written as P9, the substitution here being a form of vertical inversion. An attempt to write 158 to dictation resulted in 15. The patient lost the task by the time he reached the final digit. He wrote 984 to dictation as 934, apparently because he could not grasp the closure of the figure 3 to make an 8. Thereafter he tried to correct his error and wrote 984 as 98484, a perseverative error that violates the categorical structure of number. Reversals were also noted, as when the patient read 1023 as 1203. He continued to think that 189 was larger than 201 by the logic outlined above, but postoperatively he gave this wrong answer both in writing from dictation and when the item was presented visually. Disturbance of arithmetic operations is seen in his response that $5 \times 4 = 45$. The substitution or juxtaposition of elements for the arithmetic operation of making a larger quantity shows basic confusion of arithmetic and spatial-numerical processes. Even the most elementary one-place calculations were beyond him at this time. When asked to add $5 + 9 + 7$ he replied that 597 was the sum. He was naturally confused about the missing arithmetic signs in equations. Serial subtractions and more complex calculations were confusing, and he could not attempt them.

The 75-day follow-up evaluation revealed that the individual arabic numerals could once again be discriminated without difficulty, but the less practiced roman numerals confused him when they were mirror images of each other (IV and VI, IX and XI). He wrote 17 and 69 within the time limits, but he wrote their mirror images, 71 and 96, too slowly to receive credit. He had to analyze each number point-by-point to clarify similarities and differences, and this slowed his performance. He wrote multidigit numbers right to left on the items 14, 17, and 19. Since the numbers are read as *four*-teen, *seven*-teen, and *nine*-teen (though not emphasized in this manner), he wrote first the element he heard first (4, 7, 9), then preceded this with the place holder 1 in the tens column for the *teen* part of the number. In each case the analysis was piecemeal, since he could not make the simultaneous synthesis necessary for understanding number structure that is dependent upon the parieto-occipital area of the dominant cerebral hemisphere. He continued to compare integer elements piecemeal and again concluded that 189 was larger than 201. This time, however, he was able to recognize the correct answer when he read the item though not when he analyzed it aurally. Simple arithmetic operations were generally accurate, but two-place addition and subtraction were still beyond him if carrying was necessary. Missing arithmetic operations symbols in simple equations were recognized without error, but the first item that involved multiplication was performed too slowly for credit. Missing numbers in simple arithmetic equations were noted with difficulty, and two-place elements in the equation confused him. Serial subtraction of sevens and thirteens from 100 continued to be performed at a borderline level.

At the time of the final evaluation, 264 days postoperatively, there was no disturbance of the categorical structure of number with reading, writing from dictation, or comparison of numbers. No reversals and no mirror imaging were seen. Errors continued to occur on higher-order, multidigit calculations where there was some residual disturbance in number structure. The item $44 + 57$ was answered as 1001, since the patient did the intermediate operations $43 + 57 = 100 + 1 = 1001$. Here he became lost in the place-holder position because the intermediate calculation took all his attention. Similarly, he reasoned

that $31 - 7 = 27$ because he borrowed 1 from the tens column and then brought down the remaining 2 and 7 into the answer column. He explained that he remembered he had to carry but became confused about the procedure once he had done the intermediate step. Juxtaposition of numbers as a sum continued to occur, as when he gave $5 + 9 + 7 = 597$. Operations signs omitted from equations were inserted correctly, as were numbers in other equations, but the latter items were done too slowly. The performance on serial subtractions remained unchanged. The calculational deficits are characteristic of Luria's ''parietal acalculia'' syndrome, in which there is disturbance of the categorical structure of number and symbolic arithmetic operations. The errors are typical for patients with lesions in the left parieto-occipital area.

Memory Functions: Preoperatively, rote list learning showed adequate initial recall on the first trial but inability to predict future performance from the previous trial. He gradually became accurate in ability to predict his performance, but he could not maintain an errorless performance once he had reached that level on the next-to-last trial. There was mild confabulation across trials. Immediate sensory trace recall was marginally unstable. The patient could not recall all elements of the geometric figure on item 227. He could not reproduce a set of rhythmic beats from immediate memory, since he omitted the critical loud and soft features of the series. He made the common error of raising his third, fourth, and fifth fingers on the third position of item 229 in the familiar ''OK'' position, rather than keeping them all curled as in the examiner's example. On a list of five words given five-second exposure, he missed one of the items. Heterogeneous verbal-visual interference on item 231 led to confabulation of an element from the previous item. The correct sequence *house–tree–cat* was recalled as *house–cat–boy*. Homogeneous verbal-verbal interference on item 232 led to perseveration as well as confabulation. The first three words were recalled correctly (*man–hat–door*), but the second three (*light–stove–cake*) were confabulated as *boy–stable–horse*. Repetition of *boy* was the perseverative feature. The stable and horse confabulations apparently were associations to the distractor picture of the previous item, which shows a man on horseback with a pack of hounds embarking on a fox hunt. At sentence level, the first sentence was recalled but the second was not. Recall of a brief story of several lines (item 234) was adequate and confabulation-free. The meaningful story line seemed to have aided recall and mnestic organization. Cueing with visual aids did not seem to aid recall, which was in the brain dysfunctional range, but errors were verbal approximations to the correct answer. For example, *employment* was recalled as *labor, party* as *picnic,* and *happy* as *pleasure/fun.*

At seven postoperative days the performance on list learning was more stable, with approximately the same initial performance. The prediction was accurate in most trials, but the patient failed to progress beyond the level of 6/7 items after the second trial. Instability of the memory trace was definitely in the brain dysfunctional range across items, with the exception of the hand position item 229, which was performed correctly. All five words were recalled correctly on the five-second memorization task with immediate recall. Confabulation from previous items persisted on the heterogeneous-interference verbal learning item 231. Recall was abolished on the homogeneous-interference item (232). The two-sentence homogeneous-interference task was recalled accurately, but the paragraph-length recall confused the patient somewhat and led to confabulation. Visual cueing did not aid verbal recall on item 235 postoperatively; he had no response for most of the items.

At the follow-up evaluation on the 75th postoperative day the patient was able to make steady progress on the list-learning task to a criterion normal performance by the third trial. This performance level was maintained on subsequent trials. The immediate memory trace remained unstable on visual retention and retrieval items (226–229). Immediate recall of the five-word list after five-second exposure remained stably accurate. Confabulation with homogeneous and heterogeneous interference on verbal

learning remained unimproved. The recall of sentence- and paragraph-length material was also unchanged from the previous evaluation. Pictorial cues did not aid verbal recall.

Final evaluation of mnestic functions at 264 days postoperatively showed perfect performance on the verbal list-learning task from the outset. The sensory memory trace for nonverbal material (items 226–229) was intact, and the performance was errorless. Recall of the word list on item 230 remained intact. Confabulation continued with heterogeneous and homogeneous interference on items 231–232, as had been noted postoperatively in previous evaluations. Recall of sentences and paragraphs was again intact. Pictorial cues did not aid recall; this ability was unimproved after the operation and was poor preoperatively as well.

Higher Intellectual Functions: Preoperatively the patient's comprehension and explanation of thematic pictures was intermittently confabulated or incomplete. His ability to deal with sequencing of events was mildly disturbed, though he could grasp the overall story line logically. Interpretation of thematic texts was adequate for simple factual details but not for inferential details. For instance, he interpreted the theme of the fable of the hen and the golden eggs as "don't kill the goose." Similarly literal interpretation of idioms was seen in his interpretation of the term *iron hand* as "a good strong grip." He interpreted some proverbs appropriately, in an abstract fashion, and he made appropriate choices for multiple-choice proverbial interpretation on item 247. Definitions, analogies, comparisons, and differentiations were functionally or descriptively concrete on some items. Logical relationships were analyzed logically for the most part. Discursive reasoning on elementary arithmetic problems was accurate but showed borderline slowing. Complex arithmetic problems were beyond his ability except for the final item of the test, which he performed quickly and correctly.

One week postoperatively the patient's performance on thematic picture interpretation and sequencing was unchanged from the baseline evaluation. The concrete functional description of thematic texts was also unchanged. There was no improvement from baseline in the various concept-formation skills. Seventy-five days postoperatively the patient's performance on higher intellectual functions continued to remain stable vis-à-vis the baseline performance.

At the final evaluation the patient had learned to describe abstractly and fully the relevant elements of thematic pictures; this was a skill that had not been noted previously. The mild difficulty with sequencing remained, but this was subtle. Interpretation of proverbs and idioms remained concrete and functional, but these items are overlaid with previous learning and may have been unfamiliar to the patient, given his 10th-grade education. Concept formation on various items such as definitions, comparisons, and differentiations continued to show intermittent concreteness. Logical relationships, opposites, and analogies were performed consistently at an abstract level. The slowness on mental arithmetic calculations continued, but performance was accurate. Some modest improvement in the more complex mental calculations was noted as well.

Pathognomonic Scale: Preoperatively, the Pathognomonic scale ranked near the cutoff for organic cerebral dysfunction, as is expected from previous research on lesions in the left parieto-occipital area of the cerebral cortex, where focal lesions typically appear less severe on this scale than in other parts of the left hemisphere. The marginal preoperative level could also be predicted in part from knowledge that this was a chronic lesion. One week postoperatively there was a dramatic elevation of the Pathognomonic scale to a point four standard deviations above the mean. The sensitivity of the scale to an acute brain lesion is in accord with previous research findings. Seventy-five days after surgery the Pathognomonic scale still remained two and one-half standard deviations above the mean, but the relative decline in the scale is in accordance with the clinical improvement noted from the item analysis. This final score on the Pathognomonic index

approximates the baseline preoperative evaluation level, and the profile shows the generalized level of improvement as noted from the foregoing item analysis by functional area.

SYNOPSIS

The lack of efficient kinesthetic feedback was revealed by motor deficits in oral and manual movement. Attentional skills were markedly disturbed postoperatively. Disturbance of the efferent system was seen in motor stereotypy associated with deficient kinesthetic feedback. Tactile functions were affected primarily at modality-nonspecific higher-order secondary and tertiary integrative levels of symbolic interpretation. Sensory errors occurred primarily in graphesthesic and stereognostic recognition during the course of recovery, whereas more basic sensory functions that were dependent upon projection areas farther from the area of surgical resection were spared. Higher-order visual-perceptual errors were also the rule, particularly when there was a need to integrate logico-grammatical structures into the interpretation. Secondary visual areas were affected considerably after the surgery, with directional disorientation and confusion on higher-order perceptual tasks such as those involving plane rotation and perspective analysis. Spatial disturbances were especially apparent in reversals of letters and numbers and misarrangement of letter sequences. Particularly characteristic for the parieto-occipital lesion site was the syndrome of parietal acalculia, with profound disturbance of the categorical structure of number and symbolic arithmetic operations.

It is noteworthy that disruption of the functioning of one of the two tertiary zones of the cortex, here the temporoparieto-occipital area, had generalized effect in elevating the profile as a whole. This was to be expected, since in the adult the tertiary zones have subordinated the functioning of the primary projection and secondary association areas to the overall planning and integrative programming of the tertiary cortical zones. When this controlling function is disturbed, there is generalized disruption of higher cortical functions until the functional system can be reorganized, as happened over the postoperative recovery period. In this case the final workup showed generalized improvement of higher cortical functions to a point better than the preoperative baseline. A similar pattern occurred in the course of recovery of patient 2, who had a lesion very similar to that of this patient.

Patient 2

MEDICAL-SURGICAL BACKGROUND

Patient 2 is a 40-year-old Mexican-American male with 14 years of education. English is his only language. He was natively left-handed but was converted to use of the right hand in fifth grade. Examination with the Harris Tests of Lateral Dominance revealed mixed ambidexterity with a right hand perference at the time of the preoperative examination. The neurological history of 10 years was remarkable for left retro-orbital headache, dizziness, fainting spells, and nocturnal seizures. During the extended preoperative course there had been increasingly severe headaches and progression of dysfunction on the right side of the body. Intermittent difficulty in word finding was noted; the patient would report that he knew a word but would lose track of it before he could fully articulate it. Some paraphasic misuse of words was also noted. Serial arteriography and computed tomography scans during the course of the illness showed progressive enlargement of the left parietal arteriovenous malformation. The preoperative arteriogram revealed a "large left parietal arteriovenous malformation with feeders from the left internal, left external, and left posterior cerebral arteries. There is also contribution of the right internal carotid to the left anterior cerebral artery via a large anterior communicating artery." Postoperative CT scans and angiography showed complete obliteration of the lesion.

NEUROPSYCHOLOGICAL STUDIES

Patient 2 was examined four times with the Luria-

Nebraska Neuropsychological Battery: at three days preoperatively and at 22, 43, and 214 days postoperatively (Figure 14.2). The period between the first and second postoperative evaluations was relatively brief, since his clinical status was thought to have changed significantly during that interval.

Motor Functions: Preoperatively the patient showed borderline manual speed and fine motor dexterity in attempts to touch each finger with the thumb. Alternate fist clenching and finger extension was also done at a borderline level. Kinesthetically controlled simple movement of the hands was intact. Optic-spatial organization of the hands showed intermittent echopraxia on the first trial of items 9 and 11, both of which are done with the right hand, but in each instance the patient corrected his errors on the second trial. Dynamic organization of the hands and ex-

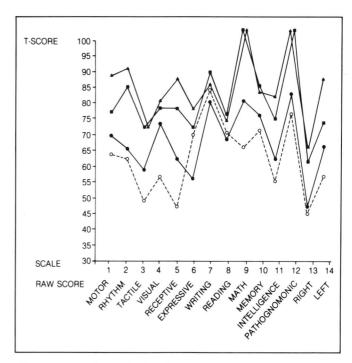

Figure 14.2.   Age and education-corrected Luria-Nebraska Neuropsychological Battery scores for patient 2. The broken line with open circles shows the preoperative scores. The solid lines show postoperative scores, with values for 22, 43, and 214 postoperative days indicated by solid squares, solid triangles, and solid circles respectively.

tension of the fingers of the other hand (item 21) showed normal performance of the left hand but slowed performance with the right hand. Simultaneity of movement was lost in alternation and led to perseverative tapping with the right hand only. The reverse sequence (2L-1R) was performed at a borderline-normal level without perseveration. Here again there was better motor control of the left hand. Complex forms of praxis that are primarily dependent upon executive frontal lobe function were errorless. Kinesthetically based oral movement and dynamic motor organization items were errorless and deft. Freehand drawing and copying of simple geometric shapes were consistently slowed into the brain dysfunctional range. Errors of figure closure, usually overlapping at the terminal junctions, accounted for the inaccuracies of detail.

At 22 days postoperatively the patient's finger dexterity remained unchanged, and extension was well within the normal range. Initial echopraxia was noted with the left hand on item 10 and with the right hand on item 13, but these errors were corrected spontaneously with a second trial on each item. Consistent echopractic errors were seen on items 17 and 19. When attempting to imitate the examiner's model of pointing with the right hand to the left eye, the patient pointed with his right hand to his right eye. When attempting to respond to the verbal command to point to his left eye with his right hand, he pointed with his left hand to his left eye. It is significant that he made consistent errors only on the more complex items that involved cross-body commands, and that he did not evidence primary confusion of left and right on other items. Dynamic organization of the hands for simultaneous alternating movements was improved from the previous workup. The right arm and hand tired much more quickly than the left, but the patient did not lose the alternating manual synchrony he had done preoperatively. The mild perseveration with the right hand on rhythmic tapping with alternate hands also had resolved. The patient could not draw the figure of item 24 postoperatively. Among the complex forms of praxis, he had lost the whole-hand movement of cutting with scissors (item 27) and simplified it to vertical movement of the index and middle fingers to indicate the cutting action of the scissor blades. Buccofacial dexterity was slightly slowed into the borderline range compared with the normal preoperative performance. The mild construction difficulty persisted, with less adequate fine motor control but more rapid performance than preoperatively. On item 51, involving the speech regulation of motor acts, the patient repeated *opposite* to himself before the first item and then proceeded instead to directly imitate the model of the examiner on every item. The salience of a direct model was too great for him to inhibit the imitative tendency, and he thus produced the wrong responses.

At 43 days postoperatively the patient's finger dexterity with the right hand had slowed barely into the brain-dyfunctional range, but his borderline speed with the left hand was unchanged. The manual flexion-extension sequence was done with borderline speed with the right hand but was normal with the left. The kinesthetic basis of movement was adequate for each hand individually, but cross-hand transfer was impaired. The patient touched the ring finger to the thumb instead of the middle finger, but he initially made the correct response with the right hand. Echopraxia was seen on the first trial with the more complex items (13 and 14), which require placing the hands in horizontal and sagittal planes, perpendicular to each other. When asked to imitate the examiner in pointing with his right hand to his left eye, the patient pointed with his left hand to his left ear. He imitated the examiner's model of pointing with his left hand to his right eye by pointing with his right hand to his right eye. He identified his right hand correctly on item 19, but then pointed with his left hand to his left eye when he was told to point to his left eye with his right hand. Dynamic organization of the hands progressed properly for three repetitions and then became desynchronized, with the hands moving independently. The rhythmic tapping of alternating beats was replaced by a single alternation sequence on item 23 and was slowed into the brain dysfunctional range on item 22. The patient still could not copy the line figure of item 24. On complex forms of praxis he showed coarse movement, as in attempts to mime the pouring of tea from a pot. Threading a needle was replaced by pointing with the index finger. The index–middle finger movements continued to replace the whole-hand scissors cutting movement. Buccofacial praxis was adequate with unlimited time, but the patient became confused and lost track of the three-stage sequence of items 32–33 when he had to perform them quickly and repetitively. Freehand drawing of simple geometric figures was errorless but was slowed into the brain dysfunctional range. Copying of the same figures continued to show the slowness of motor output, and accuracy declined to a borderline level. Impaired kinesthesia was seen on items 50 and 51, on which the patient commented "I have to figure out where my hands are." He perseveratively raised the right hand to all cues on item 50, and he made an error on the final trial of item 51 by imitating the examiner's model directly instead of giving the alternative correct response.

At the final evaluation, 214 days postoperatively, the patient showed mild slowing of the manual dexterity task of sequentially touching the digits to the thumb. Residual echopraxia remained on the crossed pointing tasks in imitation of the examiner's model and at verbal command, but in each instance the patient was able to correct these errors on a second trial. Dynamic organization of the hands for alternating flexion-extension movements was mildly slowed, but there was no desynchronization. Alternation of tapping movements similarly showed slowing but no loss of fluidity. The figure in item 24 was correctly drawn, though a few seconds too slowly to receive credit. Fine motor dexterity for complex forms of praxis was much improved, but the patient continued to use his fingers to imitate the cutting action of scissor blades when asked to demonstrate how to cut with scissors. Buccofacial praxis was adequate, but it was slowed to a borderline level on speeded repetition. Freehand and copied

drawings were done with borderline accuracy and were consistently slowed into the brain dysfunctional range. Speech regulation of motor acts was fully within normal limits.

Acoustic-Motor Organization (Rhythm): A remarkable finding at each examination from the preoperative workup to the final follow-up period was the patient's intolerance for high-pitched sounds. He would wince, grimace, withdraw, and cover his ears at the sound of the taped rhythm items, even when they were played at a lower, more muted level than normal.

Preoperatively the patient had marginal difficulty discriminating between pairs of high-pitched tones, but he was able to accurately compare groups of tones without difficulty. Reproduction of pitch relationships was marginal, and he could not sing a melodic line. Ability to distinguish rapidly presented tonal series on item 61 was borderline. Motor performance of rhythmic groups showed perseveration of the initial two-tap series when a three-tap series was required on the next trial. More complex patterns with alternating numbers of items and accentuation of groups with loud and soft taps (item 62) led to gross errors in which rhythm and accent were lost. Performance at verbal command was similar to that for the aurally presented model.

At 22 and 43 days postoperatively, pitch discrimination was diminished, and the patient made perseverative guesses when he was unsure of the answers. His intolerance for high-pitched sounds was more marked. He still could not sing a melodic line or hum notes that varied in pitch in imitation of a taped model. Tapping of rhythmic series to verbal command was errorless, but the same sort of errors made on accented tapping items preoperatively continued unabated.

At the final workup, 214 days postoperatively, he had no difficulty telling whether two sounds were the same or different, but he still had borderline trouble making such distinctions for groups of sounds. Pitch discrimination and reproduction remained marginally impaired. The patient spoke a melodic line rather than singing it as he had been instructed to do. Evaluation of groups of sounds remained marginal on some items, but the most difficult item in the series, number 61, was passed errorlessly. Motor performance of rhythmic groups in imitation of a taped model and to verbal command were errorless.

Higher Cutaneous and Kinesthetic Functions (Tactile): Preoperatively the patient misidentified the ring finger of the right hand as the middle finger. This is a common error, as the middle and ring fingers are most often confused in the tactile finger recognition task. Graphesthesia was diminished with the right hand only. The patient could not recognize a triangle drawn on the back of his right wrist. He could not tell whether the number written on his right wrist was a 3 or a 5, and he was correct but unsure whether the letter written on the back of his right wrist was an *S*. He was correct and definite in each instance for one of the same items drawn on the back of his left wrist. The other sensory findings were unremarkable.

At 22 days postoperatively there was gross confusion of the fingers and upper parts of both hands and arms. There was also confusion over which arm was being touched. Graphesthesia was bimanually diminished. A triangle drawn on the back of the right wrist could not be identified, and a triangle drawn on the back of the left wrist was misidentified as a cross. The patient could not recognize letters or numbers written on the back of either wrist. He misidentified a quarter as a nickel with his right hand, and stereognostic recognition time was slowed marginally with the left hand.

The sensory examination done 43 days postoperatively showed consistent confusion of the adjacent index, middle, and ring fingers of the right hand. The third and fourth fingers of the left hand were confused, and the left forearm was misidentified as the palm. Two-point discrimination was borderline with the right hand at 10 mm; this measure with the left hand remained within normal limits. Graphesthesia with the left hand was within normal limits for recognition of geometric figures and letters, but

not for numbers. The patient misidentified a 3 drawn on the back of his wrist as an 8. Recognition of geometric figures, letters, and numbers was consistently impaired for the right hand. Stereognosis was marginal for accuracy and recognition time with both hands. The patient called the paper clip "paper—what you put two pieces of paper...''; he seemed to have a functional grasp of the object's use but could not verbalize it clearly or name the object.

The final sensory evaluation at 214 days postoperatively revealed only residual confusion of the middle and ring fingers of the right hand. Two-point discrimination for the right hand remained borderline at 10 mm. Graphesthesia remained consistently impaired with the right hand. The only error with the left hand in this area was the continued misidentification of the number 3 as an 8 when written on the back of the left wrist. The other sensory findings were within normal limits.

Higher Visual Functions: Preoperatively the patient recognized objects presented for visual identification, but he had trouble with more subtle naming of items presented in pictures. He called a nutcracker tweezers, and a graduated cylinder part of a slide rule. He was able to recognize all the overlapping figures of item 90, but he correctly identified the dish and teakettle in the overlapping figures of item 91 only beyond the time limit. He performed the items from Raven's Progressive Matrices errorlessly, but his recognition time was slowed. Clock reading and setting were errorless, but he could not tell cardinal compass directions. He reversed north and south and east and west. Analysis of perspective on the stacked-block counting task of item 97 was disturbed only at the highest level, on the final item. He began by counting only the visible blocks, guessing first six and then seven blocks and finally attempting to include the hidden blocks with a final incorrect answer of nine. He made one error on the plane rotational analysis of the figures in item 99.

At 22 days postoperatively the errors of picture naming were unchanged. The same errors were also made on item 91, but this time the teakettle was paraphasically misidentified as a ''teapedal.'' The patient could no longer analyze the items from Raven's Progressive Matrices. He made intermittent errors on clock reading, misinterpreting 1:25 as 1:30 and being unable to read the time with the clock hands set at 10:35. He could not set the hands correctly at 12:50 on the blank clockface, but he passed the other clock-setting items correctly. He had no idea of cardinal directions. He was able to solve the most elementary of the stacked-block problems of item 97 but could solve none of the more complex ones. The plane rotational task of item 99 confused him, and he did not attempt to solve it.

At 43 days postoperatively there was no improvement in visual recognition on picture naming items. There was no simultaneous agnosia, but recognition time for overlapping figures remained excessive. Given sufficient time, however, the patient could name the figures. The items from Raven's Progressive Matrices were still too difficult for him. Clock reading was less efficient than at the last examination, and he passed no items. The patient read the clock set at 5:09 as 8:08, then corrected the error to ''eight after five'' with great effort. He began to read 1:25 as ''five . . . no,'' apparently attempting to analyze one clock hand at a time. He was able to set clock hands to appropriate times on blank clockfaces by counting around the clockface from the ''one'' position to the appropriate digit and drawing in the hands one at a time by repeating this procedure. He complained, ''I can't see,'' which Luria cites as a common expression of visual integrative difficulty in patients with lesions of the occipital association (tertiary) cortex. Cardinal directions remained confused. Analysis of perspective was considerably improved, with correct but slow responses on all items. To the plane rotational task the patient responded: ''I know how, but I can't see.'' He would not attempt the task.

The final workup showed continuance of the mild difficulty with the same picture-naming items as noted at baseline. The nutcracker was identified as clips and the graduated cylinder was functionally described as ''for measuring liquid.'' Higher visual cortex functioning was

significantly improved, with only one error on the 10 overlapping figures of items 90 and 91. The patient called the bowl a pan. The error was one of precision identification rather than basic perceptual inaccuracy. Owing to his right homonymous hemianopsia, he ignored the items on the right side of the card on the first of the items from Raven's Progressive Matrices, but he solved both correctly when he scanned the entire array. Clock reading inaccuracies persisted, with 10:35 misread as 9:35 and, more seriously, 7:53 misread as 10:35. All the blank clockfaces were correctly set to the specified times for item 95, but two of the three problems could not be solved within creditable time limits. The inability to distinguish cardinal directions remained unimproved. Intermittent errors with perspective analysis returned at this evaluation. The patient remained confused about the task demands of item 99, the plane rotational task.

Receptive Speech Functions: Preoperatively the patient showed intact phonemic hearing for repetition, writing, conditioned reflexes, and pitch change. Word comprehension for definition, repetition, identification, and simple sentence structure was also intact. Logical grammatical structures were intact for inflective and attributive case items. In the comparative constructions the patient could not comprehend item 126 about the relative sizes of an elephant and a fly before the time limit had passed. He thought that the phrases presented in the item sounded the same. He made an error in identifying the ''less light'' card of item 127. The inverted grammatical construction of item 130 was interpreted according to the usual expectation of eating before working rather than vice versa, as the item states.

At 22 days postoperatively the patient was able to repeat material adequately, but the spatial schemes of writing were seriously disturbed. As a result he failed all the phonemic writing items. He wrote an *m* in rotated fashion as the number 3, and he did not know how to make the letter *p*. Thereafter he refused to attempt the writing items because this difficulty confused and upset him. The patient's sequencing was also affected, in that he could carry out only the initial eye–nose part of the eye–nose–ear–eye–nose pointing sequence of item 109 before becoming confused. He accurately identified objects and concepts from multiple-choice pictures on items 110 and 111. He demonstrated the concept *pat* by touching the table with his open palm, but he could not define it verbally when he was asked to do so on item 112. Spatially organized language confused him greatly. He pointed to the key with the pencil when asked to do the opposite. When asked to draw a cross beneath a circle, he drew only a circle near the bottom of the space provided. When asked to draw a circle to the right of a cross, he drew another circle in the right portion of the space. When the examiner asked him where the cross was, the patient replied: "I haven't marked it down." When asked why he had not done so, the patient replied: "you said to draw the circles, that's all, one beneath and one next to *the cross*." Spatially organized grammatical comparative constructions also confused him, and he continued to say that a fly was larger than an elephant when the question was comparatively phrased. Additional questioning showed that the error was a function of the way the question was phrased, since he recognized the relative sizes of the two animals when asked to describe them individually. The comparative construction involving the "less light" comparison continued to be incorrect. Inverted grammar also led to a choice error on item 129, but not on items 130–132.

At 43 days postoperatively, phonemic hearing was intact but there was still confusion of the spatial elements of letter writing that interfered with all attempts at writing. Phonemic hearing with pitch change on item 107 was done in error.

All but the last item of the sequence of item 109 were done correctly, a great improvement from the baseline performance. On item 111 he misidentified his chin as his cheekbone. Conflicting instructions on item 117 led to inconsistent errors, with perseveration from the first response to the second one. Attributive grammatical structures were impaired. The patient identified the daughter instead of the mother when asked to point to the "daughter's mother." He said that the "father's brother" and the "brother's father" were the same person. When asked to draw a cross beneath a circle and then to draw a circle to the right of a cross, he reversed the positions in each case, drawing the figures in the order of presentation rather than in the spatial configuration requested. He continued to confuse the concepts *lighter* and *less light*, *darker* and *less dark*. He could no longer do the three-person comparison of item 128. Inverted grammatical constructions were intermittently misunderstood. Spatially organized and complex logical grammatical structures confused him, as Luria's theory of higher cortical functions predicts for a tertiary left parietal lesion.

By the final workup at 214 days postoperatively there was residual phonemic hearing difficulty, with confusion of the phonemes *s* and *l*, *g* and *d* when pairs of phonemes were dictated phonetically. The *bi–ba–bo* sequence was repeated as *ba–bi–bo*. Pitch change confused the patient on item 107, where he could not distinguish between similar-sounding phonemes. While he passed item 123 at the final examination, he did much self-questioning of which was his right hand and which was his left. When asked to draw a circle to the right of a cross, he drew the circle first and then was confused about where to place the cross. He first drew the cross to the right of the circle, then changed it to the left of the circle and clarified the solution through a self-questioning process. Comparative constructions of *less light* and *less dark* on item 127 continued to be incorrect, and the complex three-person comparison of item 128 continued to be wrong.

Expressive Speech Functions: Preoperative articulation of written phonemes, syllabic blends, and the words of items 133 through 142 was errorless. Pronunciation of blends presented on cards caused consistent difficulty. The speech sound *th* was repeated as *t*, *pl* was repeated as *p*, *str* was repeated as *sh*, and *awk* was repeated as *hack*. Errors involved phonemic approximations on the whole, usually with omission of one or more letters. For example, *laborious* was read as *laborous*. Paraphasias occurred in running speech, such as *shun* for *sun* on item 154 and *woof* for *wolf* on item 155. Response times were slowed on extemporaneous narrative and reproductive speech, but output was inadequate only on item 167, where the patient became confused. He did well when he could organize the topic himself (items 165, 169), but he became confused with too much input when he had to assimilate detailed paragraph-length material (item 167). He was unable to syntactically reorganize the elements of disarranged sentences on item 173.

The postoperative workup at 22 days showed no appreciable change in phonemic pronunciation with an aural or a written model. Reversed counting from 20 to 1 was correct until the end of the sequence, when the patient omitted the number 1 and counted 3-2-0. Extemporaneous speech was more fluid and spontaneous, and output remained within normal limits. Paraphasias were not noted at this administration. Syntactical reorganization at sentence level from disarranged words remained beyond his ability.

At 43 postoperative days paraphasias were again noted, such as *bell* for *ball, crees* for *trees, shun* for *sun.* On reversed counting from 20 to 1 the patient omitted the numbers 10 through 1. He recited days of the week in reversed order correctly for Sunday through Wednesday, then lost the task and began to recite them forward. The other findings were unchanged.

The final workup was remarkable for slow but accurate reversed counting, slowed initiation but adequate output on extemporaneous speech, and syntactical reorganization difficulty in forming sentences from disarranged words. Other expressive speech functions were within normal limits. It is remarkable that spatially complicating the task by reversing an overlearned sequence such as counting or reorganizing words to make larger sentence units led to errors, whereas tasks without the spatial component were not consistently disturbed.

Writing Functions: Preoperatively the patient had great difficulty with phonemic analysis. He could not tell the number of letters in words or their relative position in the sequence. His copying of letters was too slow to re-

ceive credit, and his signature was illegible. Writing phonemic blend sounds from dictation was impaired into the brain-dysfunctional range, and more complex spelling of unfamiliar words, as well as writing from dictation at longer unit levels such as phrases and sentences, was beyond him.

At 22 days postoperatively the performance remained much the same on the profile scaled score, but the quality of disturbance was much more serious. The patient was unable to reliably write even single letters because of his spatial disorientation. There was no significant change at 43 postoperative days. Copying and writing from dictation remained slavish even at the final workup, and there was basic confusion. The patient wrote a *t* when asked to write an *f,* then misread the letter *t* he had written as an *l.* He analyzed each letter's elements piecemeal in terms of vertical and horizontal components, and this finally produced correct identification. With a model he could copy letters in printed and script form very slowly and accurately. Without such cues his performance was severely impaired.

Reading Functions: Reading was less severely impaired preoperatively than writing, but performance was still well into the brain-dysfunctional range. Phonemic approximations were seen on a number of items: *play* for *ply, corn* for *cra, spore* for *spro,* and *clockroom* for *cloakroom.* He was able to read *insubordination* with great difficulty, but he could not finish reading the simpler but longer paragraph of item 199 within the allotted time.

Postoperatively at 22 days the foregoing deficits were more pronounced and consistent. Even letters were misread, as when *U.S.S.R.* was read successively as *U.S.R.-U.R.R.-no-U.S.S.R.* The patient complained of poor vision when presented with the paragraph of item 199 and said that it was difficult for him to read because the print was "too small." He had been reading the same size print with variable success on the preceding items. The only significant change seen at 43 postoperative days was his reading the letter array of item 190 from right to left.

By the time of the final workup the patient still evidenced basic reading deficits. Phonetic synthesis showed borderline impairment, and reading of syllables and words was excessively slow. Most serious errors occurred with novel, difficult words (hemopoiesis, astrocytoma) that would have required intact phonemic analytic and synthetic skills for decoding. Reading at brief paragraph level remained very slow and labored, but it was accurate within the patient's modest residual ability range in this area.

Arithmetic Functions: Preoperatively the patient wrote some numbers illegibly, so that the number 9 appeared to be a 1 in one instance. He wrote roman numerals slowly but accurately and showed no mirror-imaging on item 202. Arabic numberals were written with normal speed and accuracy. He wrote numbers through four-place level accurately but misread 27 as 24. The two-place addition and subtraction problems of item 215 that involved carrying were accurate when done mentally. The categorical structure of number and symbolic arithmetic operations were intact. Subtraction of serial sevens was accurate but slowed to borderline level; subtraction of serial thirteens was within normal limits for speed and accuracy.

At 22 days postoperatively the patient showed the parietal acalculia syndrome. He was confused about writing single numbers from dictation. He substituted 9 for 3, and he thought that a properly written numeral 3 was a "backward three." He could not write roman numerals for IV, IX, or XI though preoperatively he had been able to do so in the overtime period. Writing of numbers that were mirror images of each other in arabic numbers (17, 71, 69, 96) was errorless. In reading numbers he showed breakdown of the spatially based categorical structure of number, with loss of the idea of place holders in four-digit numbers. He could not read the number 9845 as a unit but rather read it as 9–845 (nine–eight hundred forty-five). He misread the number 158 as 159 and read the number 1023 as "1–02 . . . 32 . . . no, 2–3." The patient could tell which of two numbers was larger when they were dictated and when he saw them, but he was excessively slow to decide which was larger when they were presented in written form. He would not attempt the two-digit addition and subtraction problems that he had previously been able to do mentally. The concept of symbolic arithmetic operations was abolished postoperatively at this period. He would not attempt serial subtractions.

At 43 days postoperatively the patient still substituted numbers for each other when writing from dictation (confused 5 and 7), but now he recognized the error spontaneously. He continued to have trouble recognizing numbers as units, and though he wrote them correctly in most instances he often thought they were "backward." He thought his correct rendering of 69 was backward, but he did not confuse it with 96. He thought the figures 9 and 5 in the number 9845 were "backward," even though he had written them correctly. He misread the number 396 as 986. He could not read vertically arranged numbers as integers on item 209, and he had not been able to do so on the previous postoperative evaluation. This spatial reorientation was sufficiently difficult to confuse his weak spatial-analytic skills and categorical structure of number so that he reduced the integers to single digits. There was no difficulty distinguishing which of two numbers was larger with either visual or verbal presentation of the material. His difficulties with more complex arithmetic, symbolic arithmetic operations, and serial mental calculations were unchanged from the previous workup.

At the final workup less-practiced roman numerals still caused the patient some confusion when he attempted to write them from dictation, but he had no difficulty reading them on a later item. Arabic numerals were written accurately without evidence of mirror-imaging or other error. At the four-digit level the number 9845 was misread as 985 but was then reread correctly. The vertically rearranged integer sequence of item 209 was confused so that 158 was misread as 185. The number 396 was misread as 196, possibly as a perseveration from the previous item. Surprisingly, the patient was able to read 1023 correctly on the first attempt. He corrected his errors spontaneously within the time limit in each case. He was once again able to do mental two-place calculations involving carrying. Symbolic arithmetic operations were confused, as they had been previously. Serial mental calculations and more complex three-digit or three-item mental calculations still remained too difficult for the patient. The syndrome of parietal acalculia had partially resolved to a residual disturbance of the categorical structure of number, but symbolic arithmetic operations remained basically disturbed.

Memory Functions: Preoperatively the patient's rote verbal learning of unrelated words was superior but unstable. He achieved a perfect performance on the first trial of the word list presented in item 223, but he forgot the list completely on the second trial. He recalled six of the seven words on trial 3, and his performance was errorless thereafter. The immediate sensory trace was unstable for retention of visually and aurally presented material on items 226–228. The hand positions of item 229 were recalled correctly. The patient forgot one of the five words at immediate recall for item 230, but he had no difficulty with heterogeneous or homogeneous interference on verbal recall. He recalled the first of the two sentences of item 233 correctly but made an omission in recall of the second sentence. Recall of the brief story about the crow and the doves presented in item 234 was within normal limits. Visual aid did not assist recall sufficiently on item 235, and the performance ranked in the brain-dysfunctional range.

At 22 days postoperatively the verbal learning curve was initially somewhat lower, with five of seven words recalled. Performance did not improve with practice on successive trials. The immediate visual memory trace remained unstable. He passed the accented rhythmic tapping sequence of item 228 this time, but on the previously passed hand position sequence (item 229) he failed all three procedures. Recall of the five-word list of item 230 was deficient by three words postoperatively, a performance decline of 40% from the preoperative level.

Heterogeneous visual interference with verbal recall did not impair performance, but he forgot one item in the second group with the verbal-verbal homogeneous interference procedure of item 232. Recall of sentences was unchanged, but the patient was confused postoperatively by the brief story of item 234. Visual aids continued to be ineffective in aiding verbal recall, but level of performance was much more clearly into the brain dysfunctional range postoperatively, with six errors in seven items compared with two errors on this item preoperatively.

Significant changes at 43 postoperative days were selective. He again failed the accented tapping sequence of item 228, as at the preoperative baseline. The five-word sequence of item 230 was recalled errorlessly. The other performances were unchanged from the last workup.

The final evaluation at 214 postoperative days showed return of verbal learning ability to the preoperative normal baseline, but with a more stable learning curve at follow-up. The immediate memory trace remained unstable for visual retention and retrieval. Immediate recall of the five-word series was stable and errorless. Heterogeneous and homogeneous interference produced instability of verbal recall, with poorer performance after heterogeneous interference. Recall of the unrelated sequential sentences remained unimproved, but recall of the meaningfully organized brief paragraph was within normal limits. Visual cues did not aid recall and may have interfered with verbal rehearsal, as in the foregoing heterogeneous verbal-verbal interference paradigm.

Higher Intellectual Processes: Interpretation of thematic pictures and sequencing skills were intact preoperatively. Definitions were intermittently concrete with descriptive (table: "four legs and a flat piece of wood") or functional (ax and saw are alike because "they both cut") explanations of the object or concept in question. Logical relationships, opposites, and analogies were performed correctly with the exception of the second part of item 254. Here the patient confused part and whole concepts and reasoned that if the whole were a tree, the parts would be the leaves and trunk, whereas the task was to reason from the tree as the *part* to the whole as a forest or woods.

At 22 days postoperatively the patient's complex logical-grammatical structures were seriously disturbed. He interpreted the winter scene of item 237 with two people riding a horse-drawn cart and a dog looking on as follows: "this is a dog on a sled . . . and it's wintertime. When I say sled I mean horse and . . ." (no further comment). The patient was unable to do sequential reasoning adequately on the picture-arrangement items. His concrete interpretation of the theme of the fable "the hen and the golden eggs" was "don't kill the hen." Similarities, differences, opposites, and analogies also showed concreteness of reasoning postoperatively. At 43 postoperative days the patient confabulated on item 237, which presented the winter scene. He interpreted this scene as "they're riding in a snowmobile." The remainder of intellectual functions was not significantly improved at this recovery stage.

At follow-up 214 days postoperatively the patient showed recovery of ability to interpret thematic pictures, and his grasp of logical sequencing was slowed but accurate. Understanding of simple factual details remained adequate, but his grasp of unifying themes remained concrete and literal. Comparison and differentiation was consistently concrete. Logical relationships for class inclusion were appropriately abstract for inductive and deductive reasoning items, except for the second part of item 254, which had confused him preoperatively as well. With the part concept given as *trees,* he gave the whole concept as *lumber,* whereas he had previously misinterpreted it as leaves and trunk. The patient still could not deal with analogies at the final workup. To the analogy that posed the relationship of shoe:foot as hand:_____ (glove, mitten) the patient commented: "both belong to the same body, and both have five of a kind" (fingers, toes). He had lost the idea of comparing *pairs* of items to define relationships. This sort of complex language disorganization that is dependent upon teritary parietal zone functioning

was expected in light of the known area of surgical resection, and the deficit was seen at each postoperative workup.

SYNOPSIS

Like the first case, patient 2 showed a syndrome of the tertiary temporoparieto-occipital cortex of the dominant hemisphere that affected higher cortical functions generally. This is reflected in the overall elevation of the profile postoperatively and the decline of the profile as the lesion healed. Deficits consistently involved more complex forms of praxis, gnosis, and speech. The dominant right hand was implicated in echopractic errors, lack of synchrony in bimanual movements, manual perseveration, and construction difficulty. Higher-order integrative sensory deficits were similarly the rule, with sparing of more elementary skills dependent upon subordinate primary and secondary perceptual systems. Graphesthesia, finger gnosis, and two-point discrimination were all mildly impaired with the right hand. Visual perception showed slowness to process more complex material such as items from Raven's Progressive Matrices and the overlapping figures of Poppelreuter. More complex visual-spatial functions such as recognizing cardinal directions, reading and setting clocks, and analyzing plane rotation and perspective that are dependent upon the parieto-occipital zones remained impaired.

Complex logical-grammatical structures of speech were seriously disturbed, with even elementary literal and lexical forms confused early in the postoperative period. Spatially organized linguistic forms and comparative forms based upon them resolved more gradually. The categorical number structure of number and symbolic arithmetic operations were very seriously disturbed postoperatively, and significant difficulty remained in this area at follow-up. These skills depend on the spatial schemas of the dominant temporoparieto-occipital cortical zone. Inability to deal with pairs of items in logical comparisons was affected by the spatial confusion and contributed to descriptive and functional "concrete" comparisons when items were analyzed piecemeal and compared according to their characteristics.

Patient 3

MEDICAL-SURGICAL BACKGROUND
Patient 3 is a 33-year-old, right-handed, Filipino-American male with 12 years of education. English is his second language after Tagalog, but he has spoken both languages fluently since childhood and is quite articulate in English. His history is remarkable for onset four months before surgery of headache that was unrelieved by aspirin. Associated symptoms included nausea, vomiting, blurring of vision, visual hallucinations, increased urinary frequency, and a 25-pound weight gain. A preoperative CT scan revealed "a large enhancing lesion of the third ventricle that on angiography appeared avascular." The patient underwent right frontal craniotomy with transcallosal intrathird ventricular resection of the tumor, which proved to be a craniopharyngioma. In the operative report the surgeon noted that "the tumor was large, certainly bigger than a hen's egg." Postoperative and subsequent CT scans showed recurrent tumor in the suprasellar cistern. The patient underwent radiation therapy to the area of the focal residual tumor. Further surgery to remove the residual tumor mass was deferred, and the patient's case was being followed at the time of testing since he was neurologically asymptomatic and there was significant associated surgical risk with a subfrontal approach to the tumor. There are only postoperative results with the Luria-Nebraska Neuropsychological Battery for this patient, since he was treated at another hospital before he was transferred to the Palo Alto Veterans Administration Medical Center for follow-up evaluation and treatment.

NEUROPSYCHOLOGICAL STUDIES
Patient 3 was examined with the Luria-Nebraska Neuropsychological Battery 126 days postoperatively.

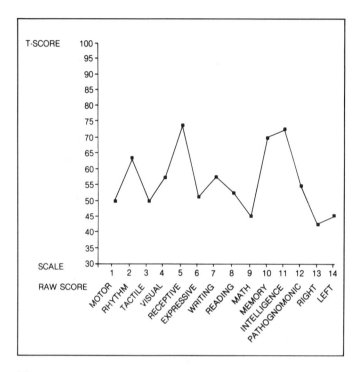

Figure 14.3.   Age and education-corrected Luria-Nebraska Neuropsychological Battery scores for patient 3. The profile shows the 126-day postoperative performance.

Motor Functions: The patient showed mild slowing in touching the fingers of the left hand with the thumb. While the performance was identical with that of the right hand on this item, the more stringent norms for the left hand gave the appearance of mild lateralized deficit. Fist-clenching, alternating finger-extension, manual kinesthesis, and manual optic-spatial organization were all within normal limits. Dynamic organization of the hands on the alternating flexion-extension task of item 21 was normal, but tapping of alternating rhythms with the hands was slowed to a borderline level (score of 1) on items 22 and 23. In performing complex forms of praxis, he simplified the whole-hand scissors-cutting pantomime to vertical movements of the index and middle fingers to indicate the action of scissor blades. On a test of buccofacial praxis he was unable to protrude his tongue and roll it up. The three-stage oral sequence of item 33 was slowed to a borderline level. Mild construction difficulty was seen in freehand drawing and copying of a circle, square, and triangle.

Acoustic-Motor Organization (Rhythm): The patient's ability to discern pitch relationships between single tones was borderline. He was completely unable to distinguish between groups of tones. Humming of tones was adequate with two-tone series and marginal with three-tone series. Attempts to sing a melodic line were adequate spontaneously but not in imitation of a taped model. He had borderline difficulty in identifying the number of sounds in groups that were presented more quickly and subtly, as on item 60, but the more elementary items 58 and 59 were done errorlessly. He had intermittent difficulty in tapping a rhythmic sequence, both in imitating an aural model and at verbal command.

Higher Cutaneous and Kinesthetic Functions (Tactile): Sensory examination was very nearly errorless. All the following modalities were intact: tactile finger identification, pinprick sensation (dorsal manual), cutaneous light pressure, two-point discrimination, tactile directionality, and proprioception. The patient mistook the number 3 written on the back of his right wrist for an 8, but performance on the other graphesthesic items was unremarkable. Stereognostic performance was errorless, but recognition time was bimanually slowed to a borderline level.

Higher Visual Functions: Naming of concrete objects was adequate, but on more subtle items presented pictorially there were naming errors. The patient could not recognize the nutcracker on item 87, and he misidentified the graduated cylinder as a ruler. He identified the egg carton as an egg holder. He had no difficulty with identification of the intentionally blurred pictures of item 88, but he could not recognize the ambiguous figures of item 89. The overlapping figures of items 90 and 91 presented no frank perceptual difficulty, but he called the teakettle a kettle and the bowl a pan, so that he earned a borderline score.

The patient could solve neither of the items from Ra-

ven's Progressive Matrices. Clock reading showed inaccuracy of detail (5:09 read as 5:07; 1:25 read as 1:20). Clock setting was within normal accuracy limits. The patient reversed east and west on the directionality task. His performance on higher-order perspective and plane rotational analysis on items 97–99 was entirely within normal limits.

Receptive Speech Functions: Phonemic repetition and reproduction were errorless for items 100–105. Phonemic discrimination at differing pitches on item 107, however, was too difficult, and the patient reported that the same phoneme repeated at a different pitch was a different letter. Care was taken to be sure he understood the task before the examples were presented. The elements of item 109 were recalled, but the sequence was wrong (eye-ear-nose-eye-ear substituted for eye-nose-ear-eye-nose). The patient pointed to his chin when asked to point to his cheekbone. When asked to define *pat* he said: "It's made of clay; you put something in it in the ground to cook it." When asked if he meant *pot,* he agreed. He could not grasp the concept of *pat* when the item was repeated.

Simple sentences, conflicting instructions, inflective, attributive, and spatially organized grammatical constructions were errorless. Some comparative constructions caused difficulty, as when the patient could not grasp item 125: "Which boy is shorter if Tom is taller than Arnie?" He made the common error of misidentifying the gray card as "less light" when presented with a black and a gray card on item 127. The three-person comparison of item 128 confused him, as did the inverted and complex grammatical constructions of items 129–132.

Expressive Speech Functions: Repetition was nearly errorless at phonemic through lexical level of items 133–142. On item 134 the patient substituted *pa* for *th,* and he substituted *mell* for *bell* on item 141. Reading phonemes caused more difficulty. The patient could not find a phonetic equivalent for *m* and *b,* and he read them as letters despite an adequate performance on the other items. He had difficulty with some of the blends as phonemic units, but he knew how to use them appropriately in words. He could not read *pl, str,* or *awk* phonetically by themselves but substituted *plateau, straight,* and *awkward.* Repeated attempts to explain the task in a testing-the-limits procedure were fruitless. On item 149 *hierarchy* was misread as the verbal paraphasia *hierarsee;* more complex items were read errorlessly. In the second part of item 155, simplication and substitution of the sentence produced: "In the edge [of the forest] . . . the hunter kills [ed] the wolf." A literal paraphasia on item 157 led to the misnaming of the candle as a *handle.* Extemporaneous speech was fluent, relevant, and coherent. Item 172 was missed because the patient altered one of the words to maintain correct grammatical form: "The *automobile* was parked inside the *garage* with a *wooden* door." He could not solve the first sentence rearrangement task of item 173, but he solved the second passage.

Writing Functions: Errors in the Writing scale involved primarily spelling and phonemic analysis. The patient thought there were three letters in *trap* and four letters in *hedge.* He could not spell *district, antarctic,* or *probabilistic.* He substituted *some* for *sun* and *rain* for *wren* from dictation. Extemporaneous writing on the topic of child-rearing was within normal limits for grammar, content, spelling, and quantity of output. All of the patient's handwriting was legible.

Reading Functions: Phonetic synthesis at syllabic level was intact, but the patient could not recognize the word *knight* when it was spelled aloud to him. He could not tell which of the letters *B, J,* or *S* was the initial for the name John. He misread *cloakroom* as *clockroom.* He was able to read hemopoiesis correctly, but he mispronounced *astrocytoma* as *atrocytoma.* His phonetic analytic skills were quite good on the whole. He substituted the more logical *he* for *she* in the sentence of item 198, which reads: "The boy went to bed, because she was ill." His time for paragraph reading was slowed but errorless on item 199.

Arithmetic Functions: The entire Arithmetic section of the battery was errorless, except for borderline performances on serial substraction of sevens and thirteens from 100, on items 221–222. On subtraction of serial sevens the

patient made one error, and he was overtime for the last two items of the series. On the thirteens he made two errors within the time limit.

Memory Functions: Performance on the word list learning task of items 223–225 was correctly predicted by the patient on each trial after the first. He showed a slow but steady learning curve that reached asymptote at a subcriterion level, with recall trials of 4-4-5-6-6 on a seven-item series with a normal criterion of two consecutive errorless trials. The immediate sensory memory trace was unstable with visually presented material. The patient omitted the diamond from the five-figure reproduction of item 227, and he could not reproduce the second and third hand positions of item 229. He showed normal ability to tap the rhythm of item 228, which provides a visual model augmented by auditory cues.

Mild confabulation was noted in attempts to remember word series on item 230, where the patient substituted *tree* for *street* at immediate recall. He made no error with heterogeneous interference on item 231. Homogeneous interference on item 232 led to failure to retrieve two of the three words in the second set after correct recall of the first set. Confabulation of details was more apparent on measures of retention and retrieval of sentences and brief paragraphs. Visual cues did not aid recall on item 235; most errors involved association of the wrong target words with the pictorial stimuli.

Higher Intellectual Functions: Understanding of thematic pictures was reduced to enumeration of details rather than identification of the unifying theme of the action taking place. The patient made minor but consistent sequencing errors on the picture arrangement items 238–241. His reasoning was concrete and literal on the proverb about the hen and the golden eggs. The patient gave the moral of the story as "you will not judge the eggs by the colors. Know everything before you kill the hen." He could not interpret idioms, but this was likely a culturally biased difficulty. He explained the proverb "don't count your chickens before they have hatched" adequately: "Don't count on anything that's not in your posession yet.'' Definitions were intermittently concrete in the functional or descriptive sense. Logical relationships phrased in the manner of items 251, 253, and 254 were confusing to the patient. He could not grasp the concept of verbal analogies.

SYNOPSIS

Patient 3 showed sparing of elementary motor functions and only selective dysfunction at the more complex levels of motor integration. Sensory examination was essentially unremarkable. Pitch and rhythmic discrimination were adequate at basic levels but broke down with longer, more complex, and more detailed aural pattern analyses. Basic phonemic discrimination was intact, but there was difficulty with interpretation of spatially organized linguistic structures that involved reversed grammar or inverted and comparative constructions. These errors have been noted in patients with right frontal lobe lesions. Retraction of the right frontal area was necessary to expose the corpus callosum for the surgical approach to the lesion in this case, and this may account for these findings. Mnestic difficulty, particularly short-term memory trace instability, was expected with a large third ventricular tumor that compressed medial temporal structures. Mild but consistent deficits with abstraction, sequencing, and concept formation account for the elevation of the Intelligence scale. The mildness of the neuropsychological deficits, given the massive size of the lesion in this area of the brain, is remarkable.

Patient 4

MEDICAL-SURGICAL BACKGROUND

Patient 4 is a 47-year-old, right-handed white male with 14 years of education. The history is neurologically remarkable for surgical repair of a lumbar meningocele eight years before the diagnosis of hydrocephalus of unknown etiology. The patient presented for treatment with severe low back pain that radiated to the lower extremities,

patchy sensory loss in the lower extremities, standing and walking intolerance followed by weakness and a tendency to stumble. Long-standing preoperative problems also involved ''dropping things from his hands, a thick type speech, and severe episodic occipital headaches.'' A CT scan was done to rule out the possibility of hydrocephalus or a Chiari malformation, and both were demonstrated radiologically. ''The CT scan showed a massive hydrocephalus with tonsillar herniations of his cerebellum to the foramen magnum and cerebellar degeneration.'' Ventriculoatrial cerebrospinal fluid shunting led to satisfactory reduction of the ventriculomegaly and resolution of the headaches. Postoperative neurological examination showed no focal weakness. A follow-up myelogram showed no evidence of residual cerebellar tonsillar herniation at the level of the foramen magnum.

NEUROPSYCHOLOGICAL STUDIES

Patient 4 was examined at one day preoperatively and at 30 days postoperatively with the Luria-Nebraska Neuropsychological Battery (Figure 14.4). In both instances he demonstrated minimal objective clinical evidence of cognitive deficit, and this impression was confirmed by the formal test results.

Motor Functions: Preoperatively, bimanual dexterity was mildly diminished for speed and coordination when touching the fingertips with the thumb in succession. This was slightly improved postoperatively. The flexion-extension sequence of fist clenching was barely into the borderline range preoperatively with the left hand only, and it remained so postoperatively. The kinesthetic basis of movement was intact, and there was no echopraxia at any time. Preoperatively the patient was able to repeat the coordinated bimanual alternating flexion-extension movements of the hands for five repetitions of the sequence before desynchronization occurred. Postoperatively he completed the sequence nine times and lost synchrony only once—a normal performance. Preoperatively, alternating rhythmic tapping of beats with the hands was borderline, and postoperatively the hand mak-

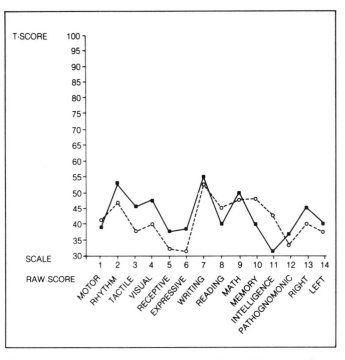

Figure 14.4.   Age and education-corrected Luria-Nebraska Neuropsychological Battery scores for patient 4. The broken line with open circles shows the preoperative profile. The solid line with solid squares shows the 30-day postoperative profile.

ing multiple taps (e.g., two right–one left) would make superfluous taps (e.g., three right–one left). Complex forms of manual praxis and buccofacial praxis were errorless. Mild construction difficulty in attempts to draw freehand and copy the simple geometric figures circle, square, and triangle remained mildly impaired postoperatively. The cerebellar disorder appeared to have contributed to this performance. Speech regulation of motor acts were errorless at all times.

Acoustic-Motor Organization (Rhythm): Preoperatively there was errorless discrimination of pitch relationships, but postoperatively there was borderline impairment on elementary and more complex group discrimination items of this kind. This appeared to be a function of concentration and attention span, which were restabilizing in the postoperative period. Humming of pitch relations

was borderline both pre- and postoperatively. The patient noted that the notes he had trouble with "sound the same," though the pitch differences were distinct. Perception and evaluation of more complex acoustic signals and reproduction of accented rhythm by loud and soft tapping remained unchanged at a borderline level from the pre- to the postoperative evaluation.

Higher Cutaneous and Kinesthetic Functions (Tactile): The sensory examinations pre- and postoperatively are remarkable only for dysgraphesthesia. The patient could not interpret letters written on the backs of his wrists preoperatively, and he had difficulty interpreting both letters and numbers postoperatively. He made no errors with simple geometric figures drawn in a similar fashion, perhaps because there were fewer alternatives and the three figures (circle, triangle, cross) were less similar than the alphabetical and numerical arrays. The other sensory findings were completely within normal limits.

Higher Visual Functions: The patient named concrete objects correctly at both examinations. Preoperatively he misidentified a picture of a graduated cylinder as a ruler or thermometer, and he persisted in the latter response postoperatively. He correctly identified the elements of item 88, but technicalities of scoring lowered his performance to a borderline level (e.g., glasses for sunglasses). He had difficulty with the first part of item 89, with its incomplete figures. There was no simultaneous or visual agnosia. He did the items from Raven's Progressive Matrices at a marginal level overall. Clock reading was errorless preoperatively, but he made one mistake postoperatively (7:53 misread as 8:53). Clock setting was errorless. He had no difficulty recognizing cardinal directions. Analysis of perspective was correct for all but the most difficult final portion of item 97, which he missed pre- and postoperatively. Plane rotational analysis on item 99 was passed errorlessly on both examinations.

Receptive Speech Functions: Preoperatively the entire section was errorless. Postoperatively the patient reported that the attributive phrases "father's brother" and "brother's father" of item 122 were the same. He also missed the first part of item 132, concluding that Mary rather than the woman from the store gave the talk. His performance was otherwise errorless.

Expressive Speech Functions: Preoperatively the entire section was remarkable only for the grammatically stilted attempt at solving item 170: "The automobile is parked in the wood garage." This error persisted postoperatively. Scattered errors were also noted. On item 134 the consonants *th* were mispronounced as *d, hierarchy* was pronounced as *hiearchry* (item 138), and *cat* was misread as *eat* on item 146 but was spontaneously corrected. There were no diagnostically contributory speech errors.

Writing Functions: Pre- and postoperative errors were confined to spelling of more complex words such as those presented by items 179, 183, and 184.

Reading Functions: Performance was unremarkable pre- and postoperatively.

Arithmetic Functions: The only errors involved minor inaccuracies due to carrying errors on the serial subtraction problems at the end of the section, items 221–222. Subtraction of serial sevens was within normal limits postoperatively and slightly improved from the preoperative level. Subtraction of serial thirteens was unchanged at a borderline level.

Memory Functions: Pre- and postoperatively the patient learned the seven-word list of item 223 to criterion, but his ability to predict his performance improved from a borderline to a normal level during his course. Form recognition was unimproved postoperatively, but form recall improved from a borderline to a normal level. Mild confabulation persisted with heterogeneous interference pre- and postoperatively. Retention and retrieval of sentences improved to a normal level postoperatively. Recall of paragraph-length material remained normal at both examinations. Logical memorizing with visual aids remained borderline at both examinations.

Higher Intellectual Functions: Understanding of thematic pictures was adequate at both examinations. Mild preoperative sequencing difficulties resolved post-

operatively. Proverb interpretations remained literal postoperatively. Quality of concept formation remained intermittently concrete. Ability to solve analogies, opposites, and logical relationships remained abstract, apparently as residuals of old formal learning.

SYNOPSIS

This patient demonstrated the reorganization of functional systems of the cerebral cortex to compensate for a slowly developing, advanced hydrocephalic process. The disorder is thought to have progressed very slowly over a number of years. There were more clinical symptoms from the cerebellar and spinal complaints than from the cerebral disorder. Special tests were necessary to demonstrate the higher-order manual motor coordination deficits and the postoperative motor improvement. There was some resolving difficulty with concentration postoperatively, at the time of the second examination. Sensory examination was remarkable only for higher-order graphesthesic errors. Visual-perceptual errors were similarly subtle and intermittent. Receptive and expressive speech and their related functions, reading and writing, were all within normal limits. Serial subtractions reflected the mild attentional difficulty seen elsewhere. Mild confabulation with interference was consistent with medial temporal dysfunction, but the subtlety of the deficits is striking given the gross level of the hydrocephalus. Higher-order concept formation that was based on old learning suffered least, though mild concreteness of reasoning was noted on novel solution items.

Patient 5

MEDICAL-SURGICAL BACKGROUND

Patient 5 is a 72-year-old white male with 14 years of education. He was admitted for evaluation of gait disturbances and bowel and bladder incontinence. One year before admission the patient had begun to experience walking difficulty that had deteriorated over a six-month period to a broad-based, shuffling gait. The past medical

history was neurologically remarkable for a right hemispheric cerebrovascular accident suffered in 1976, from
which he had made an excellent recovery. At the time of
preoperative examination the only residual of the CVA
was "minimal left-sided weakness in the arm." A CT
scan with contrast enhancement revealed "moderate to
severe enlargement of the ventricles, including the third
and fourth. The cisterns are commensurately enlarged. No
sulci are visible above the level of the lateral ventricles.
No parenchymal abnormalities are noted. Findings are
compatible with communicating hydrocephalus." A
cerebrospinal fluid indium scan was then performed that
showed "slow migration of the tracer from the basal cisterns to the parasagittal region and persistent tracer filling
of the ventricles compatible with reflux. These changes
are consistent with normal pressure hydrocephalus."
Ventricular-peritoneal shunting of cerebrospinal fluid
produced satisfactory resolution of the ventriculomegaly
at follow-up evaluation.

NEUROPSYCHOLOGICAL STUDIES

Patient 5 was examined twice with the Luria-Nebraska
Neuropsychological Battery: four days preoperatively and
114 days postoperatively (Figure 14.5).

Motor Functions: Pre- and postoperatively the patient
showed bilateral slowing of manual movements on the
tasks of touching the fingertips with the thumb in sequence
and clenching the fists. Preoperatively he could not reproduce the position of the right hand with the left hand from
kinesthetic cues alone, but this resolved postoperatively.
Echopraxia was seen on item 13 pre- and postoperatively,
since this is the first manual optic-spatial organization
item that calls for positioning the two hands simultaneously. Preoperatively the patient was able to correct the
echopractic imitation on item 14, in which the hand positions are reversed. The error was repeated postoperatively. Preoperatively crossed pointing (e.g., right hand
points to left eye) was done echopractically by imitation
but not at verbal command. This more complex task was
errorless postoperatively.

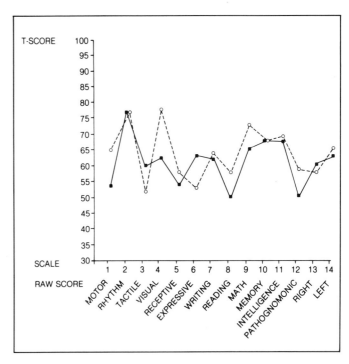

Figure 14.5.   Age and education-corrected Luria-Nebraska Neuropsychological Battery scores for patient 5. The broken line with open
circles shows the preoperative profile. The solid line with solid squares
shows the 114-day postoperative profile.

Preoperatively the patient could not do sequential hand
movements for the dynamic organization items 21–23. He
opened one hand while leaving the other open, then
opened and closed both hands together repeatedly instead
of alternately opening one hand and closing the other. He
tapped alternating patterns of beats with the hands correctly a few times and then deteriorated to random tapping. Postoperatively the flexion-extension alternation
sequence of item 21 was done at a borderline level, with no
loss of alternating synchrony. There continued to be perseverative tapping (3 right–1 left instead of 2 right–1 left)
with the right hand on item 22 only. Complex forms of
praxis were intact. Buccofacial praxis was intact, but the
rapid three-stage oral sequence of item 33 was excessively
slow at both examinations. There was mild construction
difficulty on freehand drawing and copying of figures at

both examinations. Drawing speed returned to normal post-operatively. Pre- and postoperatively the patient had an intermittent tendency to lose the task and to revert to direct imitation of the stimulus rather than producing an alternative response. In the first examination, on item 51 he tapped gently when the examiner did so; in the second examination he tapped twice when the examiner did so on item 48. He made each error on only one of the four presentations in each item. This appeared to be a function of waxing and waning concentration.

Acoustic-Motor Organization (Rhythm): Pre- and postoperatively the patient showed borderline difficulty with aural discrimination that was more evident with groups of sounds than with sound pairs. Humming of tones was normal preoperatively and borderline post-operatively. The patient was not able to sing a melodic line at either examination. He could not solve the more complex acoustic discriminations of items 60–61, and he could not do the accented tapping of the more complex sections of items 62 or 63 either with an aural model or at verbal command.

Higher Cutaneous and Kinesthetic Functions (Tactile): Preoperatively there was marginal difficulty with tactile finger identification with the right hand and definite impairment with the left hand. There was borderline impairment of two-point discrimination and graphesthesia for simple geometric figures with the right hand only. Graphesthesic interpretation of the letter *S* written on the back of the wrists was impaired bimanually. The patient misidentified a quarter as a nickel with the left hand, and his recognition time was borderline with that hand only. Postoperatively, tactile finger identification was borderline bimanually. Pinprick sensation was marginal with the left hand. Two-point discrimination and graphesthesia for geometric forms were bimanually borderline. Graphesthesia for letters written on the back of the right wrist and proprioception on the right arm were mildly impaired. The patient continued to misidentify a quarter as a nickel with his left hand. The other sensory findings were intact throughout both examinations.

Higher Visual Functions: Preoperatively the patient named objects adequately, but he misidentified the nutcracker as calipers and the graduated cylinder as a thermometer. He could not correctly identify the blurred pictures of sunglasses, and he misidentified the clear picture of them as eyeglasses. He had no difficulty recognizing overlapping figures. He could not solve the items from Raven's Progressive Matrices. Clock reading was errorless, and the clock setting for one item was overtime but correct. He reversed the cardinal directions east and west, and he could not solve the plane rotational task of item 99.

Postoperatively he misidentified a quarter as a nickel when it was visually presented. He made the same errors as before with picture naming. He had no guess about the nutcracker, and he called the graduated cylinders "measuring sticks." He could not recognize the blurred sunglasses in item 88, but this time he was correct with identification on the clear picture. He could not recognize the incomplete figures of item 89. He omitted one figure each from the overlapping figure arrays of items 90 and 91 for a borderline performance, but he made no identification errors. He still could not solve the items from Raven's Progressive Matrices. One clock reading error occurred (10:35 misread as "twenty-five to one"); clock setting remained borderline. Confusion of east and west also remained unchanged from baseline. Minor inaccuracies, usually counting errors of one or two items, led to errors on item 97. The plane rotational task of item 99 remained too difficult for the patient to attempt.

Receptive Speech Functions: Preoperatively the patient had borderline difficulty with phonemic discrimination at two- and three-item group levels. The patient was able to do the first three parts of the five-part sequence in item 109 before he lost the task. He had difficulty with the inverted grammatical constructions of items 130 and 132. The other receptive speech functions were intact. Postoperatively the phonemic discrimination difficulty resolved. The patient wrote the lower-case letter *m* with an extra loop, a form of motor perseveration not uncommon in the elderly. Conditioned reflex response to phonemic hearing on item 106 replaced the correct sequence with a simplified single alternation pattern. The item 109 sequence remained too complex for the patient to perform. He pointed to the picture of the fireplace rather than the matches on item 116 when asked which of the three figures presented was necessary for lighting a fire.

Inflective grammatical forms confused him, so that he pointed to the pencil with the comb instead of vice versa. Comparative constructions also caused some difficulty, so that he reported that Tom was shorter when asked: "Which boy is shorter, if Tom is taller than Arnie?" The three-person comparison of item 128 confused him postoperatively, whereas he had been able to guess half the solution in the preoperative workup.

Expressive Speech Functions: Preoperatively there were errors in repetition of speech sounds (*b* for *sp*, *sl* for *pl*, *ra* for *str*) and words (*see-strict* for *tree-trick*). On item 142 the patient repeated *house-ball-chair* as *house-ball-stair*. He could not provide the phonemic equivalents for *m* and *b* and instead read them as letters. He could not recall the final portion of the three-phrase sequence in item 156. He could not name the candle in item 157. When asked to name the object that protects you from the rain in item 159, he replied "roof." Extemporaneous speech was slowed to a borderline level on the descriptive task of item 164, but speech output was within normal limits. The patient could not rearrange either of the syntactically disorganized sentences of item 173.

Postoperatively the speech sound repetition errors persisted (*t* for *sh*, *ought* for *awk*, *bar* for *ball*, *out* for *house*). Repetition at sentence level produced verbal paraphasias (*blooms* for *grew*, *foliage* for *forest*—item 155). Picture-naming errors occurred on item 157. The candle still could not be identified, a guitar was misidentified as a mandolin, and a stapler was misidentified as a paperclip. The errors of syntactical reorganization on item 173 were unchanged.

Writing Functions: Pre- and postoperatively the patient was unable to spell *antarctic* from immediate memory on item 179, and he could not spell the words *physiol-*

ogy and *probabilistic* from item 184. Handwriting legibility improved postoperatively, but writing at phrase and sentence level remained in the brain-dysfunctional range.

Reading Functions: Pre- and postoperatively the patient showed minor difficulty with phonetic synthesis (*grr* for *gro*, *shone* for *stone*). Reading of words and letter abbreviations (U.N., U.S.A., U.S.S.R.) was adequate at both examinations. Phonetic approximations of even the most complex words (*astrocytoma, hemopoiesis*) were intermittently creditable. At both examinations the word *he* was substituted for *she* to make the sentence more logical in item 198. Reading at paragraph level remained borderline for accuracy, but reading speed improved postoperatively.

Arithmetic Functions: Preoperatively the patient wrote one-digit arabic numerals accurately, but he had difficulty writing the roman numerals IX and XI from dictation. He wrote 69 as 59 in arabic numerals from dictation. When writing the number 396 from dictation he placed an extra vertical loop on the three, a form of motor perseveration. He had trouble with categorical number structure at the four-digit level when he attempted to write 1023. Various attempts produced: 10-123, 123, 1023. He had no difficulty writing the number 9845 to dictation. The zero place holder seemed to cause the patient the most problems, since he had lost the concept of the need for a place holder when there was no numerical quantity. More complex arithmetic calculations on item 215 showed intermittent errors. The patient could not recognize an omitted division sign on item 218 (10 [ ] 2 = 5), but he solved the other equations with omitted signs. He could not do the multidigit mental addition problem of item 220 or the serial subtractions of items 221–222.

Postoperatively, writing of roman numerals caused the patient confusion only on the last item, XI. He also misread VI as V. The categorical number structure difficulties had resolved. Trouble with complex mathematical operations persisted, as did trouble with symbolic arithmetic operations in which signs were omitted from equations. The complex calculations of item 220 were improved to a normal level, and the patient was marginally successful at subtracting serial sevens and thirteens from 100.

Memory Functions: Preoperatively the patient showed good initial performance but little improvement with practice on a rote list-learning task. He did not reach criterion normal performance of two consecutive errorless trials, but he approached this level. Retention and retrieval of forms was normal. The immediate sensory trace was unstable, so that the patient retained the general form of the task and the solution but omitted details. He forgot one of the five figures of item 227. He tapped a monotonic series of two beats for item 228 but omitted the accented loud and soft taps on every other pair. This series also showed gross motor perseveration. The three manual positions of item 229 were all done incorrectly. Instead of raising the index and little fingers on position 1, he raised all five fingers. He raised the second, third, *and* fourth fingers for position 2, and he fanned the third, fourth, and fifth fingers of position 3 in the familiar OK gesture rather than curling the last three fingers as had been demonstrated.

In attempting immediate recall of the five words shown in item 230, he omitted one word from the sequence. There was no impairment of recall with heterogeneous interference on item 231, but the patient confabulated words from the previous items and recalled only one of six words on the homogeneous interference task of item 232. He recalled the competing sentences of item 233 correctly, but he reproduced only scattered details of item 234. Pictorial cues did not aid verbal recall on item 235, where the patient remembered only three of the seven words.

Postoperatively the recall on the rote verbal list-learning task was unchanged. Form retention and retrieval remained stable. Immediate sensory trace recall for geometric forms was unimproved, but accented tapping was errorless. The manual positioning task also improved from a grossly impaired to a borderline level. The immediate verbal recall of item 230 was slightly poorer than before, with two words missed rather than one. On item 231 he could not recall any of the three words after heterogeneous interference. He recalled the first but not the second set of three words after homogeneous interference on the subsequent items. The variation in these items from the baseline performance appeared to reflect attentional fluctuation and difficulty with concentration. This was confirmed by the continuing elevation of the Rhythm scale score (T = 80), which remained at the preoperative level. Performances on the competing sentence task of item 233 remained within normal limits. Recall of paragraph-length material on item 234 was still sketchy, and cueing with pictorial aids on item 235 led to simple description of the pictures at both administration and recall, except for the initial item that was formally cued to explain the task in the instructions.

Higher Intellectual Processes: Preoperatively the patient had borderline mastery of thematic pictures, but he omitted significant details. He also had difficulty with sequencing. On item 240 he arranged the cards B–C–D in proper order to show the progressive stages of growth of the plant, but he said that cards A and E (unplanted potato and woman digging up potatoes from fully grown plant) did not belong to the sequence. Here he was stimulus-bound to the picture of the plant rather than attending to the more inclusive growth sequence. He confabulated in item 242 and explained the comic intent of the picture sequence as ''the frog biting the stork on the leg.'' He was able to understand the intent of item 243.

Preoperatively, he understood details of thematic texts adequately in the fable about the hen and the golden eggs, but he could not grasp the moral of the story. He could not interpret idioms or proverbs adequately on his own, and he consistently gave concrete explanations in multiple-choice proverb interpretation on item 247. Definitions, comparisons, and differentiations were all at a concrete, descriptive level. Analogies were analyzed at a borderline level.

Postoperatively the description of thematic pictures was improved, with more attention to detail and story line. Sequencing was still significantly impaired, but there was now a consistent attempt to include all elements of the sequence in a coherent story. The patient could not interpret item 242, which he also missed at baseline, but he recognized that he was confused by the item and he did not confabulate an answer. Interpretation of idioms was improved, and proverb interpretation was more abstract though his spontaneous attempts at solution were incorrect. Multiple-choice explanations of proverbs were chosen errorlessly. Definitions were typically concrete. Logical relationships were more consistently correct and abstract than at baseline. Analogy comprehension continued to be borderline.

SYNOPSIS

Motor examination showed persistent impairment of manual dexterity, with improvement of kinesthesia and resolution of some echopractic errors postoperatively. Coordination of the hands showed postoperative improvement as well. The mild construction difficulty persisted, but motor output speed was improved from baseline. Attention and concentration skills remained significantly impaired and unchanged at the two examinations, with a Rhythm scale score three standard deviations above the mean. Sensory dysfunction remained mild and selective throughout the patient's course. Visual-perceptual functioning improved during the postoperative period. The perceptual improvement was due to a generalized increase in accuracy and speed of response rather than to dramatic reversals of preoperative deficits. This is consistent with the pathological process in this case and with the generalized pressure reduction on the brain postoperatively.

Speech, reading, and writing functions showed modest improvement postoperatively, consistent with the changes seen in other functions. Calculations showed breakdown of higher integrative activity only at the highest levels, with resolution of the number structure deficits postoperatively. Short-term memory instability heightened by interference procedures persisted at follow-up. Inductive reasoning was improved postoperatively, and concept formation was more abstract. Sequencing was still im-

paired, but the patient had a better grasp of the task, and he was not as stimulus-bound as he had been previously. Accessibility of old learning such as idiomatic and proverbial interpretation was improved from baseline. Logical reasoning was somewhat more coherent as well.

General Overview

This series of surgical cases was chosen to demonstrate the sensitivity of the Luria-Nebraska Neuropsychological Battery in a variety of situations involving neoplastic, cerebrovascular, and hydrocephalic problems. Two cases from each of the latter categories were chosen to demonstrate individual similarities and differences in syndrome analysis. The tumor resection case obtained postoperatively (patient 3) shows the value of postoperative evaluation alone when preoperative workup is not possible. This situation often occurs with an emergency admission or a transfer case such as this one. The profile elevation in each case corresponded well with the patient's clinical status. The detailed syndrome analyses based on Luria's theoretical model of cerebral functioning supplemented the formal quantitative scoring that was summarized on the test profiles. Full understanding of the patient as an individual in his natural complexity requires item analysis of the deficit performances and the means by which they are generated.

The effects of functional system reorganization are particularly evident in patient 4, whose very slowly developing massive hydrocephalus produced no striking cognitive deficit or postoperative change despite the severity of the physical pathology. Patients 1 and 2, in contrast, showed dramatic generalized postoperative impairment with a discrete surgical resection in the left parieto-occipital tertiary zone of the cerebral cortex. Complete reorganization of their functional systems to a point where only the effects of the focal lesion were evident took many months. Patient 3 showed quite specific mnestic and linguistic deficits associated with the site of the lesion and possibly the surgical removal. Patient 5 evidenced modest generalized improvement that was reflected more in the item analysis than in the formal quantitative scoring shown by the profile. In each case the test performance was understandable in light of the history and the surgical procedures. Integration of all available information in each case was necessary to arrive at a clear impression of the clinical syndrome.

15. Subcortical Dysfunction

While much of traditional neuropsychological assessment and the specific research on the Luria-Nebraska has concentrated on the effects of cortical disorders, it is important to remember that subcortical disorders may also affect performance on tests which are traditionally labeled as tests of cortical dysfunction such as the Luria-Nebraska. This chapter is intended to review briefly the possible effects of subcortical disorders on the Luria-Nebraska, on the basis of our own clinical experience as well as research findings in subcortical disorders. It is not our intention to provide a review of the literature on subcortical disorders or their effects on the Luria-Nebraska, but rather to alert the reader to the possible roles of these disorders which may cause relatively massive impairment on the Luria-Nebraska in some cases, or none at all in cases where the problems are limited to areas not covered on the battery. Much more research is necessary before we can understand the effect of subcortical disorders on the test battery.

Essentials of Subcortical Anatomy and Function

The central nervous system comprises the spinal cord and the brain. Although certain behaviors are entirely controlled at the spinal cord level, the brain is of primary importance to behavior. It can be divided into hindbrain, midbrain, and forebrain. While this distinction can be made clearly using anatomical evidence, functional differentiation is more complex. However, the less complex the behavior, the more likely that it will be influenced by the hindbrain and midbrain; the more complex the behavior, the more likely that it will be controlled by the forebrain.

HINDBRAIN

Anatomically, the hindbrain connects the brain to the spinal cord. It comprises the medulla, which feeds directly into the uppermost segments of the spinal cord, the pons, which is immediately above the medulla, and the cerebellum, a convoluted structure that protrudes from the back of the pons.

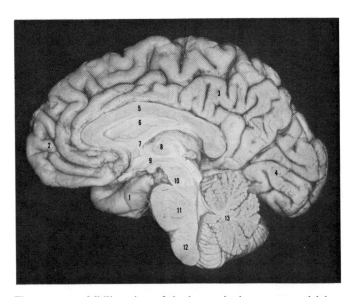

Figure 15.1. Midline view of the human brain: 1, temporal lobe; 2, frontal lobe; 3, parietal lobe; 4, occipital lobe; 5, corpus callosum; 6, septum pellucidum; 7, fornix; 8, thalamus; 9, hypothalamus; 10, midbrain; 11, pons; 12, medulla; 13, cerebellum.

FOREBRAIN

The most recent phylogenetic addition to the nervous system, the forebrain, is in the uppermost segment of the brain. Although this large area contains numerous nuclei and structures, the most important include the hypothalamus, thalamus, limbic system, and cerebral cortex.

The hypothalamus has been implicated in various behaviors but is most often associated with sex, hunger, thirst, and aggression. Traditionally, the thalamus has been thought to be involved with sensory relay. Considerably more elaborate is the limbic system, which includes the hypothalamus, thalamus, hippocampus, amygdala, septal area, corpus callosum, and portions of the frontal lobe. Originally this system was implicated in olfactory functions, but later evidence indicated that it was involved with emotional and affective behavior. The cerebral cortex, by far the most complex of brain structures, thinly covers the entire surface of the brain and is involved with numerous higher-order activities.

Effects of Subcortical Dysfunction

SENSORY

Visual: After transduction occurs at the optic receptor level, impulses are transmitted by cranial nerve II, the optic nerve. The nerve partially decussates before entering the brain and terminating in the lateral geniculate nucleus of the thalamus. From here, optic radiations eventually reach the visual cortex of the occipital lobe.

Damage to any point within this system alters visual behavior. Congestion due to tumors or masses at the receptor level may lead to papilledema. After deterioration of central vision, perhipheral vision diminishes gradually to complete blindness. Lesions or pressure on the visual pathway usually results in visual-field deficits. Deficits of the visual field, scotomas, may be manifested in problems with perception of light, visual acuity, and color fluctuations. Additionally, pituitary-gland tumors or other diseases affecting forebrain structures will often lead to inter-

Its anatomical position ensures a critical role for the hindbrain, since all sensory and motor impulses travel through this area. These impulses are monitored and integrated by various nuclei of the hindbrain, including the reticular formation. The cerebellum, which is not centrally located, is involved with feedback of motor behavior.

MIDBRAIN

Immediately above the pons is the midbrain, which contains the tectum (i.e., colliculi), substantia nigra, and various cranial nerve nuclei. Like the hindbrain, these structures play an important part in monitoring and integrating sensory and motor activity. At this level, however, differentiation of activity becomes more pronounced because the auditory reaction and visual orientation substrates are located in the tectum. The substantia nigra is involved with the motor system.

ference with the peripheral visual process. Oculomotor movement, controlled by the abducent, trochlear, and oculomotor cranial nerves, may be severely disturbed by damage to nuclei of these nerves. Also, dysfunction may manifest itself in lack of optic reflexes, vertigo, or altered posture of the head.

The Luria-Nebraska Neuropsychological Battery's section on visual assessment includes naming visually identified objects, visual-spatial perception and organization, and dimensional analysis. Although these are typically cortical activities, symptoms referable to optic receptors or pathways may account partially or exclusively for decreased performance. Subcortical disorders may mimic cortical symptoms. Interference with visual pathways (especially when accompanied by damage to the corpus callosum) may lead to a cessation of visual input to one hemisphere, causing deficits related to the visual functions of that hemisphere.

Owing to the visual pathway's centralized location within the forebrain as well as its transverse course through the brain, it is not surprising to find visual deficits secondary to many subcortical disorders.

Auditory: After processing sound waves at various receptor levels (e.g., inner ear), auditory signals enter the lower brainstem before they course through the midbrain and terminate in the medial geniculate body of the thalamus. This structure, in turn, forwards auditory impulses to the auditory cortex of the temporal lobe.

Noises in the ear—tinnitus—or deafness may indicate dysfunction of the canal, the cochlea, or the acoustic cranial nerve. Infections of the canal are common and can cause numerous dysfunctions. Some have theorized a relationship of such disorders to learning problems.

The Luria-Nebraska places emphasis on receptive speech and rhythm skills, not simply auditory behavior. Clearly, however, dysfunction of auditory receptors or pathways will affect complex cortical processes. Since all items involve hearing as a prerequisite, careful attention must be given to determining whether the impairment is attributable to hearing or to speech. Evaluation of pro-

gressive hearing loss and tinnitus should be considered when there is impairment on the Speech and Rhythm scales of the Luria-Nebraska.

Somesthetic Sensation and Proprioception: While the categories of somesthetic senses—pressure, pain, warmth, and cold—have been considered too broad, the central circuits for these sensations are better defined. Touch and pressure sensations are transduced by different receptors peripherally before being transmitted in the posterior white columns of the spinal cord to the thalamus. The substantia gelatinosa of the spinal cord carries peripherally processed sensations of pain and temperature to the reticular formation and thalamus.

Cerebellar lesions may affect fine tactile sensations. Hemisection of the spinal cord, Brown-Sequard syndrome, leads to loss of tactile, pain, and temperature sensations contralaterally. Thalamic damage may lead to the thalamic syndrome: excessive activity increasing the painful quality of all somesthetic senses.

Proprioceptive cues from the internal environment, are derived from the labyrinthine and kinesthetic senses. Transduction for the former occurs in the inner ear, while receptors in the limb process information for the kinesthetic sense. In both cases information is transmitted initially to the hindbrain, where the information is distributed to various cranial nerves, the cerebellum, and the reticular formation.

Cerebellar lesions may disrupt proprioceptive feedback and consequently cause problems with fine postural adjustment. Also, damage to the vestibular portion of the eighth cranial nerve leads to vertigo and unsteadiness of gait.

Like somesthetic activity, proprioception is assessed by the Tactile scale of the Luria-Nebraska. The later items on this scale tend to reflect kinesthetic sensation. Gross impairment of cerebellar origin may influence these measures. Since the individual's gait is not observed as part of the standard Luria-Nebraska, it is difficult to accurately assess any labyrinthine dysfunction without supplemental testing.

MOTOR

Although controversy surrounds the pyramidal/extrapyramidal dichotomy of the motor system, it appears that such a dichotomy can be easily made anatomically. Impulses initiated in the Betz cells of the motor cortex travel down the internal capsule to form the first portion of the pyramidal tract. From here most of the fibers continue to the medulla and cross before forming the corticospinal tract of the spinal cord. The extrapyramidal tract takes a less direct approach by first coursing to the basal ganglia. After leaving this area it joins the pyramidal tract in the internal capsule. However, it is influenced by cerebellar activity and eventually forms its own descending system in the spinal cord.

The basic functional difference between these two systems appears to be that the pyramidal tract controls fine movement such as writing while the extrapyramidal tract controls movement of larger muscles. Lesions or disturbances of the cortex, pathway, or nuclei involved in these systems will significantly alter motor behavior. For example, Parkinsonian tremors appear to be a function of basal ganglion impairment. Vascular lesions often occur near or on the motor pathways and result in initial flaccid paralysis and eventual hyperreflexia. Finally, cerebellar lesions or diseases such as multiple sclerosis not only affect motor performance but may result in double vision and headaches. Subcortical lesions may affect voluntary movements as well as being manifested at rest, and can affect both fine and gross motor control.

Although elevation of the motor scale of the Luria-Nebraska is often seen with nonfrontal damage, this scale affords increased sensitivity to the motor strip. Similarly, this appears true for subcortical dysfunction. That is, this scale is sensitive to a variety of subcortical impairment but appears selective to disruption of motor pathways. Disruption of basal ganglion activity would affect items involving precise movements, whereas rapidly alternating movements show impairment with cerebellar damage. Pyramidal damage should generally elevate the score for fine motor items on the Motor scale and affect the Writing scale as well.

LEARNING

Owing to the plasticity of the brain and the extensive neural feedback system involved in learning, the search for anatomical substrates has all but been replaced by a more physiological orientation. Recent investigations have concentrated mainly on cortical activity. Research and clinical evidence suggests, however, that certain subcortical structures play an important role in learning.

Ablation of the caudate nuclei of the basal ganglia results in delayed responding, while damage to the septal area leads to hyperresponsiveness. Two additional forebrain structures, situated adjacent to the temporal cortex, appear to be involved in learning. The hippocampus appears involved in complex responses, and the amygdala may be involved in generalization of behavior. Also, the corpus callosum plays an integral part in transferring the neural composites of learning from one hemisphere to the other. Even though no specific scale of the Luria-Nebraska measures learning performance directly, all scales are affected, since numerous items require association formation. Thus, one might look for a general elevation of scales emphasizing associations, such as Motor scale, if damage encompasses one of these structures. Additionally, cultural or educational deprivation owing to long-standing minimal brain dysfunction could significantly elevate numerous scales. Discrete damage to one area, however, may only affect one scale.

MEMORY

Few areas of the brain besides the cerebral cortex have been implicated in memory. The following forebrain structures do appear to be involved: hippocampus, thalamus, and hypothalamus.

Bilateral destruction of the hippocampi may result in an inability to form new long-term memories (but will not interfere with immediate recall when there have been no interfering stimuli) or to recall past events which occurred prior to the injury. Korsakoff's encephalopathy, a disease causing observable partial retrograde amnesia in addition to an inability to form new memories, results from destruction of portions of the thalamus and hypothalamus.

Since the Memory scale of the Luria-Nebraska evaluates recall of short-term memory, disruption of the hippocampus, thalamus, or hypothalamus could elevate this score.

EMOTION

Despite the lack of an adequate operational definition of emotion, it appears that numerous limbic structures are implicated in emotional and affective behavior. The septal area, amygdala, hypothalamus, and thalamus, which all have extensive neuronal interaction, play important roles in emotional activity.

Generally these structures are involved with either aggression or affective reactions. Destruction of the thalamus will often result in overreaction to emotionally laden stimuli. Also, patients with limbic damage may display overtly aggressive behavior and changes in affect similar to those seen in some psychiatric patients.

Although no scale of the Luria-Nebraska directly assesses limbic integrity, general test-taking behavior may suggest limbic impairment. Extensive disruption of these structures will affect most scales, owing to their anatomical placement as well as their interconnections. The most important clue to such damage, however, is the patient's aggressive and uncooperative manner.

CONSCIOUSNESS

The operational definition of consciousness is even more elusive than that of emotion. However, disturbances of consciousness are important in determining the reliability of neuropsychological findings as well whether such findings are a function of structures implicated in consciousness.

Clinical evidence in conjunction with extensive experimental findings suggests that the reticular formation is associated with general activation or arousal. Whether lower brainstem structures are critical for consciousness has yet to be clearly elucidated. Also, there is evidence that disturbances outside the reticular formation alter consciousness. Even with these limitations, it still appears that the reticular formation is important at least in regulating levels of consciousness.

Traditionally, simple scales (e.g., Glasgow Coma Scale) have been used to assess levels of consciousness in severe injuries. The Luria-Nebraska, however, may provide a more comprehensive approach if the patient is conscious. Considering that more simplistic behavior tends to be regulated by lower brainstem structures, the test administrator should look for such signs as alteration of wakefulness and attention. Pretest interviews should aid in determining potential disruption. Clearly, one most also consider that significant elevations of all scales do not necessarily reflect extensive cortical damage. When extensive damage is recorded, careful attention must be given to whether the observed results are strictly cortical or a function of extensive subcortical damage.

CASE I

B. R. is a 60-year-old, right-handed female with a history of tertiary syphilis. She has a seventh-grade education and her premorbid IQ is estimated to be at least borderline.

As can be seen from her Luria-Nebraska profile (Figure 15.2), there is evidence of at least moderate cerebral dysfunction. Of particular importance is that the Motor scale is highly elevated while the Tactile scale demonstrates only minimal elevation. The Tactile scale is in fact one of the two best scores on the entire profile. It is the extreme Motor scale elevation that suggests subcortical involvement in this case. As Luria (1973) has noted, approximately 20% of the motor strip area is composed of sensory cells, and roughly 20% of the sensory strip area is composed of motor cells. Thus, if the dysfunction causing

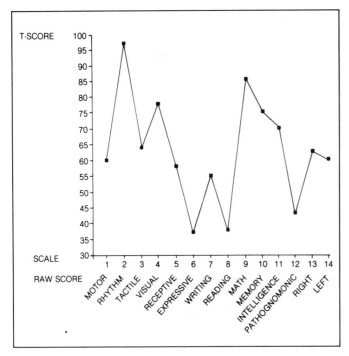

Figure 15.2.   Luria profile for Case 1 (B. R.)

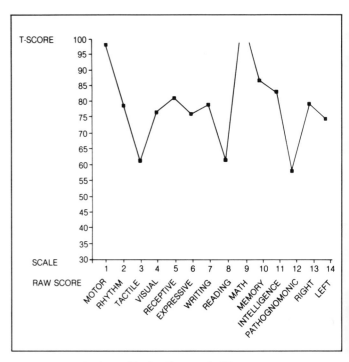

Figure 15.3.   Luria profile for Case 2 (G. W.)

the poor motor performance were exclusively cortical, one would expect the Tactile scale to be more elevated, especially given the overall poor performance demonstrated on the rest of the profile. Since it is unlikely that this profile represents a series of highly circumscribed lesions, it is reasonable to suspect at least some subcortical involvement.

CASE 2

G. W. is a 24-year-old, right-handed white male who was born prematurely. Medical tests confirmed temporal lobe damage extending to subcortical areas. He has an IQ in the dull normal range and a seventh-grade education.

This Luria-Nebraska profile (Figure 15.3) shows elevations on the Rhythm and Memory scales. Both of these skills are thought to be temporal lobe functions. An analysis of the items missed on these two scales reveals that most require short-term memory or the ability to learn

new information relatively rapidly. It is likely, therefore, that the subcortex is contributing, at least in part, to the poor performance on these two scales.

The profile points up the difficulty of discriminating between cortical and subcortical damage. In this case it is obvious that the cortex is involved by the history alone. However, the clinician should be aware of the potential involvement of subcortical structures in all brain injuries, since this offers important considerations for rehabilitation planning. For example, bilateral hippocampal injuries may make the retention of new information very difficult (see Chapter 10). If a patient has incurred such an injury, one must consider alternate strategies for dealing with new information.

CASE 3

R. C. is a 32-year-old, right-handed male with no significant medical history before he was found unconscious in a wooded area. Examination suggested that he had been severely beaten over the frontal area with a large blunt object. Extensive frontal lobe damage was detected, as was vascular hemorrhaging of the limbic areas.

This profile (Figure 15.4) demonstrates the drastic effect such an injury produces on the Luria battery. Luria (1966, 1973) has ascribed wakefulness, or a general level of activation, to both subcortical (reticular activating system) and cortical (frontal) structures. As is clearly evident, all scales on this profile demonstrate profound dysfunction that is probably due in large part to the generalized cerebral trauma. However, with such extreme elevations one must certainly consider the possibility of subcortical damage, most likely in the reticular activating system.

CASE 4
C. H. is a 37-year-old right-handed white female with no significant medical history before she had difficulty getting out of bed one morning. She was taken to the hospital,

where she eventually developed a left hemiparesis. A CT scan revealed a lesion in the right internal capsule, probably due to a cerebrovascular accident. At the time of evaluation, approximately two weeks after the onset of the hemiparesis, the patient was beginning to improve and had regained some movement and control of the left side of her body.

The Luria-Nebraska profile (Figure 15.5) is well within normal limits with the exception of the Motor and Right Hemisphere scales. The Right Hemisphere scale is, of course, elevated owing to the left hemiparesis. This profile clearly demonstrates that there is little if any cortical involvement. Therefore, even without the confirmatory evidence of the CT scan, one would suspect either a subcortical or a peripheral lesion. The profile shows that the battery can detect a very circumscribed subcortical lesion. Cases like this are, however, relatively rare, and the clinician generally can expect to find more scales elevated.

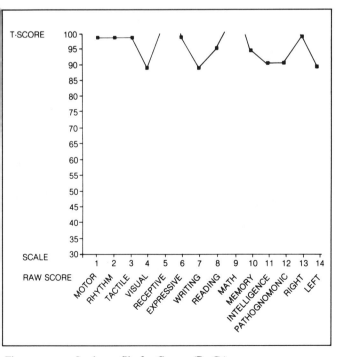

Figure 15.4. Luria profile for Case 3 (R. C.)

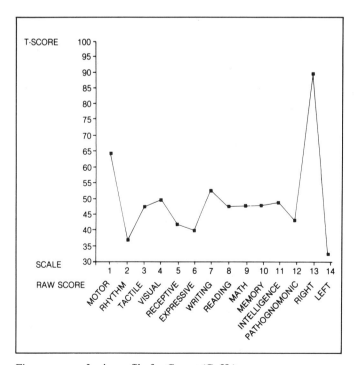

Figure 15.5. Luria profile for Case 4 (C. H.)

CASE 5

The following case was adapted from Newlin and Tramontana (in press) with permission of the authors. N. B. is a 16-year-old, left-handed male who was admitted to a psychiatric hospital for behavioral and mental changes coinciding with the onset of a malignant subcortical brain tumor approximately two years earlier. Apart from a history of obesity and chronic enuresis, the patient's premorbid status was essentially unremarkable until about the age of ten. At that time a carcinoma of the spine was diagnosed, but it was successfully treated with radiation therapy without apparent sequelae. He did experience some anxiety and feelings of rejection associated with his family's reaction to his illness but reportedly was able to resolve these problems rather well. However, he had not yet reached puberty at age 16—a condition possibly related to the earlier radiation treatment for his spinal tumor, but more probably attributable to the proximity of his subsequent brain tumor to the pituitary gland.

In March 1978 a neurological evaluation was prompted by complaints of a recent deterioration in his mental status, vomiting, and pain in the lumbar region of his spine. A CT scan of the head was performed at that time, and slice 3A is illustrated in Figure 15.6. This CT scan

(with intravenous iodine contrast) revealed an area of high density within the right anterior portion of the basal ganglia, occupying the head of the caudate nucleus on the right side and extending into the internal capsule. The tumor was diagnosed as a possible medulloblastoma, a fast-growing malignant tumor usually originating from the archicerebellum. Figure 15.7 illustrates the anatomy of this CT scan slice, with selected subcortical structures indicated, and Figure 15.8 shows a lateral representation of the site of the lesion and the location of the CT scan slice illustrated in Figure 15.6.

The patient was treated with radiation and chemotherapy through November 1978. Another CT scan was performed in March 1979, and a slice corresponding to the earlier one shown in Figure 15.6 is illustrated in Figure 15.9. This scan revealed bilateral atrophy of an iatrogenic nature (probably secondary to radiation therapy), with dilated ventricles and widened sulci. The tumor apparently had resolved completely.

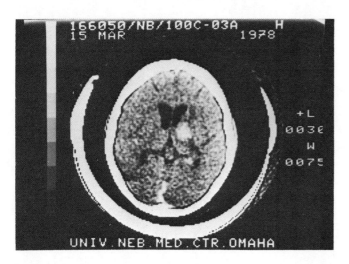

Figure 15.6.   CT scan (slice 3A) showing the tumor within the right anterior portion of the basal ganglia.

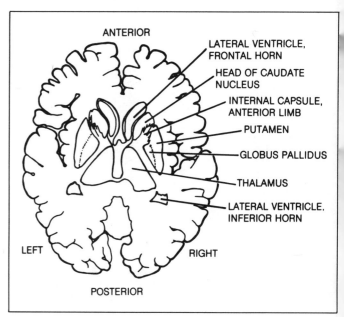

Figure 15.7.   Identification of selected subcortical structures corresponding to the CT scan slice shown in Figure 15.6.

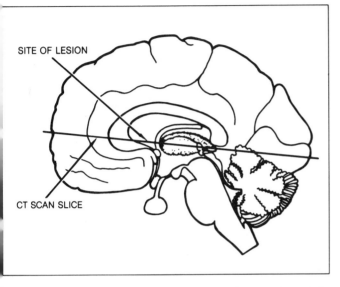

Figure 15.8.   Lateral perspective locating the site of the lesion and the level from which the CT slice was drawn.

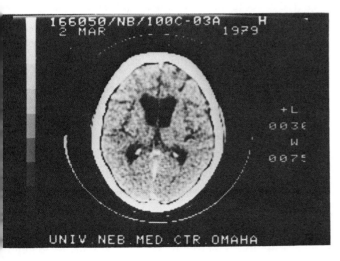

Figure 15.9.   Subsequent CT scan (slice 3A) showing resolution of the tumor after treatment.

Despite the stabilization of the patient's neurological status, the personality changes that appeared with the onset of his brain tumor persisted. He was psychiatrically hospitalized by November 1979, presenting symptoms characterized by hyperarousal and a failure in goal-directed regulation of behavior, cognition, and affect. His symptoms at the time of admission included distractibility, behavioral disinhibition, and vocal perseveration, together with clang associations, flight of ideas, and rapid speech. Further indications of heightened arousal and motor overflow were mannerisms such as twiddling his fingers and shaking his legs, and difficulty in sitting in one place for an extended period. Short-term and recent memory were impaired; he would often reintroduce himself to persons he had already met, and he also showed a tendency to confabulate in recounting details of his distant past. He displayed a superficial congeniality and an apparently carefree attitude along with "silly" or hypomanic affect. Taken together, his psychiatric symptomatology was similar to that of a hyperactive child. Treatment with Ritalin was, in fact, initiated and resulted in some apparent improvement. A trial of Lithium was later also tried because of the patient's hypomanic affect, but it was soon discontinued because there was no positive response. He was discharged to his family after approximately two months of inpatient care, and there has been no report of significant changes in his overall status since that time.

The Luria-Nebraska results are shown in Figure 15.10. Since the patients' critical level is 61; scores above this are considered abnormal. With this it appears that basic sensory, motor, and spatial functions were largely intact, as evidenced by the absence of significant elevations on the Motor, Tactile, and Visual scales of his profile. However, considering that the patient was left-handed and that the Right and Left scales were standardized on primarily a right-handed population, the relative impairment of the right hemisphere over the left was probably even greater than is reflected in the T score difference of 10 points shown here. Although there was no evidence of overall motor impairment, inspection of the

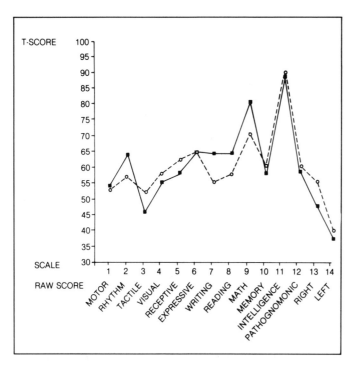

Figure 15.10.   Luria profile for Case 5 (N. B.): *solid line* = raw scores; *broken line* = age- and education-corrected.

individual items on the Motor scale did reveal a specific dysfunction of the left upper extremity and thus raises the possibility of right frontal involvement. The elevation of the Motor scale over the Tactile scale and of Expressive Speech over Receptive Speech also is compatible with an inference of predominantly anterior dysfunction.

Other indications of impairment included the patient's very pronounced elevations on the Arithmetic and Intelligence scales as well as lesser elevations on the Rhythm, Writing, Reading, and Memory scales. To an extent, some of these could be taken as an indication of disrupted academic achievement brought about by the patient's medical condition. It is doubtful, however, that they primarily reflect the effects of diffuse cortical damage, since in some instances the elevations considerably exceeded the degree of damage indicated in the modest elevation of the Pathognomonic scale (a composite scale consisting of the items in the battery found to be most sensitive

to brain damage). It is more likely that on these scales, where performance greatly depended on focused attention or on the efficient execution of higher cognitive functions, much of the patient's impairment resulted from a breakdown in the regulatory and inhibitory functions of attention, which rendered him highly susceptible to interference and distraction. Taken together with the previous findings, this would implicate prefrontal cortical impairment (especially in considering his disproportionately poor performance on the Intelligence scale) and raise the possibility of subcortical involvement as well.

It appears that the neuropsychological effects of the patient's subcortical lesion were primarily reflected in his difficulty in regulating attention and his susceptibility to interference in complex tasks. The results giving additional indication of prefrontal dysfunction along with mild right premotor involvement certainly suggest that the tumor had infiltrated or exerted significant pressure effects on these cortical areas. However, the similarity of his results to what would be expected with prefrontal impairment alone poses an interpretive problem for the clinical neuropsychologist, in that the results could easily have been taken to indicate only frontal lobe dysfunction.

In retrospect, the features of the case that might have signaled subcortical involvement had the neurological information not been available were the patient's pronounced distractibility and hyperarousal. These were seen in his difficulty on tasks such as the Rhythm and Arithmetic scales of the Luria-Nebraska and were most apparent in qualitative observations of his behavior during testing. Although disrupted attentional processes can certainly occur with prefrontal cortical impairment, the practicing neuropsychologist should at least consider the possibility of subcortical involvement in patients who otherwise appear to exhibit prefrontal dysfunction, especially when hyperarousal and distractibility are the most salient features in the history and test performance and when evidence of motor impairment is largely absent. Research is needed to determine whether these or other features provide a reliable means of distinguishing prefrontal from subcortical dysfunction. At present, however, the use of conjuctive neurodiagnostic methods such as CT scan assessment appears to be necessary for accurate differentiation.

Of course, contrasting the effects of prefrontal dysfunction and various forms of subcortical impairment often may be only a forced and artificial distinction, in that there is a highly intimate and integrated relationship between these neuroanatomical regions in the regulation of goal-directed behavior, cognition, and affect. Luria (1966, 1973) proposed that the prefrontal cortex may in fact be viewed as a tertiary (integrating) zone of the limbic system, with its extensive descending pathways that inhibit or otherwise regulate emotion and arousal. In the case presented here, the proximity of the lesion to both frontal lobe and anterior limbic structures suggests that a number of these descending pathways had been disturbed or destroyed, with a resultant loss of inhibitory control. Luria has also noted that anterior limbic lesions tend to be associated with disturbed consciousness and confabulation; both were observed in this patient's psychiatric status. Although the precise behavioral functions of the basal ganglia—consisting of the caudate nucleus, putamen, globus pallidus, and corpus striatum—are obscure, they often are classified as part of the extrapyramidal motor system and appear to play a role in the control of movement (Thompson, 1967). Luria, however, has implicated the caudate nucleus in selective attention, and he sees it and other parts of the basal ganglia as involved in the control of cortical tone and activity level. It was clear in this patient, whose tumor had specifically occupied the head of the caudate nucleus on the right side, that the level of arousal and activity was high and there were marked problems in selective attention.

Thus the psychiatric, neurological, and neuropsychological aspects of this case can be integrated through the theoretical writings of A. R. Luria. The similarity of the patient's psychiatric status to the syndrome of childhood hyperactivity is particularly interesting, not only because it follows from a neuropsychological conceptualiza-

tion of the case based on Luria's theory, but also because it suggests a possible neuroanatomical locus of dysfunction that can mimic the disorder and perhaps play a role in its pathogenesis. In this regard Gorenstein and Newman (1980) have drawn parallels between behavioral syndrome in rodents, characterized by an inability to delay gratification, induced by anterior limbic (septal) lesions, and disinhibitory psychopathology in humans such as psychopathy and hyperactivity. Also, Pribram and McGuinness (1975) have further implicated the caudate nucleus and other structures of the basal ganglia in the control of "activation," defined as a tonic state of arousal and selective attention. Finally, in light of this patient's disturbed, hypomanic affect and his primarily right-hemispheric impairment, it is interesting that Newlin and Golden (1980) have emphasized the presence of right hemisphere dysfunction in manic-depressive patients, a pattern of findings congruent with other research suggesting right hemispheric specialization in the processing of affect.

Systematic application of comprehensive neuropsychological methods to children and adolescents with psychiatric disorders have begun (Tramontana, Sherrets, & Golden, 1980), and it is important that others follow. This case has illustrated some of the interpretive problems posed when subcortical brain pathology is involved and has pointed toward a possible role of particular structures along frontolimbic pathways in the syndrome of hyperactivity—an intriguing avenue for future research.

Summary

While relatively few subcortical disorders are directly related to behavior assessed on the Luria-Nebraska Neuropsychological Battery, damage to any subcortical structure may impair traditionally more complex behaviors regulated by the cortex.

Generally, subcortical damage will generate numerous elevated scales. Although the Pathognomonic scale does not appear to exhibit very high scores for disorders like those discussed in this chapter, the Arithmetic scale appears to be significantly increased after subcortical dysfunction. In general, it appears that owing either to the diffuseness of many subcortical injuries or to the scales themselves, the Right and Left Hemisphere scales rarely show clinically significant differences for subcortical disorders.

We have attempted to increase the clinician's understanding of the effects of subcortical impairment on behavior as well as of complications due to both cortical and subcortical dysfunction. Historically, neuropsychology has been oriented toward complex behaviors modulated by the cerebral cortex. This chapter suggests that many of these activities are initiated, influenced, or regulated by subcortical structures. Consequently, careful attention must be paid to test scores as well as to patterns of responding, and one must relate such findings to potentially useful historical or medical evidence suggesting subcortical impairment.

Appendix A:
Luria-Nebraska Items

Motor Functions

SIMPLE MOVEMENT: HANDS
1. Using your right hand, touch your fingers in turn with your thumb as quickly as you can while you count them.
2. Same as #1 with left hand.
3. Do as I do. Clench your right hand and then stretch your fingers repeatedly until I ask you to stop.
4. Same as #3 with left hand.

KINESTHETIC BASIS OF MOVEMENT: HANDS
5. With your eyes closed, place your right hand in the same position I place it in. (Press patient's thumb against fifth finger for 2 seconds.)
6. Same as #5 with left hand.
7. With your eyes closed, place your right hand in the same position I place your left hand in. (Thumb and middle finger are placed against each other for 2 seconds.)
8. Same as #7 with left hand.

OPTIC SPATIAL ORGANIZATION: HANDS
9. Do as I do. Place the right hand under the chin with fingers bent.
10. Same as #9 with left hand.
11. Right hand fingers extended in sagittal plane touching chin.
12. Same as #11 with left hand.
13. Right hand held horizontal to vertical left.
14. Left hand held horizontal to vertical right.
15. Raise the right hand.
16. Raise the left hand.
17. Right hand points to left eye.
18. Left hand points to right eye.
19. Point to your left eye with your right hand.
20. Touch your right ear with your left hand.

DYNAMIC ORGANIZATION: HANDS
21. Do as I do. Change the position of your two hands at

the same time. First you are to clench your right hand and at the same time extend the fingers of your left hand. Then I want you to reverse the position of your two hands over and over.

22. Do as I do. With your hands in front of you, tap your right hand twice and your left hand once, changing smoothly from one hand to the other like this. Do it as fast as you can until I tell you to stop.
23. Same as #22, but reverse order of hands.
24. Draw this pattern without lifting your pencil from the paper.

COMPLEX FORMS OF PRAXIS

25. Pretend you are holding a teapot in your hand and show me how to pour and stir tea.
26. Show me how to thread a needle.
27. Show me how to cut with scissors.

SIMPLE MOVEMENT: ORAL

28. Puff out your cheeks.
29. Stick out your tongue as far as possible and keep it there until I tell you to put it back in your mouth.

KINESTHETIC MOVEMENT: ORAL

30. Stick your tongue out and roll it up.
31. Place your tongue between your upper teeth and upper lip.

DYNAMIC ORGANIZATION: ORAL

32. I am going to ask you to make three movements with your mouth. Do as I do. First I want you to show your teeth, then stick out your tongue, then place your tongue between your lower teeth and lower lip. Now I want you to do those three movements.
33. Now do those three movements rapidly several times until I tell you to stop.

INTEGRATIVE ORAL PRAXIS

34. Show me how to chew.
35. Show me how to whistle.

SELECTIVITY OF MOTOR ACT

36. Without lifting your pencil from the paper, I want you to draw the best circle you can.
37. Time for #36.
38. Without lifting your pencil from the paper, I want you to draw the best square you can.
39. Time for #38.
40. Without lifting your pencil from the paper, I want you to draw the best triangle you can, and make all three sides equal.
41. Time for #40.
42. Copy this figure as best you can without lifting your pencil from the paper (circle).
43. Time for #42.
44. Copy this figure (square).
45. Time for #44.
46. Copy this figure (triangle).
47. Time for #46.
48. If I knock on the table once, you knock twice; if I knock twice, you knock once.

SPEECH REGULATION OF MOTOR ACTS

49. If I say *red,* squeeze my hand; if I say *green,* do nothing.
50. If I knock once, raise your right hand; if I knock twice, raise your left hand.
51. If I knock hard, you knock gently; if I knock gently, you knock hard (demonstrate intensity).

Acoustic-Motor Organization (Rhythm)

PERCEPTION OF PITCH RELATIONSHIPS

52. Now you are going to hear two tones on a tape recording. Tell me whether the tones you hear are the same or different.
53. Again, you will hear two tones. Tell me which is higher, the first tone or the second tone.
54. Now you will hear two groups of sounds. There will be about four tones in each group. I want you to tell

me whether the two groups of tones you hear sound the same or different.

REPRODUCTION OF PITCH RELATIONSHIPS AND MUSICAL MELODIES

55. Listen to these tones, then hum them.
56. Listen to this melody. Will you please sing it?
57. Please sing the first line of "Home on the Range."

PERCEPTION AND EVALUATION OF ACOUSTIC SIGNALS

58. Tell me how many beeps you hear.
59. How many beeps are there all together in these groups?
60. How many beeps are there in each of these groups?
61. In the next groups some of the beeps are loud and some are soft. Tell me how many beeps there are in each group.

MOTOR PERFORMANCE OF RHYTHMIC GROUPS

62. You will now hear a rhythm on the tape. When I tell you the rhythm is over, I want you to tap with your hand the rhythm you heard on the tape.
63. Please make a series of: two taps; three taps; two taps; two strong and three weak taps; three weak and two strong taps; a series of two taps followed by three taps.

Higher Cutaneous and Kinesthetic Functions (Tactile)

CUTANEOUS SENSATION

For all the tests in this section the subject should be blindfolded.

64. Tell me where I am touching you. (Touch subject with eraser end of pencil, *alternating between right and left*.) Right side performance.
65. Left side performance.
66. Am I touching you with the point or with the head of a pin? Right hand performance.
67. Left hand performance.

68. Is this a soft or a hard touch? Right hand performance.
69. Left hand performance.
70. How many points do you feel? Right hand performance.
71. Left hand performance.
72. In what direction am I touching you, up or down your arm? Right arm performance.
73. Left arm performance.
74. I am going to trace either a cross, a triangle, or a circle on your wrist. Tell me what I am tracing. Right hand performance.
75. Left hand performance.
76. (On back of wrist.) What number is this? (3) Right hand performance.
77. Left hand performance.
78. (On back of wrist.) What letter is this? (s) Right hand performance.
79. Left hand performance.

MUSCLE AND JOINT SENSATION

80. Now I will put your left arm in a certain position; try to put your right arm in the same position.
81. Now I will put your right arm in a certain position; try to put your left arm in the same position.

STEREOGNOSIS

82. Feel this object and tell me exactly what it is. (Quarter, eraser, key, paperclip.) Right hand errors.
83. Right hand time.
84. Left hand errors.
85. Left hand time.

Visual Functions

VISUAL PERCEPTION: OBJECTS AND PICTURES

86. What do you call this object? (Pencil, eraser, rubber band, quarter.)
87. What is this picture supposed to be? (Handbag,

purse or pocket book; nutcracker; vial, glass, measuring glass, test tube, rain gauge, or graduated cylinder; camera [and lenses]; egg carton.)

88. What is this picture supposed to be? (Book, any book; book; sunglasses, glasses, spectacles; sunglasses, glasses, spectacles; sunglasses.)

89. What is this picture supposed to be? (Telephone; man's profile, man's face.)

90. What objects can you make out in this picture? (Pail, bucket; paintbrush, brush, baster; rake; scissors, shears; hatchet, ax.)

91. What objects can you make out in this picture? (Coffeepot, teapot, teakettle; fork; bottle; glass, wire basket; bowl, dish, saucer, basin.)

92. The upper part of this card has a design with a piece missing. Put your finger on the piece with the design that will complete the pattern of the large design.

93. Time for #92.

SPATIAL ORIENTATION

94. Tell me exactly what time these clocks tell. (7:53; 5:09; 1:25; 10:35.)

95. Draw the hands of a clock if the time is 12:50; 4:35; 11:10.

96. If this compass were on a map, which way would be north? east? west?

INTELLECTUAL OPERATIONS IN SPACE

97. This drawing shows a stack of blocks. When I show you the card again, tell me how many blocks make up the stack. Be sure to include both the blocks you see and those you don't see.

98. Time for #97.

99. At the left of this paper there is a square with a circle in one corner. Notice the heavy dark line on one side of the square. This is the base line. Now look at these squares and notice that each square has a circle in one corner and the bottom of each square is a heavy line, the base line. By using the base line as a refer-

ence point, you can tell which square is just like the sample. Now I want you to circle the letter under the square that is just like the sample. Now look at sample 2. This is the same type of problem, but the heavy base line is on the left side of the square. To solve the problem you have to turn the sample square in your head so that the base line is on the bottom as it is here. Now do the rest of these by circling the letters under the correct squares.

Receptive Speech

PHONEMIC HEARING: REPETITION AND WRITING

100. Repeat exactly the sound that you hear (*b, p, m*).

101. Now I am going to say some sounds and I want you to write down the letter of the alphabet that the sound represents (*b, p, m*).

102. Now I am going to say two sounds. After I say them I want you to repeat them right after me (*m-p, p-s, b-p, d-t, k-g, r-l*).

103. I am again going to repeat two sounds as I just did before. I want you to write down the letters represented by the two sounds rather than saying them aloud (*m-p, p-s, b-p, d-t, k-g, r-l*).

104. Now I will say three sounds. After I complete them, repeat them after me (*a-o-a, u-a-i, m-s-d, b-p-b, d-t-d, bi-ba-bo, bi-bo-ba*).

105. I am going to say three sounds. After I have finished the three sounds I want you to write down the letter represented by each sound. (*a-o-a, u-a-i, m-s-d, b-p-b, d-t-d*). Now I am going to say several more sets of three sounds. This time I want you to write down all the letters that go with the sounds you hear, not just the first letter (*bi-ba-bo, bi-bo-ba*).

PHONEMIC HEARING: CONDITIONED REFLEX

106. If you hear *ba*, please raise your right hand; if you hear *pa*, please raise your left hand.

PHONEMIC HEARING: PITCH CHANGE

107. I want you to tell me whether the letters you hear are the same or different: *b–p* (pronounced at same pitch); *b–b* (pronounced at different pitches).

WORD COMPREHENSION: DEFINITIONS

108. Will you please point to your: eye, nose, ear.

WORD COMPREHENSION: EFFECT OF REPETITION

109. I want you to point to these, in this order: eye-nose-ear-eye-nose.

WORD COMPREHENSION: IDENTIFICATION

110. I want you to point at: the shoe; the candle; the stove.
111. Will you point at: your knee; your elbow; your cheekbone.
112. What does (*word*) mean? (*cat; bat; pat*).

SIMPLE SENTENCES: PHRASES

113. Point to the picture that shows: typewriting; mealtime; summer.

SIMPLE SENTENCES: INSTRUCTIONS

114. Put your hand on your head; wiggle your feet.
115. Tell me whose watch this is. Whose is this?
116. Show me what is used to light a fire.

SIMPLE SENTENCES: CONFLICTING INSTRUCTIONS

117. Here are a gray card and a black card: If it is night now, point to the gray card; if it is day now, point to the black card. This time, if it is day now, point to the black card; if it is night now, point to the gray card.

LOGICAL GRAMMATICAL STRUCTURES: INFLECTIVE

118. Point at the pencil; point at the key.
119. Point with the key toward the pencil; point with the pencil toward the key.

120. Point to the pencil with the key; now point to the comb with the pencil.

LOGICAL GRAMMATICAL STRUCTURES: ATTRIBUTIVE

121. Show me, by pointing, who is the daughter's mother.
122. Will you tell me whether the "father's brother" and the "brother's father" are two persons or the same person?

LOGICAL GRAMMATICAL STRUCTURES: SPATIAL RELATIONSHIPS

123. Draw a cross beneath a circle; now draw a circle to the right of a cross.
124. Which statement is correct: "Spring comes before summer" or "Summer comes before spring."

LOGICAL GRAMMATICAL STRUCTURES: COMPARATIVE CONSTRUCTIONS

125. Which boy is shorter, if Tom is taller than Arnie?
126. Which statement is correct: "A fly is bigger than an elephant" or "An elephant is bigger than a fly"?
127. Look at these cards. Which of the two is lighter? Which of the two is less light? Which of the two is darker? Which of the two is less dark?
128. Tell me which girl is lightest, if Mary is lighter than Jane but darker than Sue? Which of the girls is darkest, if Mary is lighter than Jane but darker than Sue?

LOGICAL GRAMMATICAL STRUCTURES: INVERTED GRAMMATICAL CONSTRUCTIONS

129. If Arnie hit Tom, which boy was the victim?
130. If I had lunch after I cleaned house, what did I do first?
131. Is the following sentence said by a disciplined or an undisciplined person? "I am unaccustomed to disobeying rules."

LOGICAL GRAMMATICAL STRUCTURES:

COMPLEX STRUCTURES

132. Listen to this sentence: "The woman who worked at the store came to the school where Mary studied to give a talk." Tell me who gave a talk. Tell me what Mary was doing.

Expressive Speech

Stimulus items 133–142 may be repeated by examiner.

ARTICULATION OF SPEECH SOUNDS

133. Repeat after me: *a* (as in *late*); *i* (*light*); *m* (*milk*); *b* (*baby*); *sh* (*shine*).
134. *Sp* (*spot*); *th* (*thaw*); *pl* (*plate*); *str* (*string*); *awk* (*awkward*).
135. *See–seen; tree–trick.*

REFLECTED (REPETITIVE) SPEECH: SINGLE WORDS

136. *House; table; apple.*
137. *Hairbrush; screwdriver; laborious.*
138. *Rhinoceros; surveillance; hierarchy.*
139. *Cat–hat–bat.*
140. *Streptomycin; Massachusetts Episcopal.*

REFLECTED SPEECH: SERIES OF WORDS

141. *Hat–sun–bell; hat–bell–sun.*
142. *House–ball–chair; ball–chair–house.*

ARTICULATION OF SPEECH SOUNDS

143. Say the sounds that go with these letters: *a, i, m, b, sh.*
144. *Sp, th, pl, str, awk.*
145. Read these words: *see–seen; tree–trick.*

REFLECTED (REPETITIVE) SPEECH: SINGLE WORDS

146. Read these words: *cat; dog; man.*
147. *House; table; apple.*
148. *Hairbrush; screwdriver; laborious.*

149. *Rhinoceros; surveillance; hierarchy.*
150. *Cat–hat–bat.*
151. *Streptomycin; Massachusetts Episcopal.*

REFLECTED SPEECH: SERIES OF WORDS

152. *Hat–sun–bell.*
153. *House–ball–chair.*

REFLECTED SPEECH: SENTENCES

Repeat these sentences.

154. The weather is fine today. The sun shines and the sky is blue.
155. The apple trees grew in the garden behind a high fence. In the edge of the forest, the hunter killed the wolf.
156. The house is on fire, the moon is shining, the broom is sweeping.
157. What objects do these pictures represent? (Guitar; table; can opener; candle; stapler.)
158. What parts of the body do these pictures represent? (Foot, ankle; forearm, elbow, arm; finger, fingernail, any finger.)

NOMINATIVE FUNCTION OF SPEECH:

NAMING FROM DESCRIPTION

159. What do you call the object with which you fix your hair each morning? (Comb, hairbrush, or brush.) What do you call the object that shows you what time it is? (Watch, clock, or any timepiece.) What do you call the object that protects you from the rain? (Umbrella or raincoat.)

NARRATIVE SPEECH: FLUENCY

AND AUTOMATIZATION OF SPEECH

160. Count from 1 to 20 out loud.
161. Count backward from 20 to 1.
162. Tell me the days of the week.
163. Say the days of the week backward starting with Sunday.

PREDICTIVE SPEECH: REPRODUCTIVE FORMS

164. Tell me what's happening in this picture. Response time.
165. Number of words in first 5 seconds.
166. I am going to read this short story out loud. Follow along carefully, because when I'm through I'm going to take the card away and then you'll have to tell the story back to me in your own words. Response time.
167. Number of words in first 5 seconds.

NARRATIVE SPEECH: PREDICTIVE FORMS

168. Please make up a short speech about the conflict between the generations. Response time.
169. Number of words in first 5 seconds.

COMPLEX SYSTEMS OF GRAMMATICAL EXPRESSION

170. A word is omitted in this sentence (on cards). Fill in with a word that you find suitable.
171. Time for #170.
172. Make up a sentence that includes the three words on this card.
173. The words on this card can make a sentence if they are arranged correctly. I want you to arrange them so they do make a sentence.
174. Time for #173.

Writing

PHONETIC ANALYSIS

175. How many letters are there in: *cat, trap, banana, hedge.*
176. What is the second letter in *cat?* What is the first letter in *match?* What is the third letter in *hedge?* Which letter in *stop* comes after *o?* Which letter in *bridge* comes before *g?*

COPYING AND WRITING: SIMPLE

177. Copy these letters in your own handwriting: *B, L, L, D, B.*

178. Copy these in your own handwriting: *pa, an, pro, pre, sti.*
179. I will now show you a card that has three words on it for 5 seconds. When I remove the card, I want you to write the words: *match; district; antarctic.*
180. Please write your first and last names.

COPYING AND WRITING: COMPLEX FORMS

181. Write the letters that I say: *f, t, h, l.*
182. Now write these sounds: *ba; da; back; pack.*
183. Now write these words: *wren; knife.*
184. Write: *physiology; probabilistic.*
185. Now write these words and phrases: *hat–sun–dog; all of a sudden; last year before Christmas.*
186. Write a few sentences about your main ideas on bringing up children.
187. Number of words written for #186.

Reading

PHONETIC SYNTHESIS

188. What sound is made by these letters: *g–r–o; p–l–y?*
189. What word is made by these letters: *s–t–o–n–e; k–n–i–g–h–t?*

READING: ANALYSIS AND PERCEPTION OF LETTERS

190. Tell me what you see here: *K, S, W, R, T.*
191. Which of these letters, *B, J,* or *S,* stands for *John?*

READING: SYLLABLES AND WORDS

192. Read these sounds: *po; cor; cra; spro; prot.*
193. Read these words: *juice; bread; bonfire; cloakroom; fertilizer.*
194. Read these letters: *U.N., U.S.A., U.S.S.R.*
195. Read these words: *insubordination; indistinguishable.*
196. Read these words: *astrocytoma; hemopoiesis.*

READING: PHRASES AND WHOLE TEXTS

197. Read these sentences: The man went out for a walk.

There are flowers in the garden.

198. Read these sentences: The sun rises in the west. The boy went to bed because she was ill.
199. Read this story out loud.
200. Time for #199.

Arithmetic

COMPREHENSION OF NUMBER STRUCTURE:
WRITING AND RECOGNIZING FIGURES

201. Write down the numbers I say: 7-9-3; 3-5-7.
202. Write down these roman numerals: IV and VI; IX and XI.
203. Write down the regular numbers: 17 and 71; 69 and 96.
204. Write: 27, 34, 158, 396, 9845.
205. Write: 14, 17, 19, 109, 1023.
206. Read these numbers: 7-9-3; 3-5-7.
207. Read these numbers: IV, VI, IX, XI; 17, 71, 69, 96.
208. Read these numbers: 27, 34, 158, 396, 9845.
209. There are three numbers on this card arranged from top to bottom. Read each number as a whole number: 158; 396; 1023.

COMPREHENSION OF NUMBER STRUCTURE:
NUMERICAL DIFFERENCES

210. Tell me which number is larger: 17 or 68; 23 or 56; 189 or 201.
211. Look at this card and show me, by pointing, which of the top two numbers is the larger. Which of the bottom two is larger? 189 or 201; 1967 or 3002.

ARITHMETIC OPERATIONS: SIMPLE

212. Now I will ask you to solve some problems; you may write them down if you like. How much is: 3×3; 5×4; 7×8?
213. How much is: $3 + 4$; $6 + 7$?
214. How much is: $7 - 4$; $8 - 5$?

ARITHMETIC OPERATIONS: COMPLEX

215. How much is: $27 + 8$; $44 + 57$; $31 - 7$; $44 - 14$?
216. On this card the numbers are arranged up and down. Add them in your head: $5 + 9 + 7$.
217. In your head, subtract the number above from the one below on this card: $24 - 18$.

ARITHMETIC OPERATIONS: SIGNS

218. What is the missing sign in each of these—a plus, a minus, or some other sign? $10\ (\ )\ 2 = 20$; $10\ (\ )\ 2 = 12$; $10\ (\ )\ 2 = 8$; $10\ (\ )\ 2 = 5$.
219. What is the missing number? $12 - (\ ) = 8$; $12 + (\ ) = 19$.
220. What is the answer to the top problem on this card? Figure the answer in your head. Now do this bottom problem: $27 + 34 + 14$; $158 + 396$.

ARITHMETIC OPERATIONS: CONSECUTIVE SERIES

221. I want you to count backward from a hundred by sevens like this: $100 - 93 - 86$, and so on.
222. Now I want you to do the same thing, but this time start at 100 and subtract 13 each time.

Memory

No stimulus repetitions are allowed for any item in this section.

THE LEARNING PROCESS: SERIES OF UNRELATED WORDS

223. I am going to say seven words. After I finish saying them, I want you to repeat as many of them back to me as you can remember: *house–forest–cat–night–table–needle–pie.* You remembered ( ) words out of the seven on that trial. I am going to say the same seven words again, and I want you to try to recall as many as you are able to again when I finish. But before I begin I want you to tell me how many words

you think you'll remember this next time, after I finish saying them.

224. Sum of (predicted minus actual) divided by (trials minus one), multiplied by 100.

225. Were two correct trials in order achieved on #223?

RETENTION AND RETRIEVAL: FORM RECOGNITION

226. I am going to show you a card with some pictures on it. You will have 5 seconds to examine it, and then I will remove it. Now I want you to count to 100 out loud. (After 30 seconds say), Is the picture on this card the same as or different from the one on the card I showed before?

RETENTION AND RETRIEVAL:
IMMEDIATE SENSORY TRACE RECALL

227. I am going to show you a card; look at it carefully. When I remove the card I want you to draw as much from it as you can remember.

228. Now I am going to tap a rhythm with my hand on the table. Listen carefully, because when I finish I want you to tap the same rhythm. Make sure that you have the same number of taps I have and that you tap the same loud and soft taps I do.

229. I am going to put my hand in three positions. I want you to remember what positions my hand made, because I will then ask you to make the same positions.

230. Now I am going to show you a card. You will have five seconds to examine it, and then I will remove it. I want you to repeat the words written on the card after I remove it: *house; moon; street; boy; water.*

RETENTION AND RETRIEVAL OF WORDS

231. *Heterogeneous Interference*
I want you to remember some words I am going to say: *house-tree-cat.*
Now look at this picture. What do you see? (Have patient describe the picture for 15 seconds.) What were the words? (*House-tree-cat.*)

232. *Homogeneous Interference*
Now I'm going to say some more words; try to remember them: *man-hat-door.*
Now try to remember these words: *light-stove-cake.*
What were the words I said first? What were the words I said second?

RETENTION AND RETRIEVAL:
SENTENCES AND PARAGRAPHS

233. Now I want you to remember two sentences I am going to say: The sun rises in the east. In May the apple trees blossom.
What was the first sentence? What was the second sentence?

234. Now I am going to read a short story. Listen carefully, because when I am finished I want you to say the story back to me.

LOGICAL MEMORIZING: RECALLING BY VISUAL AID

235. Now I am going to show you some pictures. With each picture I am going to say a word. When I finish, I will show you the pictures, and I want you to say the word I said with each picture: *energy; employment; party; happy; family; project; pollution.*

Intellectual Processes

UNDERSTANDING OF THEMATIC PICTURES

236. Look carefully at this picture and then tell me what is happening in it.

237. What is happening in this picture?

238. These pictures are in the wrong order. I want you to put them in the right order so they make sense.

239. Time for #238.

240. These pictures also are in the wrong order. Put them in the right order so they make sense.

241. Time for #240.

242. What's comical about the story in these pictures?
243. What's comical about these pictures?

UNDERSTANDING OF THEMATIC TEXTS

244. Listen carefully to the story I tell you; when I have finished I am going to ask some questions about it (hen and golden egg story).
245. What is meant by these expressions: "iron hand"; "green thumb"?
246. Explain to me what is meant by the saying "Don't count your chickens before they have hatched."
247. On the top of this card there is a saying. Below are three possible explanations of it. Which is the correct one? ("Strike while the iron is hot"; "Still waters run deep.")

CONCEPT FORMATION: DEFINITION

248. What do these words mean? *table; island*.

CONCEPT FORMATION:

COMPARISON AND DIFFERENTIATION

249. In what way are *table* and *sofa* alike?
     In what way are *ax* and *saw* alike?
250. What is the difference between: a fox and a dog; a stone and an egg?

CONCEPT FORMATION: LOGICAL RELATIONSHIPS

251. The word *table* belongs to the group of objects called *furniture*.
     What group does (*rose; carp*) belong to?
252. If we start with the group *animals,* then a *horse* will be a member of the group. Give me an example of a member of these groups: *vehicles; tools*.
253. If we consider a table as a whole, then the legs will be part of the whole; can you tell me what are the parts of the whole *knife?*
254. If we start with the part *wall* then the whole will be *house*. What will the whole be of these parts; *pages; trees?*

CONCEPT FORMATION: OPPOSITES

255. The opposite in meaning to the word *healthy* is *sick*. What is the opposite of: *high; fat?*

CONCEPT FORMATION: ANALOGIES

256. What word has the same relationship to *good* as *high* has to *low?*
     What word has to the same relationship to *wide* as *fat* has to *thin?*
     What word has the same relationship to *hand* that *shoe* has to *foot?*
257. Which word of the four I will now say does not belong to the same group as the other three? *spoon-table-glass-plate; cigar-wine-cigarette-tobacco*.

DISCURSIVE REASONING:

ELEMENTARY ARITHMETIC PROBLEMS

258. Peter had two apples and John had six apples. How many did they have together?
259. Time for #258.
260. Jane had seven apples and gave three away. How many did she have left?
261. Time for #260.
262. Mary had four apples and Betty had two apples more than Mary. How many apples did they have together?
263. Time for #262.

DISCURSIVE REASONING:

COMPLEX ARITHMETIC PROBLEMS

264. A farmer had ten acres of land; from each acre he harvested six tons of grain; he sold one-third to the government. How much did he have left?
265. Time for #264.
266. There were 18 books on two shelves; there were twice as many on one shelf as on the other. How many books were there on each shelf?
267. Time for #266.

268. A pedestrian walks to the station in 15 minutes, and a cyclist rides there five times faster. How long does the cyclist take to get to the station?

269. Time for #268.

Appendix B:
Methodology from Correlational
Study and Factor Analysis

The following methodology sections from the original factor analysis and correlational study are provided for readers who want more information on the procedures employed.

Correlational Studies (Golden and Berg, 1980a–d), 1981(a–c), & in press.

METHOD

Subjects for the studies consisted of 338 patients, tested on the complete Luria-Nebraska Neuropsychological Battery. Of these patients, 70 were diagnosed as normal, 70 carried psychiatric diagnoses, usually schizophrenia or a personality disorder, and the rest carried diagnoses of brain damage. The patients with brain damage fell into the following categories: head trauma, neoplasms, cerebrovascular disorders, degenerative diseases, multiple sclerosis, congenital brain dysfunction, and alcoholism or other drug-related or metabolic disorders. Patients were not chosen to meet any specific criteria except that they had completed the entire Luria-Nebraska Neuropsychological Battery. Average age of the patients in this study was 40.38 years ($SD = 17.2$ years), with an average educational level of 10.9 years ($SD = 2.3$ years). The population was about evenly divided by sex, with 180 males and 158 females. The sexual composition of the three groups did not differ significantly according to a chi-square test, nor did the groups differ significantly in age or education according to two F tests.

All patients in the study were administered the Luria-Nebraska Neuropsychological Battery according to the instructions in the original manual (Golden, Purisch, & Hammeke, 1979). All items initially were scored on a 0, 1, 2 system according to objective criteria recorded in the test manual. Scores of 0 generally indicated normal performance, while a score of 1 represented borderline performances and a score of 2 indicated performance characteristic of brain damage. As would be expected using this type of system, intercorrelations between all items are positive. Further details on the scoring of specific items may be found in the test manual.

Factor Analysis (Golden, Sweet, Hammeke, Purisch, Graber, & Osmon, 1980)

METHOD

A sample of 270 subjects, equally divided among normal controls, psychiatric patients, and brain-damaged patients, was used. The average age of each of the three patient groups was 41.3 years (*SD* = 15.3 years) for the normal patients, 39.6 years (*SD* = 14.8 years) for the psychiatric patients, and 42.1 years (*SD* = 15.7 years) for the neurological patients. Patients in the normal group had no history of brain damage but had been admitted to a hospital with some condition other than brain dysfunction. Most of the psychiatric patients were admitted with a diagnosis of schizophrenia. Approximately 10% of the sample had a diagnosis of personality disorder. All patients were admitted to a psychiatric hospital at the time of testing. Average number of hospitalizations for the group was 4.6, and the patients had an average history of 15 years since their first admission to a psychiatric hospital.

For the neurological group, there was an average of 5.6 years since the onset of their neurological conditions. Of the patients in the sample, 40 had lateralized injuries, 20 to the left hemisphere and 20 to the right hemisphere. Of the neurological patients, 50 had diffuse disorders. The primary diagnostic categories were vascular disorders, 25 cases; head trauma, 20 cases; degenerative disorders, 10 cases; tumors, 8 cases; congenital disorders, 8 cases; chronic alcoholism with atrophy identified by CT scan, 9 cases; multiple sclerosis, 6 cases; and Parkinson's disease, 4 cases. All patients in all groups were able to follow directions, and in no case did the patient get less than 40% of the items correct overall. No patient who was unable to finish the testing in its entirety was included.

All patients were tested with the Luria-Nebraska Neuropsychological Battery according to the directions given in the test manual (Golden, Purisch, & Hammeke, 1979). Their performance on each item was reported as a scaled score (0, 1, 2) according to normative data in the test manual. A score of 0 generally indicates no significant deficits, a score of 1 borderline deficits, and a score of 2 significant deficits on the item or scale being measured. Items on each scale were assigned theoretically according to the work of Luria and Christensen.

For each scale the items were subjected to a factor analysis using the Statistical Package for the Social Sciences (SPSS) program (Nie et al., 1975). A principal components analysis with communalities on the diagonal and iteration to the most ideal solutions was employed. The results were obliquely rotated into the simplest factor structure, with the number of factors to be rotated for each scale determined by the Screen Test. The simplest solution that maximized the number of factors falling into the hyperplane was adopted.

References

Ajax, E. T. Acquired dyslexia. *Archives of Neurology,* 1964, *11,* 66.

Bay, E. Zum Problem der taktilen Agnosie. *Deutsche Zeitschrift für Nervenheilkunde,* 1944, *1–3,* 64–96.

Bender, M. D., Postel, D. M., & Krieger, H. P. Disorders of oculomotor function in lesions of the occipital lobe. *Journal of Neurology, Neurosurgery, and Psychiatry,* 1957, *20,* 139.

Benson, D. F., Segarra, J., & Albert, M. L. Visual agnosia-prosopagnosia. *Archives of Neurology,* 1974, *30,* 307.

Benson, D. F., & Wier, W. F. Acalculia: Acquired anarithmetica. *Cortex,* 1972, *8,* 465.

Botez, M. I., & Wertheim, N. Expressive aphasia and amnesia following right frontal lesion in a right-handed man. *Brain,* 1959, *82,* 86.

Brain, W. R. Visual disorientation with special reference to lesions of the right cerebral hemisphere. *Brain,* 1941, *64,* 244.

Butters, N. Amnesic disorders. In K. M. Heilman and E. Valenstein (Eds.), *Clinical neuropsychology.* New York: Oxford University Press, 1979.

Butters, N., & Brody, B. A. The role of the left parietal lobe in the mediation of intra- and cross-modal associations. *Cortex,* 1969, *4,* 328.

Carmon, A., & Benton, A. L. Tactile perception of direction and number in patients with unilateral cerebral disease. *Neurology,* 1969, *19,* 525.

Christensen, A. L. *Luria's neuropsychological investigation.* New York: Spectrum, 1975.

Chusid, J. G. *Correlative neuroanatomy and functional neurology* (15th ed.). Los Altos: Lange, 1973.

Cohn, R. Dyscalculia. *Archives of Neurology,* 1961, *4,* 301.

Corkin, S. Tactually guided maze learning in man: Effects of unilateral cortical excisions and bilateral hippocampal lesions. *Neuropsychologia,* 1965, *3,* 339.

Corkin, S., Milner, B., & Rasmussen, T. Somatosensory thresholds: Contrasting effects of postcentral gyrus and posterior parietal lobe excisions. *Archives of Neurology*, 1970, *23*, 41.

Critchley, M. *The parietal lobes*. London: Arnold Publishers, 1953.

Cumming, W. J. K., Hurwitz, L. J., & Perl, N. T. A study of a patient who had alexia without agraphia. *Journal of Neurology, Neurosurgery, and Psychiatry*, 1970, *33*, 34.

Curtis, B. A., Jacobsen, S., & Marcus, E. M. *An introduction to the neurosciences*. Philadelphia: W. B. Saunders, 1972.

DeJong, R. N., Itabashi, H. H., & Olson, J. R. Memory loss due to hippocampal lesions: Report of a case. *Archives of Neurology*, 1969, *20*, 339.

DeRenzi, E., & Faglioni, P. The relationship between visuo-spatial impairment and constructional apraxia. *Cortex*, 1967, *3*, 327.

DeRenzi, E., Faglioni, P., & Scotti, G. Tactile spatial impairment and unilateral cerebral damage. *Journal of Nervous and Mental Disease*, 1968, *146*, 468.

Douglas, R. J., & Pribram, K. H. Learning aids and limbic lesions. *Neuropsychologia*, 1966, *4*, 197.

Drachman, D. A., & Arbit, J. Memory and the hippocampal complex. *Archives of Neurology*, 1966, *15*, 52.

Drachman, D. A., & Ommaya, A. K. Memory and the hippocampal cortex. *Archives of Neurology*, 1964, *10*, 411.

Drewe, E. A. The effect of type and area of brain lesion on Wisconsin Card Sorting Test performance, *Cortex*, 1974, *10*, 109.

Fontenot, D. J., & Benton, A. L. Tactile perception of direction in relation to hemispheric locus of lesion. *Neuropsychologia*, 1971, *9*, 83.

Gazzaniga, M. S., Glass, A. V., Sarno, M. T., & Posner, J. B. Pure word deafness and hemispheric dynamics: A case history. *Cortex*, 1973, *9*, 136.

Geschwind, N. Disconnexion syndromes in animals and man. *Brain*, 1965, *88*, 237, 585.

Golden, C. J. *Diagnosis and rehabilitation in clinical neuropsychology*. Springfield, Ill.: Charles C. Thomas, 1978.

Golden, C. J. *Clinical interpretation of objective psychological tests*. New York: Grune and Stratton, 1979.

Golden, C. J. The Luria-Nebraska Neuropyschological Battery and computed tomography (CT) scan results. Symposium presented at American Psychological Association annual convention, 1980.

Golden, C. J., & Berg, R. A. Interpretation of the Luria-Nebraska Neuropyschological Battery by item intercorrelation: The Writing scale. *Clinical Neuropsychology*, 1980, *2* (1), 8. (a)

Golden, C. J., & Berg, R. A. Interpretation of the Luria-Nebraska Neuropsychological Battery by item intercorrelation: The Motor scale (items 1–24). *Clinical Neuropsychology*, 1980, *2* (2), 66. (b)

Golden, C. J., & Berg, R. A. Interpretation of the Luria-Nebraska Neuropyschological Battery by item intercorrelation: Items 25–51 of the Motor scale. *Clinical Neuropsychology*, 1980, *2*, 105–108. (c)

Golden, C. J., & Berg, R. A. Interpretation of the Luria-Nebraska Neuropsychological Battery by item intercorrelation: The Rhythm scale. *Clinical Neuropsychology*, 1980, *2*, 153–156. (d)

Golden, C. J., & Berg, R. A. Interpretation of the Luria-Nebraska Neuropsychological Battery by item intercorrelation: The Tactile scale. *Clinical Neuropsychology*, 1981, *3* (1), 25–29. (a)

Golden, C. J., & Berg, R. A. Interpretation of the Luria-Nebraska Neuropsychological Battery by item intercorrelation: The Visual scale. *Clinical Neuropsychology*, 1981, *3* (2), 22–26. (b)

Golden, C. J., & Berg, R. A. Interpretation of the Luria-Nebraska Neuropsychological Battery by item intercorrelation: The Receptive Speech scale. *Clinical Neuropsychology*, 1981, *3* (3), 21–27. (c)

Golden, C. J., & Berg, R. A. Interpretation of the Luria-Nebraska Neuropsychological Battery by item intercorrelation: The Expressive Speech scale. *Clini-*

cal Neuropsychology, in press.

Golden, C. J., & Berg, R. A. Interpretation of the Luria-Nebraska Neuropsychological Battery by item intercorrelation: The Reading scale. *Clinical Neuropsychology*, in press.

Golden, C. J., & Berg, R. A. Interpretation of the Luria-Nebraska Neuropsychological Battery by item intercorrelation: The Arithmetic scale. *Clinical Neuropsychology*, in press.

Golden, C. J., & Berg R. A. Interpretation of the Luria-Nebraska Neuropsychological Battery by item intercorrelation: The Memory scale. *Clinical Neuropsychology*, in press.

Golden, C. J., & Berg, R. A. Interpretation of the Luria-Nebraska Neuropsychological Battery by item intercorrelation: The Intellectual Processes scale. *Clinical Neuropsychology*, in press.

Golden, C. J., Hammeke, T. A., & Purisch, A. D. Diagnostic validity of a standardized neuropsychological battery derived from Luria's neuropsychological tests. *Journal of Consulting and Clinical Psychology*, 1978, *46*, 1258.

Golden, C. J., Hammeke, T., Osmon, D., Sweet, J., Purisch, A., & Graber, B. Factor structure of the Luria-Nebraska Neuropsychological Battery IV: Intelligence and Pathognomonic scales. *International Journal of Neuroscience*, 1981, *13*, 87.

Golden, C. J., Moses, J. A., Jr., Fishburne, F. J., Engum, E., Lewis, G. P., Wisniewski, A. M., Conley, F. K., Berg, R. A., and Graber, B. Cross-validation of the Luria-Nebraska neuropsychological battery for the presence, lateralization, and localization of brain damage. *Journal of Consulting and Clinical Psychology*, 1981, *49*, 491–507.

Golden, C. J., Osmon, D. C., Moses, J. A., & Berg, R. A. *Interpretation of the Halstead-Reitan.* New York: Grune and Stratton, 1981.

Golden, C. J., Osmon, D. C., Sweet, J., Purisch, A., & Hammeke, T. Factor analysis of the Luria-Nebraska Neuropsychological Battery III: Writing, arithmetic, memory, left and right. *International Journal of Neuroscience*, 1980, *11*, 309.

Golden, C. J., Purisch, A. D., & Hammeke, T. A. *The Luria-Nebraska Neuropsychological Battery: A manual for clinical and experimental uses.* Lincoln: University of Nebraska Press, 1979.

Golden, C. J., Purisch, A., Sweet, J., Graber, B., Osmon, D., & Hammeke, T. Factor analysis of the Luria-Nebraska Neuropsychological Battery II: Visual, Receptive, Expressive, and Reading scales. *International Journal of Neuroscience*, 1980, *11*, 227.

Golden, C. J., Sweet, J., Hammeke, T., Purisch, A., Graber, B., & Osmon, D. Factor analysis of the Luria-Nebraska Neuropsychological Battery: I. Motor, Rhythm, and Tactile scales. *International Journal of Neuroscience*, 1980, *11*, 91.

Gorenstein, E. E., & Newman, S. P. Disinhibitory psychopathology: A new perspective and a model for research. *Psychological Review*, 1980, *87*, 301.

Greenblatt, S. A. Alexia without agraphia or hemianopsia: Anatomical analysis of an autopsied case. *Brain*, 1973, *96*, 307.

Gur, R. C., Packer, I. K., Hungerbuhler, J. P., Reivich, M., Obrist, W. D., Amarnek, W. S., & Sackeim, H. A. Differences in distribution of gray and white matter in human cerebral hemispheres. *Science*, 1980, *207*, 1226.

Hammeke, T. A., Golden, C. J., & Purisch, A. D. A standardized, short, comprehensive neuropsychological test battery based on the Luria neuropsychological evaluation. *International Journal of Neuroscience*, 1978, *8*, 135.

Hebb, D. O. Intelligence, brain function and theory of mind. *Brain*, 1959, *82*, 260.

Hecaen, H., & Albert, M. L. *Human neuropsychology.* New York: John Wiley, 1978.

Hecaen, H., & Angelergues, R. Agnosia for faces—prosopagnosia. *Archives of Neurology*, 1962, *7*, 92.

Hecaen, H., Angelergues, R., & Hocillier, S. Les variétés cliniques des acalculies cours des lésions rétrolandique: Approche statistique de problème. *Review of Neurology,* 1961, *105,* 85.

Heimburger, R. F., & Reitan, R. M. Easily administered written test for lateralizing brain lesions. *Journal of Neurosurgery,* 1961, *18,* 301.

Henschen, S. E. Clinical and anatomical contributors on brain pathology (trans. W. F. Schaller). *Archives of Neurology and Psychiatry,* 1925, *13,* 226 (originally published 1919).

Isaacson, R. Hippocampal destruction in man and other animals. *Neuropsychologia,* 1972, *10,* 47.

Jerger, J., Lovering, L., & Wertz, M. Auditory disorders following bilateral temporal lobe insult: Report of a case. *Journal of Speech and Hearing Disorders,* 1972, *37,* 523.

Kimura, D. Some effects of temporal lobe damage on auditory perception. *Canadian Journal of Psychology,* 1961, *15,* 156.

Kimura, D. Right temporal lobe damage. *Archives of Neurology,* 1963, *8,* 264.

Kinsbourne, M., & Warrington, E. K. The developmental Gerstmann syndrome. *Archives of Neurology,* 1963, *8,* 490.

Kinsbourne, M., & Warrington, E. K. Disorders of spelling. *Journal of Neurology, Neurosurgery, and Psychiatry,* 1964, *27,* 224.

Kløve, H., & Reitan, R. M. Effects of dyspraxia and spatial distortion on Wechsler-Bellevue results. *Archives of Neurology and Psychiatry,* 1958, *80,* 708.

Lackner, J. R., & Teuber, H.-L. Alternatives in auditory fusion thresholds after cerebral injury in man. *Neuropsychologia,* 1973, *11,* 409.

Lansdell, H. Relation of extent of temporal removals to closure and visuo-motor factors. *Perceptual and Motor Skills,* 1970, *31,* 491.

Levin, H. S. The acalculias. In K. M. Heilman and E. Valenstein (Eds.), *Clinical neuropsychology.* New York: Oxford University Press, 1979.

Levy, J., & Reid, M. Variations in writing posture and cerebral organization. *Science,* 1976, *194,* 337.

Lewis, G. P., Golden, C. J., Moses, J. A., Osmon, D. C., Purisch, A. D., & Hammeke, T. A. Localization of cerebral dysfunction by a standardized version of Luria's neuropsychological battery. *Journal of Consulting and Clinical Psychology,* 1979, 47(6), 1003.

Lhermitte, F., & Beavois, M. F. A visual speech disconnection syndrome. *Brain,* 1973, *96,* 695.

Luria, A. R. Brain disorders and language analysis. *Language and Speech,* 1958, *1,* 1.

Luria, A. R. *Higher cortical functions in man.* New York: Basic Books, 1966.

Luria, A. R. *Traumatic aphasia.* Paris: Mouton, 1970.

Luria, A. R. Memory disturbances in local brain lesions. *Neuropsychologia,* 1971, *11,* 417.

Luria, A. R. *The working brain: An introduction to neuropsychology.* New York: Basic Books, 1973.

Luria, A. R., Pribram, H., & Homskaya, E. D. An experimental analysis of the behavioral disturbance produced by a left frontal arachnoidal endothelioma (meningioma). *Neuropsychologia,* 1964, *2,* 257.

Malmo, H. P. On frontal lobe functions: Psychiatric patient controls. *Cortex,* 1974, *10,* 231.

McFie, J. The diagnostic significance of disorders of higher nervous activity. In P. J. Vinken and G. W. Bruyn (Eds.), *Handbook of clinical neurology,* vol. 3. New York: John Wiley, 1969.

McFie, J. The other side of the brain. *Developmental and Medical Child Neurology,* 1970, *12,* 514.

McKay, S., & Golden, C. J. Empirical derivation of experimental scales for lateralizing brain lesions. *Clinical Neuropsychology,* 1979, *1,* 1. (a)

McKay, S., & Golden C. J. Empirical derivation of experimental scales for localizing brain lesions using the Luria-Nebraska Neuropyschological Battery. *Clinical Neuropsychology,* 1979, *1,* 19. (b)

McLardy, T. Memory functions in hippocampal gyri but not in hippocampi. *International Journal of Neuroscience,* 1970, *1,* 113.

Meier, M. J., & French, L. A. Some personality correlates of unilateral and bilateral EEG abnormalities in
psychomotor epileptics. *Journal of Clinical Psychology*, 1965, *21*, 3. (a)

Meier, M. J., & French, L. A. Lateralized deficits in complex visual discrimination and bilateral transfer of rem-
iniscence following unilateral temporal lobotomy.
Neuropsychologia, 1965, *3*, 261. (b)

Meyer, V. Cognitive changes following temporal lobectomy for relief of temporal lobe epilepsy. *Archives of
Neurology and Psychiatry*, 1959, *81*, 299.

Meyer, V., & Yates, A. J. Intellectual changes following
temporal lobectomy for psychomotor epilepsy. *Journal of Neurology, Neurosurgery, and Psychiatry*,
1955, *18*, 44.

Milner, B. Psychological defects produced by temporal
lobe excision. In H. C. Solomon, S. Cobb, and W.
Penfield (Eds.), *The brain and human behavior*. Baltimore: Williams and Wilkins, 1958. (a)

Milner, B. Psychological deficits produced by temporal
lobe excision. *Research Publication of the Association for Research in Nervous and Mental Disease*,
1958, *36*, 244. (b)

Milner, B. Laterality effects in audition. In *Interhemispheric relations and cerebral dominance*. Baltimore:
Johns Hopkins University Press, 1962, p. 177.

Milner, B. Effects of different brain lesions on card sorting. *Archives of Neurology*, 1963, *9*, 90.

Milner, B. Visually guided maze learning in man: Effects
of bilateral hippocampal, bilateral frontal and unilateral cerebral lesions. *Neuropsychologia*, 1965, *3*,
317.

Milner, B. Visual recognition and recall after right temporal lobe excision in man. *Neuropsychologia*, 1968,
6, 191.

Milner, B. Interhemispheric differences in the localization
of psychological processes in man. *British Journal of
Psychology*, 1971, *27*, 272.

Neff, W. A., & Goldberg, J. M. Higher functions of the
central nervous system. *Annual Review of Psychology*, 1960, *22*, 499.

Newlin, D. B., & Golden C. J. Hemispheric asymmetries
in manic-depressive patients: Relationship to hemispheric processing of affect. *Clinical Neuropsychology*, 1980, *2*, 163.

Newlin, D. B., & Tramontana, M. G. Neuropsychological findings in a hyperactive adolescent with subcortical brain pathology. *Clinical Neuropsychology*, in
press.

Nie, N. H., Hull, C. J., Jenkins, J. G., Steinbrenner, K.,
and Bent, D. H. *Statistical package for the social
sciences* (2d ed.). New York: McGraw-Hill, 1975.

Penfield, W., & Mathieson, G. Memory. *Archives of
Neurology*, 1974, *31*, 145.

Penfield, W., & Milner, B. Memory deficit produced by
bilateral lesions in the hippocampal zone. *Archives of
Neurology and Psychiatry*, 1958, *79*, 475.

Piercy, M., & Smyth, V. O. G. Right hemisphere dominance for certain non-verbal intellectual skills. *Brain*,
1962, *85*, 225.

Pribram, K. H., & McGuinness, D. Arousal, activation,
and effort in the control of attention. *Psychological
Review*, 1975, *82*, 116.

Purisch, A. D., Golden, C. J., & Hammeke, T. A. Discrimination of brain damaged and schizophrenic patients with a standardized version of Luria's neuropsychological tests. *Journal of Consulting and Clinical
Psychology*, 1978, *46*, 1266.

Reitan, R. M., & Davison, L. A. *Clinical neuropsychology: Current status and applications*. New York: John
Wiley, 1974.

Roland, P. E. Astereognosis. *Archives of Neurology*,
1976, *33*, 543.

Rubens, A. B., & Benson, D. F. Associative visual agnosia. *Archives of Neurology*, 1971, *24*, 305.

Russell, W. R., & Espir, M. L. E. *Traumatic aphasia*.
London: Oxford University Press, 1961.

Scoville, W. B., & Milner, B. Loss of recent memory after bilateral hippocampal lesions. *Journal of Neurology, Neurosurgery and Psychiatry,* 1957, *20,* 11.

Semmes, J. Hemispheric specialization: A possible clue to mechanisms. *Neuropsychologia,* 1968, *6,* 11.

Semmes, J., Weinstein, S., Ghent, L., & Teuber, H. L. *Somatosensory changes of the penetrating head wounds in man.* Cambridge: Harvard University Press, 1960.

Sperry, R. W. Mental unity following surgical disconnection of the cerebral hemispheres. *Harvey Lecture Series,* 1968, *62,* 293.

Teuber, H. L. Space perception and its disturbances after brain injury in man. *Neuropsychologia,* 1963, *1,* 47.

Thompson, R. F. *Foundations of physiological psychology.* New York: Harper & Row, 1967.

Tramontana, M. G., Sherrets, S. D., & Golden, C. J. Brain dysfunction in youngsters with psychiatric disorders: Application of Selz-Reitan rules for neuropsychological diagnosis. *Clinical Neuropsychology,* 1980, *2,* 118.

Warrington, E. K., & James M. Disorders of visual perception in patients with localized cerebral lesions. *Neuropsychologia,* 1967, *5,* 253.

Warrington, E. K., Logue, V., & Pratt, R. T. C. The anatomical localization of selective impairment of auditory short-term memory. *Neuropsychologia,* 1971, *9,* 337.

Wheeler, L. Predictions of brain damage from an aphasia screening test: an application of discriminant functions and a comparison with a non-linear method of analysis. *Perceptual and Motor Skills,* 1963, *17,* 63.

Wheeler, L., & Reitan, R. M. Discriminant functions applied to the problem of predicting cerebral damage from behavioral tests: A cross validation study. *Perceptual and Motor Skills,* 1962, *18,* 681.

Zangwill, O. L. Psychological deficits associated with frontal lobe lesions. *International Journal of Neurology,* 1966, *5,* 395.

Zurif, E. B., & Ramier, A. M. Some effects of unilateral brain damage on the perception of dichotically presented phonemic sequences and digits. *Neuropsychologia,* 1972, *10,* 103.

Subject Index

Author Index